Imitation Artist

Imitation Artist

Gertrude Hoffmann's Life in Vaudeville and Dance

Sunny Stalter-Pace

NORTHWESTERN UNIVERSITY PRESS
EVANSTON, ILLINOIS

Northwestern University Press
www.nupress.northwestern.edu

Printed in the United States of America

10 9 8 7 6 5 4 3 2 1

Library of Congress Cataloging-in-Publication Data

Names: Stalter-Pace, Sunny, 1977– author.
Title: Imitation artist : Gertrude Hoffmann's life in vaudeville and dance / Sunny Stalter-Pace.
Description: Evanston, Illinois : Northwestern University Press, 2020. | Includes bibliographical references and index.
Identifiers: LCCN 2019023401 | ISBN 9780810141919 (paperback) | ISBN 9780810141926 (cloth) | ISBN 9780810141933 (ebook)
Subjects: LCSH: Hoffmann, Gertrude. | Gertrude Hoffmann Company—History. | Dancers—United States—Biography. | Choreographers—United States—Biography. | Modern dance—United States—History. | Vaudeville—United States—History.
Classification: LCC GV1785.H57 S83 2020 | DDC 792.8092 [B]—dc23
LC record available at https://lccn.loc.gov/2019023401

To Paula Pace, who is the absolute best reader
a girl could write for

CONTENTS

ILLUSTRATIONS

ACKNOWLEDGMENTS

My first thanks go to Gianna Mosser. Her faith in this project and her early chapter feedback were indispensable. I am also grateful for the editorial work of Trevor Perri, Patrick Samuel, and Anne E. Gendler at Northwestern University Press. Brian Ostrander, Therese Malhame, and Maia Melissa Rigas helped me carve a path through a bibliographical thicket. My two anonymous readers provided generous and formative feedback.

For their help in getting the day-to-day work of writing done, I am indebted to Facebook writing group members past and present, including Anne Boyd Rioux, Pamela Toler, Susan Rudy, Rebecca Noel, Elizabeth De Wolfe, Theresa Kaminski, Jessica Parr, Lourdes Aviles, and Scottie Kersta-Wilson. Will Burch, Kaden Ivey, Raye Hendrix, and Robert Brissey provided research assistance. Thanks to the Auburn University College of Liberal Arts for a Competitive Professional Improvement Leave and photography. The Auburn University English Department's Research and Development Committee provided much-needed summer funding. So many colleagues at Auburn University listened, encouraged, and contributed to this project. Particular thanks are due to Chantel Acevedo, Paula Backscheider, Chase Bringardner, Alicia Carroll, Jeremy Downes, Emily Friedman, Ben Fagan, Ernest Gibson, Erich Nunn, and Hilary Wyss.

The Modernist Studies Association is my intellectual home. I am grateful to be in conversation with Alix Beeston, Melissa Bradshaw, Marsha Bryant, Pamela Caughie, Sarah Cornish, David Chinitz, Debra Rae Cohen, Julia Daniel, Anne Fernald, Katherine Fusco, Ben Johnson, Catherine Keyser, and Megan Minarich, among others. Colleagues in theater and performance studies welcomed me, read chapters, recommended presses, and otherwise helped shape this book. Thanks to Elin Diamond, Rhonda Garelick, Anthea Kraut, and Marlis Schweitzer.

I am thankful for the candor and generosity shown by relatives of the subjects in my book. Thanks to Ian McIniss, Trudy Brennan, and Susan Rix. I am also grateful to Terry Wiegmann and Goran Strigulica for their support and shared enthusiasm.

This book was made possible because of a wonderful archive and its equally wonderful archivists. Thanks to all the people who have worked on conserving, cataloging, and sharing the Gertrude and Max Hoffmann Papers and the Max and Gertrude Hoffmann Photograph Collection, both housed in Special Collections and Archives at the Z. Smith Reynolds Library, Wake Forest

University. My gratitude to Megan Mulder and Tanya Zanish-Belcher could only be expressed through a spectacular extravaganza. The Wake Forest University Provost's Grant Award funded the research trip that made this book possible.

Evidence of Gertrude Hoffmann's life and work is housed in archives across the United States. Thanks to the many people who helped me piece it together, including Eric Colleary at the Harry Ransom Center; Alla Roylance and Diana Smith-Bowers at the Brooklyn Public Library; Patricia Keats at the Society of California Pioneers; Edward Sykes Comstock at the University of Southern California Cinematic Arts Library; the Shubert Archive staff, with special thanks to Sylvia Wang; Terence Phillips in Special and Area Studies Collections, George A. Smathers Libraries, University of Florida; and especially Barbara Cohen-Stratyner, formerly of the New York Public Library for the Performing Arts (who remains Gertrude Hoffmann's first champion).

Although this book involved extensive in-person archival research, that work was supported by digital archives and research tools including the California Digital Newspaper Collection, Illinois Digital Newspaper Collections, Old Fulton New York Postcards, Hathitrust, the Internet Archive, and the Media History Digital Library.

Thanks to the editors of academic journals where I worked out some of these ideas in earlier forms. Specifically, early versions of the writing in chapters 6 and 8 appeared in *Theatre Symposium* 2017, volume 25. Thanks to the publisher of that work, the University of Alabama Press, for permission to reprint it. Some writing from chapter 8 first appeared as part of a *Modernism/modernity* PrintPlus cluster. Parts of chapter 15 appeared in the Shubert Archive's newsletter, *The Passing Show*.

My friends have helped me think through this project and distracted me from it when necessary. Thanks are due to Rachel Benoit, Doris Bremm, Amy Minster, and Steph Padilla, whose shadowbox of Gertrude Hoffmann photographs hangs next to my desk. My family has kept me grounded and shared my joy. Love to Jill, Mike, Gram, Chad, Casey, Sim, Arthur, and Paul.

Introduction

Gertrude Hoffmann was a lifelong performer. She began her career in San Francisco in the late 1890s; she last appeared onstage in New York City in the 1930s, once in a nightclub revue with her troupe the Gertrude Hoffmann Girls, and once performing a parody of a German modern dancer. During this forty-year stretch, she sang, danced, choreographed, produced, and directed. Even after her long career had effectively ended, she still filled her journals with ideas for skits, monologues, and stage routines for former Hoffmann Girls.

These later diaries, some written while she was in her seventies, show a woman reflecting on the beginnings of her career, trying to follow back her extraordinary life to its inception. One was written in response to Edward R. Murrow's 1959 *Person to Person* interview with the playwright Moss Hart, in which Murrow asked Hart when he first knew he wanted to work in the theater.[1] Hoffmann transcribes Murrow's question and Hart's reply.[2] She then writes her response to the same question, beginning with "The above brought to my memory." She recollects seeing *Ali Baba, or Morgiana and the 40 Thieves*, a comic-orientalist extravaganza that toured the United States in the late nineteenth century. "From the moment that curtain went up," she writes, "Kittie Hay began producing in the theatre." Hoffmann responds to the question someone else was asked in order to imagine herself as a part of that tradition. Throughout her life, copying gave her a way into the theater, and it helped her find her voice.

She remembers seeing *Ali Baba* through a producer's eyes, understanding how and why different elements brought about different audience reactions. She perceived theatrical productions in terms of their total stage picture as well as the component parts that made up the whole: "They gave at least 3 ballets—about 40 or 50 girls—I began a mental photo of each ballet, costumes, detail, all—."[3] Her near-photographic recall of costumes and choreography would serve her well later in her career, when she made a name for herself as a mimic of stage personalities and as an imitator of dances she had seen in Europe.

It did not take long for Gertrude Hoffmann to move from producing in her head to producing on the stage. While still in her teens, she adapted and performed in popular plays for her husband Max Hoffmann's small stock company. After they had a son (Max junior), Gertrude began working for theatrical producer Oscar Hammerstein, the grandfather of the lyricist and librettist who shared his name. Later in her career, she produced and directed her own revues. When she was too old to star in them herself, she continued to stage dance numbers for the Hoffmann Girls, touring Europe with them and sending them across the United States.

Her continued adherence to the exoticism and spectacle of the Victorian popular stage made her anathema to modernist theater critics, whose love for the orientalism of the Ballets Russes and Max Reinhardt's pageants was only matched by their hatred of old-fashioned American theatrical effects. When the theater began strictly enforcing the distinction between highbrow and lowbrow, Gertrude Hoffmann brazenly mixed the two. Her true genius revealed itself whenever she imitated high culture. These imitations disclosed the populist impulse behind her work: both to share it with a broader audience and to mock its overseriousness.[4]

Scholars have noted Hoffmann's importance at different points in the history of American performance including her early work as a dance director, her performance as Salome, her imitations, and her pirated Russian ballet.[5] Those highlights do not give a sense of the full sweep of her life. Hoffmann's career in the entertainment industry spanned decades that seemed like centuries, from Victorian pantomime extravaganzas and vaudeville through the rise of film, radio, and television. She learned how to imitate the most popular theater of the moment, a skill that served her well during her life but led to her loss of reputation and near-erasure from theater and dance histories. Now is the time for her reintroduction to the stage. In an era when remakes, remixes, and reboots dominate, we have room in our theater history for a woman who elevates imitation to an art.

Part I

✦

Learning How to Copy, 1883–1906

Chapter 1

✦

A Ballet Girl in San Francisco

In the late nineteenth century, San Francisco had a vibrant theatrical culture.[1] Operas and legitimate dramas were presented in elegant surroundings at the Baldwin Theatre and the Grand Opera House. The Tivoli Opera House put on light opera before a diverse crowd. Its season ran year-round, making it the only opera company continuously in production apart from Milan's La Scala.[2] The Orpheum Theatre presented the most important vaudeville acts of the day, including the Four Cohans, Eddie Foy, and W. C. Fields. With great venues, eager audiences, and remarkable performances, why is the city's performance history so unfamiliar?

San Francisco's theatrical history remains obscure for the same reason as Gertrude Hoffmann's: both were too popular and too hybrid. At a time when cultural hierarchy was separating highbrow from lowbrow, San Francisco was best known for extravaganzas and pantomimes that mixed the two.[3] Even their serious operas featured the marching girl choruses more common on the burlesque stage. The performance culture of late nineteenth-century San Francisco was built around genres and business structures that have come to be associated with the Victorian era and rejected in the modern. Stock companies and actor-managers were central to the nineteenth-century actors' theater, while playwrights were granted far more importance in the twentieth century.[4] The Works Progress Administration (WPA) confirms this logocentric bias with a damning claim: "It must be remembered that San Francisco contributed practically nothing of worth to the development of the native American drama."[5] This claim is true only if we distinguish between drama (on the page) and theater (on the stage). San Francisco may not have contributed many twentieth-century playwrights, but it more than made up for it with its performers and spectacles.

Gertrude Hoffmann's parents were both migrants to San Francisco. John Hay came from Maine, and Catherine Brogan from Ireland. They had eight children: Mamie, Nellie, John Robert, George, Margaret, Mary, Rose, and Catherine Gertrude. Catherine Gertrude Hay was born on May 7. The rest is complicated. Her original birth certificate was lost due to the great San Francisco earthquake of 1906. It is an educated guess that she was born in

1883, as her age was given as seventeen on the census of 1900 when she still lived at home.[6] The 1883 date cannot be compared to the first census on which her name would appear: the 1890 census records were mostly destroyed by a fire in 1921.[7] On other documents, Hoffmann gave her birth year as anywhere between 1879 (on her marriage certificate) and 1887 (in the 1930 census). Hoffmann's birthdate shows she refused to be pinned down to a fixed identity. Even when she was the "right" age to appear onstage, she played characters from other times and re-performed acts originated by other people. Gertrude Hoffmann was perpetually anachronistic.[8]

Gertrude Hoffmann's early life has not been studied much beyond the myths she fostered in the press. Stories about Hoffmann's career in San Francisco call her "Kitty Hayes" or sometimes "Kittie Hayes." Even the most authoritative and recent reference works list her last name as Hayes.[9] Figure 1.1 shows a picture of young Gertrude Hoffmann in a high-necked jacket and a ridiculous hat. She has wide-set, heavily lidded eyes, a large nose, and a friendly, faintly ironic mouth. This is Hoffmann as a girl, when she was called Kitty Hay.

As with her birthdate, her education is difficult to pin down. Hoffmann's formal education seems to have taken place at some combination of Catholic and public schools. No matter where she attended, Hoffmann would have found a classroom where play, physical activity, and performance were valued. Exercise and movement culture played an important role in the nineteenth-century classroom. Reformers such as Catherine Beecher insisted upon the importance of physical education for girls.[10] By the 1880s, Steele Mackaye and Genevieve Stebbins disseminated the movement systems of François Delsarte to the American public.[11]

She was introduced to this type of movement culture even before her formal education began. A later diary entry describes her "first remembrance of body action."[12] Gertrude was taken by the oldest girl in her family and remembers feeling self-conscious because all the other children were there with their mothers. Whether to overcome her embarrassment or because of her fearlessness, she volunteered to lead the group of children doing exercises:

> Believe it or not—I distinctly remember someone—the teacher—asking for one to lead calisthenics or something akin to motion dancing. I—in my baby way—said I would lead and I did—then we started the hunt for Easter eggs. Again, I distinctly remember that I was absolutely serious on the hunt, I remember that the teacher had some kind of a mirror or something that she flashed all over the school room—prompting us on where we might find eggs.[13]

This memory sets the scene for much of Hoffmann's kinesthetic life as a producer and performer. Her dance does not begin as an expression of interior emotion. She imitates a model, and she teaches her peers. She is both proud

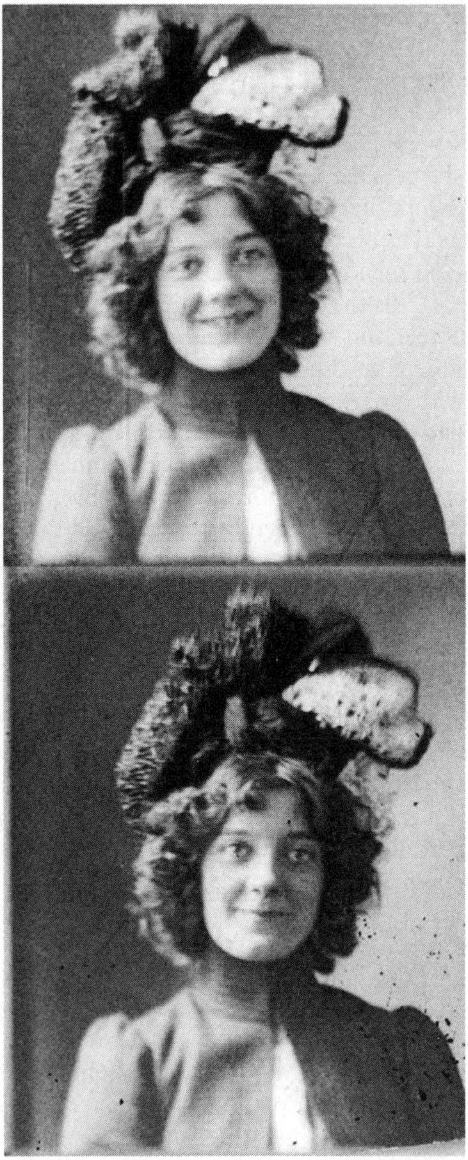

FIGURE 1.1. Gertrude Hoffmann as a girl. Max and Gertrude Hoffmann Photograph Collection, Special Collections and University Archives, Wake Forest University, Winston-Salem, N.C.

to be a leader and somewhat embarrassed by her "baby way" of demanding focus. At the kindergarten, this activity was followed by an Easter egg hunt, where the teacher flashing a mirror both directs the students' attention and turns their classroom into a glittering space for serious play.[14] Gertrude Hoffmann's life as a performer can be understood through these related impressions. As soon as she gets her first stage role, she becomes a teacher, leading the phalanx of girls in a light opera through their marches. Once she has a backstage role, she takes on the jobs that direct the audience's attention, first by staging dances and then by designing whole productions.

Throughout the 1890s the Hay family lived in downtown San Francisco, first on Stockton Street and then on Geary Street, both near Union Square Park. The Union Square neighborhood was (and continues to be) an upscale area, though one with a commercial character. The *WPA Guide to San Francisco* describes a part of town where "department stores have for so many decades been custodians of public taste—their founders being patrons of the arts and *bon vivants*."[15] Nearby stores sold perfume, clothing, jewelry, and books. Gertrude grew up surrounded by the commodity culture of the Gilded Age. She associated conspicuous consumption with elegance and sophistication throughout her life.

Hoffmann moved through San Francisco's theatrical neighborhoods from a young age, fantasizing about her future as a performer. She often went to the butcher and dairy on Market Street with instructions and money from her mother, stopping at the stores along the way. At first, this was window shopping: she determines at one jewelry store that after her career success she will have a gold or silver dresser set. She has similar daydreams at the shoe store—"my passion," she says. After she begins appearing in shows, salesmen there allow her to browse stock in their back drawers for discounted pumps and slippers to supplement her chorus costumes.[16]

The shops in Gertrude's neighborhood sold the accessories of stardom and portraits of the stars themselves. She lived a few blocks away from Elite Photography and Louis Thors Studios, two of San Francisco's most important studios for celebrity portraits.[17] Her diaries mention seeing pictures of the actresses Catherine Miskel-Hoyt and Julia Marlowe. She admired Marlowe for her Cupid's-bow mouth and dimpled chin.[18] One of those photography studios was run by a relative, her paternal aunt Mary Fitzsimmons Hay. Hay was a partner in a ferrotype studio located at 342 Kearny Street, a short walk from the stretch of Market Street where actors and other local celebrities would often promenade after Saturday matinees.[19] A descendant of Hoffmann speculates that her aunt's job may have offered Gertrude a sense of bohemian possibility.[20]

Mary Hay was one of many female business owners in the Union Square neighborhood.[21] Gertrude's mother Catherine was another. Catherine was representative of female business owners in late nineteenth-century San Francisco, typically first-generation immigrants who were married or had been.[22]

She was born in Ireland and came to the United States in 1862; she worked as a dressmaker. Perhaps Hoffmann's facility as a manager of people and of money—first as a dance director and then as a producer—was fostered by these examples.

Mary and Catherine both worked in fields dependent on the theater. Catherine made two long pink-velvet dresses for the singer Truly Shattuck's debut San Francisco performance on July 15, 1894. Gertrude's diary says this performance took place at the Wigwam Theater, while newspaper advertisements locate it at the People's Palace Music Hall, suggesting she conflated the theater nearest to their house with one a few blocks farther away.[23] Perhaps Catherine fashioned costumes for performers at the Wigwam as well.

The youngest child in a large, working-class family, Gertrude Hoffmann was eager to prove her maturity. She remembers that she "begged to be allowed to do housework" as a small girl.[24] She swept the hall and steps using tea leaves to help gather the dust, filled in scratches on the wood floor with a matchstick, and cleaned the windows with wet newspaper. In one of the few negative comments about her mother, Hoffmann recalls "Mama's daily examination—my inward rage."[25] Elsewhere in her journals, she remembers her mother making her sweep "every crevice and corner" as her introduction to routine and attention to detail.[26]

Part of that discipline arose from necessity. John and Catherine Hay separated when Gertrude was young. Catherine appears to have filed for divorce in 1893, since a John Hay was jailed for contempt of court in December of that year when he could not pay the $65 child support for the duration of divorce proceedings.[27] After the divorce, Catherine lived with five of the children, who were either mislabeled in the census or consciously took on the surname Hayes; John lived with his sister's family and his second-oldest daughter, Nellie, keeping his surname of Hay.[28] Catherine seems not to have criticized him in his absence: "I heard little ever against my father," Gertrude writes, "—in fact nothing except about the monthly payments being cut down."[29] The Hayes family lost one parent's income after the divorce, and child support payments were later lowered as well.

Gertrude was eager to get a paying job and contribute more than house cleaning. She recounts sneaking the newspaper to the bathroom and perusing the want ads. She found a want ad for dancers to support the Royal Lilliputians, a German troupe of little people who toured the U.S. performing comic variety shows. Their 1895 show, *Humpty Dumpty Up to Date* needed "200 Young And Handsome Ladies [. . .] Those who can dance preferred."[30] She auditioned for their 1897 offering called *The Merry Tramps*, using her experience attending performances to pad her resume. Instead of telling the Lilliputians' manager Carl Rosenfeld that she had seen *Ali Baba* and the Kiralfy Ballet, she said that she appeared in them.[31] She was cast in the show at the age of fourteen.

The Merry Tramps was an example of the popular theatrical form that dominated the late nineteenth-century U.S. stage, the spectacular extravaganza.

Elizabeth Kendall defines this hybrid form as "a loose fantastical pantomime plot geared to the display of theatrical marvels."[32] The U.S. spectacular extravaganza tradition developed in the wake of *The Black Crook* (1866). A smash hit that toured widely and ran for more than five hours, *The Black Crook* combined a fairy-tale plot with a Faustian bargain, songs and dances by a scantily clad female chorus, and jaw-dropping scenery transformations. The shows that made an impression on Gertrude at a young age—*Ali Baba*, Christmas pantomimes at the Tivoli Theatre, the Kiralfy Ballet—were all examples of the form. Hoffmann produced her own versions of the spectacular extravaganza well into the twentieth century.

Tied to the extravaganza is the most common of its cast members, the ballet girl. Her function in this type of show falls somewhere between that of an extra and a chorus girl, involving dance in the broadest way. The shows required a huge number of girls, who did not require much in the way of rehearsal. While the stars of shows toured from place to place, a new bunch of ballet girls was hired in each city. Elizabeth Kendall describes a typical process for hiring ballet girls: "They called at the stage door and were fitted into tutus and drilled in lines to stand obediently, or walk and turn as coryphées, without having the least idea of what ballet dancing was about."[33] Hoffmann would have gone through a very similar process at the Baldwin Theatre for her *Merry Tramps* part. Work as a ballet girl showed her the theatrical power of women moving in unison.

Hoffmann played a (small) dramatic role at the Baldwin Theatre in the summer of 1897, as page to Mary Mannering's Flavia in *The Prisoner of Zenda*. The review in the *San Francisco Call* points out that the show "even to the smallest role was well acted."[34] She took great pride in embodying her chorus parts in a realistic manner saying, "We were taught to live the characters—even tho we were choristers."[35] Gertrude Hoffmann stood out in the crowded field because she brought a serious commitment to those roles. In a later newspaper article, a fellow San Francisco native Anita Loos told a story of Hoffmann's determination: "The only bit of 'business' she had was running down a flight of stairs. But Miss Loos says that Miss Hoffman practiced that run downstairs until, on the opening night, she made it one of the hits of the play."[36]

By that winter, Hoffmann returned to a more spectacular show, the Christmas pantomime at the Orpheum Theatre called *The Birth of the Pearl*. Though just as extravagant as *Ali Baba* and *The Merry Tramps*, this show is better understood as a pantomime because of its timing—at Christmas—and its appeal to a broader audience, including children. While the pantomime at the Tivoli that year was a burlesque on Mother Goose that hewed closer to the English tradition, *The Birth of the Pearl* was what Gillian Anderson calls a "pantomime ballet."[37] This theatrical form carries on today with Christmas performances of *The Nutcracker*.

The show was by all accounts an extravagant and gorgeous one. The action took place on the deck of an ocean liner, at the bottom of the sea, and in fairyland.[38] This third-act setting was striking, with undersea fairy caves decorated with jewel-toned stalactites.[39] The ballet master Monsieur de Filippi imitated a frog with his dance, and Madame de Filippi performed a gavotte. They were supported by a corps of 125 dancers dressed as deep-sea divers, pearls, and mermaids—some of whom flew above the audience in an aerial ballet.

Hoffmann's next apprenticeship took place at the Tivoli Opera House. She joined the Tivoli chorus in 1898, probably in the spring since she lists their Easter burlesque on *Ali Baba* among her credits.[40] The Tivoli opened in 1875 as a beer garden with an orchestra. It developed into a beloved San Francisco institution. The Tivoli's fortunes were buoyed by the craze for the *H. M. S. Pinafore*.[41] Gilbert and Sullivan's operetta opened at the Tivoli on July 7, 1879, and was revived for the next two decades.[42] The theater's Christmas pantomime also played to reliably full houses. Hoffmann appeared in the 1898 pantomime *The Yellow Dwarf*, based on the fairy tale by Madame d'Aulnoy.

Hoffmann's time at the Tivoli showed her how to produce a dependable product that appealed to a broad audience. The Tivoli chorus was well-rehearsed, the orchestra was talented, and the stock company did justice to its material. Ticket prices were low, but the quality was high enough that wealthy San Franciscans attended as well. "The Tivoli," says a history of the theater in the 1890s, "was the most democratic house of amusement in the world."[43] While American culture separated into highbrow and lowbrow strains during the early twentieth century, Gertrude Hoffmann continued to produce shows that appealed to a broad audience like the one drawn by the Tivoli.

Hoffmann became a favorite in San Francisco theater circles. She sold flowers and programs at fundraisers, a duty assigned to the most popular and charming chorus girls.[44] One of the fundraisers was a benefit for California Volunteers returning from the Philippines.[45] San Franciscans supported the Spanish-American and Philippine-American wars for several reasons. The bay served as a debarkation point for fighting in Manila. The Hearst newspaper the *San Francisco Examiner* drummed up patriotism with its coverage. Even local governmental leaders saw the U.S. annexation of the Philippines as an economic opportunity.[46]

The theater community both supported and celebrated these martial forays. They disseminated news from wire reports and newsreels, put on war plays, and interpolated patriotic music into shows.[47] The benefit where Hoffmann sold programs took place in the Orpheum Theatre, which was decorated for the occasion in bunting and "twinkling red, white, and blue lights."[48] A week later, she rode a fraternal organization's float in a military parade, dressed as Columbia, the female icon of the United States before the Statue of Liberty.[49]

She was chosen to play as a page at a Mardi Gras ball for San Francisco's well-to-do. A newspaper article titled "Chorus Goes into Society" sets up the two chorus girls—Hoffmann and Irene Duval—as figures of fun, both naive and sexualized.[50] The story begins with the conceit that Ed Greenway, the wealthy man inviting them to perform at the ball, is their "sponsor" bringing them into society as "debutantes." He meets them in the Tivoli's "wine room" and asks them to participate in the ball. Gertrude appears ready for the Mardi Gras in an illustration accompanying the article: she sports a mask and beauty mark, posing saucily with her hands behind her head. It does not seem that Hoffmann got to attend: a follow-up article suggests that Irene Duval played the role of page with her friend Josie Davis instead.[51]

Then the two girls respond to the same questions: How did it happen? Will you wear tights? How long would you like to stay at the party? The *San Francisco Call* quotes Hoffmann (here, going by the name Gertrude Hayes) at length:

> "There's a man named Greenway," Miss Hayes explained, "who runs society. He saw me from the front and said the Mardi Gras couldn't be a success without me. Irene Duval tried to do me out of it, because I got mad because she couldn't keep step with me. But she couldn't fool the leader, and I'm being measured for the tights. I ain't a bit nervous about it. I'm just as good as the rest of 'em, only I haven't got the money. I came out in an Orpheum ballet and I'm climbing surely to the top. I expect to remain throughout the evening and have lots of fun."[52]

This monologue highlights Hoffmann's ambition, bravado, and lack of then-conventional feminine modesty.[53] She sounds like a plucky working-class boy from the Horatio Alger novels that were still being published. She is canny enough to understand the way her interview is being framed: she does not need to make her debut in society because she already "came out in an Orpheum ballet." The stage may be hierarchical in the same way that society is, but at least it's a meritocracy. Later in her career, though, Hoffmann noted that this interview made her sound "like a ruffian."[54]

Sometime in the spring of 1899, Hoffmann ascended another rung on the ladder. "In those days," she says in a 1911 interview, "it was the ambition of nearly every girl to get into the chorus at the Grand Opera House."[55] The theater was then the largest in San Francisco, with a "wide marble lobby and 4 or 5 balconies."[56] It was renovated over the winter, with its seating capacity expanded and three thousand electric lights installed. The Australian diva Nellie Melba was booked to open the season, after which comic opera was presented with a stock company.[57]

Gertrude Hoffmann and her sister Rose were among the youngest to audition. The music director called for someone to begin by singing the scale of notes. "As I remember," Gertrude writes, "everyone of the girls held back, blushed, pushed each other to go first."[58] Eager to begin the process, she volunteered. Rose roared with laughter, less at her sister's daring (which cannot have been a surprise by this point), than at the thin, babyish Do-Re-Mi to come. Gertrude was a graceful dancer, but she was a weak singer. She was hired despite this: "Most all were engaged," her diary notes. Gertrude and Rose continued to make each other laugh during their rehearsals until December 1899, when Rose married a machinist who worked at another San Francisco theater, and "retired from the stage."[59]

The Grand Opera House provided rigorous training that formed the bedrock of Gertrude Hoffmann's musical and theatrical education. The music director Selli Simonson and the stage director Charles Jones were strict disciplinarians who expected total professionalism from even the lowliest ballet girl. Hoffmann recounts their training process, marveling at the quick turnaround that Simonson expected for his chorus: they began learning music on Monday and were expected to perform their parts off book by Thursday.[60] Jones developed Hoffmann's interest in directing large groups of synchronized women, producing the kind of stage pictures that first struck her in the Christmas ballet pantomimes. Like Delsarte-inspired teacher Genevieve Stebbins, Jones created routines that "mixed military movement with the conventionally feminine poses of sentiment."[61] Jones was "a great producer of marches," Hoffmann says, who taught his chorus to "march with precision and power."[62] "This is a quality lacking in all theatrical producers I have since known," she writes. Since those theatrical producers included some heavy hitters—Florenz Ziegfeld among them—it is safe to say that Jones was her inspiration for training chorus members and planning revues.

Once trained by these men, Hoffmann sang and danced in the chorus supporting the Southwell Comic Opera company, whose engagement began on April 1, 1899, with *The Black Hussar*. The director of the company tried to give Hoffmann a small part in *Erminie*, which opened two weeks later, but girls from the Southwell company felt one of their ranks deserved the part and seem to have gotten her cut. In her diaries, Hoffmann claims to have been surprised, saying, "I did not seem to know enough of even child life + its so-called jealousy to realize what was going on with the others against me."[63] Hoffmann continued to perform at the Grand Opera House well into 1900, with small parts in *The Queen's Lace Handkerchief* and *The Girl from Paris*. One review observes that in the latter show, she "made a decided hit in the Spanish fandango."[64] This observation takes up two lines of a six-line review, suggesting that her performance was a high point.

Dancing in a Latin style became her specialty. In December 1899 she played a Mexican dancer in the world premiere of *Mother Earth* at the Alcazar.[65] That play was penned by Francis Powers, who also wrote San Francisco's major contribution to realism, the Chinatown-set drama *The First Born*. When Florence Roberts starred in *Sapho*, also at the Alcazar, Hoffmann appeared as Toto the Spanish dancer. She performed a graceful solo during a first-act scene at a masquerade ball.[66] That performance, in June 1900, seems to be the point when other major theatrical personalities recognized her star quality. "That girl is worth watching," remarked the Alcazar producer Fred Belasco from the wings. Belasco was the brother of the New York City producer David and a powerful and respected actor-manager in his own right. Florence Roberts agreed.[67]

Roberts and Hoffmann got off on the wrong foot. According to Hoffmann, the music director Charles Bryant wanted to cast her as Toto from the start, while Roberts preferred a wealthy classmate of Hoffmann's. As with the drama regarding her first part at the Grand Opera House, she claims ignorance: "I was unaware of just what was going on," she writes, and "stood listening and as I remember not even realizing they were battling over me."[68] Hoffmann likes to take this narrative position in her diaries, both acting as though butter would not melt in her mouth and giving us the reasons for the fights she claimed not to notice. From a young age, she seldom wanted to focus on anything other than the performance itself. Roberts offered an olive branch, sending over her maid to help Hoffmann dress on opening night.[69] As an actress who made her name on the San Francisco stage, Florence Roberts was invested in supporting local talent.

The summer she performed in *Sapho*, Hoffmann concluded that her popularity in San Francisco had peaked; to achieve greater success, she needed to move to New York City. She asked the stock company producers Dunne and Ryley for a contract, but they turned her down. She did not have much support at home: Catherine Hay did not even want her daughter to perform in Stockton, California, a ferry ride away. Finally, she was cast in the last Dunne and Ryley production of the summer season, the George Ade play *The Night of the Fourth*. The show was booked for Oscar Hammerstein's Victoria Theatre in New York City. Once Hoffmann got a contract, Florence Roberts payed her fare east.[70]

Hoffmann was at a turning point, moving away from operettas and legitimate dramas and toward modern, ragtime-inflected musical comedy shows. *The Night of the Fourth* was a farce comedy, with the thinnest of plots on which to hang the antics of the comic duo J. Sherrie Mathews and Harry Bulger.[71] Bulger plays a retired iceman who travels to the country for the summer and buys all the town's fireworks so they cannot disturb him on the Fourth of July. He stores them all in the basement of the Summer Rest Hotel where he is staying and, since it is a farce comedy, a stray firecracker sets them off.[72] Mathews took the role of a fast-talking lawyer who spars with Bulger's character and sues him for damages. Hoffmann and seven other chorines played punningly named roles, all variations on a theme: Miss Construe, Miss Lead, Miss Fortune, and so on. In the New York City production, Hoffmann played Miss Judge.

In 1900 Hoffmann left a city associated with Victorian stagecraft and traveled to one that became associated with modern theater. Where critics have stressed the ruptures between Victorian and modern performance, though, I want to highlight their continuities. Hoffmann carried with her the training, themes, techniques, and ideals of her early career. Her experience on the fin-de-siècle San Francisco stage, with its spectacular, often orientalist pantomimes and large-scale movement of girl choruses, laid the groundwork for her later revues and other interventions in the popular understanding of modernist theater.

She left a theatrical community where she had made an impact. The *San Francisco Dramatic Review* bade her farewell two times: once, on June 30, as Kitty Hayes, and again on August 18, as Gertrude Hayes.[73] Throughout her life, Gertrude Hoffmann kept in touch with friends from this era. Polly Tupper, who shared the stage with her at the Alcazar, enjoyed a long and successful stage career as Mary (sometimes Maryverne) Tupper Jones. She and Gertrude kept in close contact. Once she went on the road with *The Night of the Fourth*, though, Gertrude Hoffmann met the most consistent presence throughout the rest of her life—her future husband Max.

Chapter 2

✦

Teaming Up with Max Hoffmann

The Dunne and Ryley Company put on its farewell performance in San Francisco on August 12, 1900. The cast, now including a teenage Gertrude Hayes, headed east. For five months, they performed *The Night of the Fourth* on the road. On this tour she met the man who would become her partner, collaborator, and husband of sixty-three years. They were both multitalented performers whose talent and taste ran the gamut from highbrow to lowbrow. In the early days, Max was the more famous of the two, while Gertrude needed to prove herself. Then the roles reversed: she popularized his songs, and he arranged her shows. They were, to use a contemporary term, a power couple.

Max Hoffmann was born on December 8, 1873, in Gnesen, Poland. The region was then a part of Prussia, though at other points in its history it was occupied by Russia and annexed into Nazi Germany. Hoffmann did not live in Gnesen long; as a child, he immigrated to the United States and lived in the upper Midwest, most likely in Wisconsin. He seldom talked about his family in interviews or in his few extant journals. He worked in Hurley, Wisconsin, and Ironwood, Michigan, mining towns across state lines from one another. "I made friends with the station agent in Hurley," Hoffmann writes, "and he gave me a charity ticket through to Chi."[1]

His history begins in earnest when he moves to Chicago in the 1890s as a "kid piano player."[2] Seeing the 1930s gangster movie *In Old Chicago* led him to reminisce about his time playing music in saloons during the Gay Nineties. His first job was at a bar charmingly named the Bucket of Blood. Hoffmann was paid in beer for the first three hours of his shift; 11:00 P.M. to midnight he earned "all the beer I wanted and two bucks."[3] Competition for patrons was fierce in this part of the city, and piano playing helped draw them in: "The piano was in the rear, by the street door. Just across the street was the Blue Moon. They also had a piano by the door. It was pounded by a fellow named Burt Green. Later married Irene Franklin. Who ever played the loudest, won."[4] After paying his dues, Max moved to the Casino Theater on North Clark Street. He was hired as a pianist and bouncer. The pay was better, $20 a night and a $5 drink ticket. The bouncer part of the job came with some real risks: Hoffmann's nose was broken with brass knuckles. He once feared being shot in a brawl until he was "assisted by the fists" of a friend who was a boxer.[5] When Max Hoffmann began working at the Casino, the second-billed act starred Bert Williams and George Walker, who would reshape musical theater with their African American Broadway shows such as *In Dahomey*. "I became infatuated with colored rhythm about this time," Hoffmann writes in his journal.[6]

James Weldon Johnson's *The Autobiography of an Ex-Colored Man* notes that this was the era when the live performance of improvised ragtime songs "made its way to Chicago," where "several of these improvisations were taken down by white men."[7] Max took part in that trend. While playing clubs at night, he held a day job with the sheet-music publisher M. Witmark and Sons, where he arranged popular songs in the new syncopated style. Max wrote a ragtime accompaniment to the published version of the black performer Ernest Hogan's hit song, with the ugly title of "All Coons Look Alike to Me."[8] According to music historians, this was "the first publication to call itself a 'rag.'"[9] The Hogan song was a racist form of popular music known as the "coon song." These were Tin Pan Alley songs whose lyrics were written in clichéd approximation of African American dialect, and whose sheet-music covers were festooned with stereotypical images of black life. "Hello Ma Baby" is perhaps the song from this era most familiar to contemporary readers.

Hoffmann's work adapting ragtime revealed his skill at copying, riffing, and arranging. These abilities served him well for the rest of his long career as a composer and songwriter. He followed the trends in music of the period, during which piano players applied the ragtime style to unsyncopated songs during live improvisations.[10] These were not the songs of Scott Joplin, say, which were original compositions for piano written in that musical style. Max published several compositions that "ragged" preexisting songs and even traveled to Minnesota to perform his "Rag Medley" as part of an informal concert held by the musical instrument retailer W. J. Dyer and Bro.[11] Perhaps most important for the history of musical theater, he claimed to have arranged the music for Bert Williams and George Walker's appearance in the Victor Herbert operetta *The Gold Bug*.[12] This was Max's earliest experience of blending together highbrow and popular music in the same show, a skill that he drew on throughout his career. His familiarity with ragtime would complement his wife's background: Gertrude was trained in an old-fashioned form of popular entertainment, while Max learned a new form and helped spread it to the masses.

Work with the Witmarks put Max Hoffmann in contact with many of the most important musicians and songwriters of the era. He was even more well-connected once he took a job leading the orchestra at the Olympic Theatre, a vaudeville house at Clark and Randolph Streets in the Chicago Loop. He collaborated with Charles K. Harris, who wrote the sentimental megahit

"After the Ball."[13] He helped Paul Dresser take down the music for "On the Banks of the Wabash," though Dresser's brother, the novelist Theodore Dreiser, claimed credit.[14] Hoffmann was in such high demand that he hired musicians for the Olympic orchestra pit who could also help him work on Witmark arrangements.[15]

Like many theaters before the advent of air-conditioning, the Olympic Theatre closed in the summer.[16] During these free months, Hoffmann moonlighted as a musical director for traveling theater companies.[17] One of those companies was Dunne and Ryley's. Billed as "Herr Max Hoffman," he conducted the orchestra for their stops in Eau Claire, Wisconsin, and St. Paul, Minnesota, in the summer of 1900.[18] These shows took place as the company traveled west on the way to their ten-week stint in San Francisco; they performed Charles H. Hoyt's farce *A Rag Baby* along with their variety acts. Hoffmann rejoined the company for their eastern tour, likely during the Minnesota dates in September 1900.[19] Here Max's and Gertrude's stories intersected.

Max was a decade older than Gertrude, handsome and tall. With his foreign mien and his authority before the orchestra, perhaps he reminded her of Selli Simonson, the music director at the Grand Opera House. Gertrude was pert and fresh, with an undeniable star quality and an eagerness to learn every aspect of putting on a show. Accounts of Gertrude and Max's courtship come from newspaper stories several years after the fact: one story calls their relationship a "mixture of romance and business."[20]

The Night of the Fourth company arrived in New York City in January 1901. Gertrude was struck by the energy and sophistication of the burgeoning theatrical district then known as Longacre Square. When the Dunne and Ryley company played at the Victoria Theatre, a few restaurants and theaters were clustered around Forty-Second Street and Broadway. She recalls being impressed by "The 3 in 1—Three Theatres under one roof . . . all owned, the entire block, by the very handsome Sire Bros.—Nice men."[21] Nearby restaurants included Shanley's and Rector's, the "lobster palaces" that served an excess of food and cocktails to the celebrities of the day. Aside from a few nightspots, there was not much excitement that far north in Manhattan. "At that time, 1900–1901," she writes in her journal, "the square was like a country village."[22] Indeed, Oscar Hammerstein transformed a horse stable on Seventh Avenue into his Victoria Theatre.

Gertrude Hoffmann's later career in New York City was tied to the fortunes of both Times Square and the Hammerstein theatrical empire. That took a few more years, since *The Night of the Fourth* fizzled out. The show had strong credentials: its author George Ade was a Chicago newspaperman then famed for his "Fables in Slang"; Mathews and Bulger were well-known comedians.[23] But its New York run was by all accounts a failure. Ade's name was removed from the publicity. Reviews were dismissive: "Folks who are fond of this sort of entertainment," said a *New York Times* review, will "like this piece very much and will tell their friends so. Those who do not like high kicking, 'coon' songs and dances, pantomimic jokes, and strident music hall voices would best stay away."[24] The show ran for two weeks. The show's failure made little difference to Gertrude, who by her account was fired early in the New York run.[25] Again she blamed a jealous competitor, a "showgirl with influence" who wanted her part.[26]

While the New York show of *The Night of the Fourth* failed, one stop on their tour was a rousing success. Gertrude Hoffmann was a "favorite of the audiences" in Richmond, Virginia, when the show played at the Academy of Music. [27] They remembered her there as the "girl in lavender," a moniker still used to describe her in Virginia papers more than a decade later.[28] That lavender dress cost $6, according to her diary.[29] She was committed to spending her money on stage clothes that added to her star quality.[30] Leading ladies were expected to dress well onstage, and they paid for their own costumes.[31]

Gertrude Hoffmann returned to Richmond in March 1901 to make her vaudeville debut at the Bijou Theatre, singing one of Max's songs from *The Night of the Fourth*. In late March and early April 1901, Gertrude performed at the Wells vaudeville houses in Richmond and Norfolk.[32] On April 7, Max and Gertrude married.[33] They joined the Bijou Musical Comedy Company, a stock company managed by Jake Wells. Max was hired as musical director of the company, while Gertrude staged the dance numbers and performed. Gertrude remembered working thirteen- or fourteen-hour days. She writes, "We worked from 10 to 11 or 12 everyday except Sun. on which we rehearsed."[34] This was a common schedule in traveling theatrical companies: the stock actress Gladys Hurlbut calls it "the most sweatshop kind of work I ever heard of."[35] Their pay for these long days? "$50.00 for two idiots," Gertrude wisecracks.[36] She romanticized her work in San Francisco in later interviews, but never her time in stock.

Wells ran both the Academy of Music and the Bijou; he planned to send the company on a circuit of theaters in the Southeast, returning to Richmond with a new show every six weeks. A former baseball player and manager, Wells parlayed his experience with American amusements into a multimedia empire.[37] From his Richmond home, he managed theaters in Virginia, Georgia, Alabama, and Tennessee. Contemporary scholars emphasize how Wells shaped his theatrical programs to adhere to the region's values and attitudes. In the post-Reconstruction era, in the capital of the Confederacy, this meant catering to fantasies about white cultural dominance and the "Lost Cause."[38] Jake and his brother Otto carefully defused antitheatrical prejudices in the region, arguing that they were in favor of "civic concern and uplift."[39] The "Wells circuit" of theatrical (and then cinematic) venues shaped the entertainment experience in the new South.

Throughout 1902, the Bijou Musical Comedy Company made circuits around the Southeast, from Virginia to Georgia and back. Every time they returned they presented a new play. The circuit extended into Alabama and

Tennessee as Wells took control of theaters in the area. Over the next few years, the company changed names, incorporated new members, and lost old ones. For example, when they performed in Washington, D.C., in 1901, they were billed as "Chase's Musical Comedy Company." When performing straight vaudeville, they were sometimes billed as Max Hoffmann's Troubadours, and later the Dixie Troubadours—a name that plays up their connection to the South and to minstrelsy. Regardless of their name they worked steadily, performing comedies that were modern (but not too sophisticated) along with polite vaudeville-style acts.[40]

Because *The Night of the Fourth* was such a hit, the Hoffmanns made their Richmond debut with another Mathews and Bulger vehicle, *At Gay Coney Island*.[41] They followed with a number of farces by Charles H. Hoyt, whose plays anticipate the frothy musical comedies of the early twentieth century. Gertrude and Max interpolated up-to-date music in the shows, often music written by Max himself.[42] Max Hoffmann's name came to be associated with an updated ragtime sound: when the Bijou Comedy Company performed *What Happened to Jones?* in Atlanta, they were advertised as presenting the playwright George "Broadhurst's Great Success (Hoffmanized)."[43] From mid-1901 to mid-1903, Gertrude Hoffmann was the company's dance director and costume designer. In her words, she "staged [the] entire musical end" of their shows.[44] Some plays were easier to transform than others: most of the texts were straight plays, though Hoyt's *A Trip to Chinatown* was a musical to begin with. The Hoffmanns were early practitioners of the now-standard form of adaptation, where intellectual property that is popular in another form is made into a musical. While these shows may not have been integrated, stand-alone works of art in the same way as, say, *Wicked*, they should be understood as part of the same tradition.

Stock company tours were punctuated with occasional visits to New York City, where Gertrude Hoffmann performed solo numbers in vaudeville and farce comedies. As "Max Hoffmann's Troubadours," they finished their season in Richmond on July 12, 1902. The Hoffmanns stayed in New York City that summer. Gertrude was cast in *The Sweet Girl*, a one-act play written by Sydney Rosenfeld.[45] The *Evening World* describes it as "a mosaic of popular songs strung on a thread of dialogue."[46] Max Hoffmann's songs were included in the show.[47]

After a few weeks performing in *The Sweet Girl* in Manhattan, the Hoffmanns traveled to Brooklyn on Labor Day weekend 1902 to help open the fall season at the Orpheum Theatre. Gertrude appears on the top of the bill with her fellow Bijou company member Little Chip and the New York Theater Ballet, the corps that performed on the New York Theater mainstage and the Cherry Blossom Grove. This seems to have been another staging of Gertrude's number from *The Sweet Girl*, a song called "My Zulu Lu."[48]

The second-billed act was one whose importance to African American theater cannot be overstated: Bob Cole and J. Rosamond Johnson, the brother and sometime collaborator of James Weldon Johnson. Their composition "Under the Bamboo Tree" was just interpolated in Marie Cahill's show *Sally in Our Alley*, where it would become a smash hit.[49] (Gertrude Hoffmann worked with Cahill in 1905, originating and staging dance numbers for her show *Moonshine.*) "Under the Bamboo Tree" is now best known as sung by Judy Garland and Margaret O'Brien in *Meet Me in St. Louis*. Cole and Johnson probably performed it at this Brooklyn show as well, since it had long been a part of their vaudeville set. Scholars have discussed how "Under the Bamboo Tree" pushes back against stereotypes by focusing on universal human emotions and minimizing exoticism and dialect.[50] "This is in effect a Western courtship transplanted to Africa," says David Chinitz.[51] The performance used similar techniques: Cole and Johnson did not perform in blackface as Bert Williams and George Walker did, and they dressed elegantly.

"My Zulu Lu" and "Under the Bamboo Tree" share imagery and a basic structure: Zulu warriors and jungle maids court in a primitive but royal setting. Though New York audiences may have fancied themselves more sophisticated than those in the South, they took equal pleasure in the Hoffmanns' whitewashed sound and performance style. The presence of the New York Theater Ballet for this musical number suggests it evoked primitive exoticism using strategies Gertrude had learned as a ballet girl in Victorian extravaganzas. It is unclear whether Gertrude and Little Chip donned blackface for this performance. In the same period, Gertrude sang and appeared on the sheet music for "Sadie My Creole Lady," a song that debuted in the Bijou version of *What Happened to Jones?* On the cover of the song's sheet music in figure 2.1 an illustration of the titular Sadie seems to make coy eye contact with the viewer. An inset photograph of "Miss Gertrude Hoffmann" shows her propped on one elbow, reading on a bench. This is no modest ingenue: she posed in such a way that her legs, clad in striped tights, are exposed up to the knee. She seems to be a safe substitute for the "dusky belle" of the song who keeps the speaker "waiting in the cotton fields."[52]

Gertrude Hoffmann did not have a strong voice or a large body like May Irwin or Sophie Tucker, the white women associated with "coon shouting" in that era.[53] She was nearer in her approach to Lillian Russell and Anna Held, attractive leading ladies of the day who used dialect songs to heighten their "sexual naughtiness and their comic breadth."[54] Her white femininity played off the perceived blackness of the music. Max's songs flirted with racial and ethnic otherness, and Gertrude's staging reconnected it to all-American (i.e., white) womanhood.

White musicians and performers have long appropriated African American culture; that history spans blackface minstrelsy, ragtime, rock and roll, and contemporary hip-hop. The Hoffmanns borrowed contemporary arrangements taken from black music and presented the new product as their own, "Hoffmannized" hybrid. Throughout the rest of their careers, they continued to draw on these strategies: Gertrude imitated blackface comedians in her

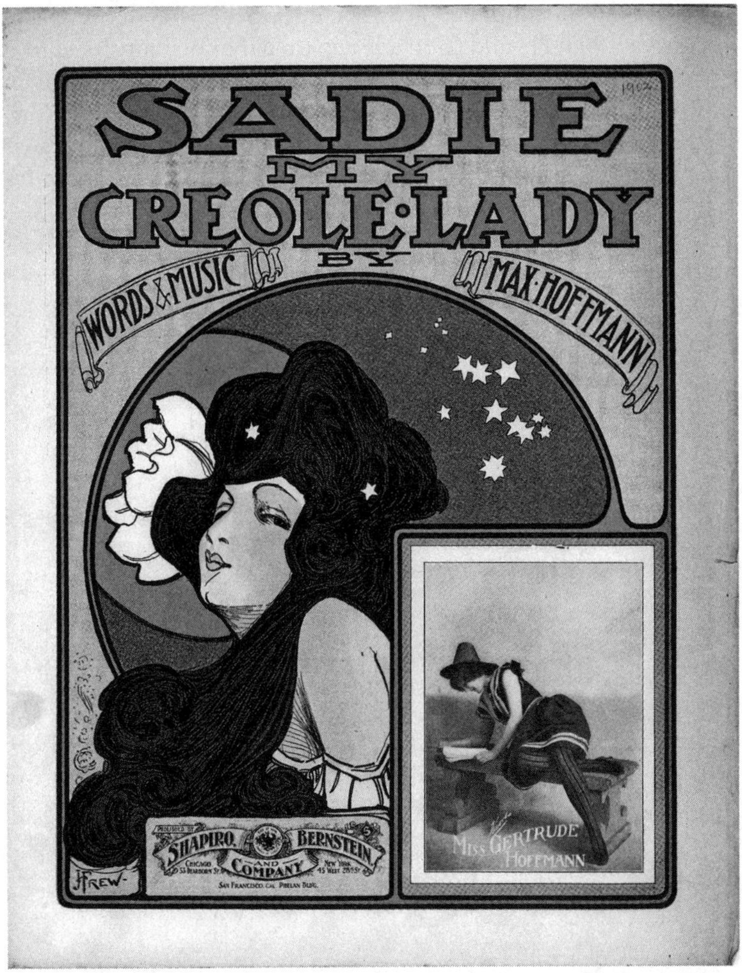

FIGURE 2.1. "Sadie My Creole Lady" sheet music with an inset photograph of Gertrude Hoffmann. Historic American Sheet Music, David M. Rubinstein Rare Book and Manuscript Library, Duke University.

act, and Max championed ragtime well past its prime. Gertrude Hoffmann would make her name in the years to come with her copies of foreign performances, but it is vital to note that imitating African American performance lies at the foundation of the Hoffmanns' career as a musical team.

After a summer performing in New York City, Gertrude and Max returned to the South and the Bijou Musical Comedy Company. They returned to Virginia in December for a different kind of engagement. Their son Max Jr. was born in Norfolk on December 13, 1902. It was time for a change.

Max Hoffmann Sr. continued as music director for the Bijou through the early months of 1903. He and Gertrude departed the company in April of that year. By May, Max was hired to write and conduct the music for the new Rogers Brothers show.[55] At the same time, Gertrude returned to New York City, this time as a stage manager and dance director for Oscar Hammerstein. She developed a talent first practiced in the choruses of San Francisco: training and arranging groups of women.

Chapter 3

✦

A Woman Stage Manager

Gertrude Hoffmann's work as a stock company dance director and stage manager made fiscal sense; she was the music director's wife, and she could perform as well. By summer 1903 she was sufficiently skilled and prepared to do her work in the high-stakes world of New York theater. She returned to the Hammerstein theater complex where she performed in *The Night of the Fourth.*[1] Oscar Hammerstein hired her for $25 a week. She continued to perform on occasion. For the most part, though, she worked behind the scenes.

It was the age of the roof garden theater.[2] At the turn of the twentieth century, several performance spaces opened atop theaters in midtown Manhattan.[3] These seasonal production venues opened for the summer. Audience members were whisked to the roof by that modern innovation, the elevator. They found themselves in a carefree world, often made up to look like another locale. The Paradise Roof Garden that topped Hammerstein's Victoria Theatre included a "Swiss Farm" with windmill and waterwheel, live animals, and a costumed milkmaid.[4] The windmill can be seen in the background of figure 3.1. Roof gardens were, in a sense, a way to take a vacation without leaving the city. Though they were not skyscrapers, theater roofs were tall enough that patrons felt cooler even on the most sweltering summer nights. These theater spaces presented breezy, fun shows that patrons usually watched while eating and drinking. "Summer audiences care little for serious entertainment," *Theatre Magazine* advises, since "the slightest mental effort makes them perspire, and a respite from the dramatic form will be granted by every manger alive to his own interest."[5] In these unserious venues, Hoffmann learned how to translate her theatrical vision into reality.

The first production on which she worked as a dance director was *Punch, Judy, and Co.*, an operetta written by Oscar Hammerstein and staged on the Paradise Roof through the summer of 1903. Gertrude brought together the skills she practiced on her southeastern tours with the ones she remembered from her days in San Francisco. She directed perhaps a dozen cast members on the Wells theatrical circuit. In Hammerstein's show, she directed a chorus of sixty.

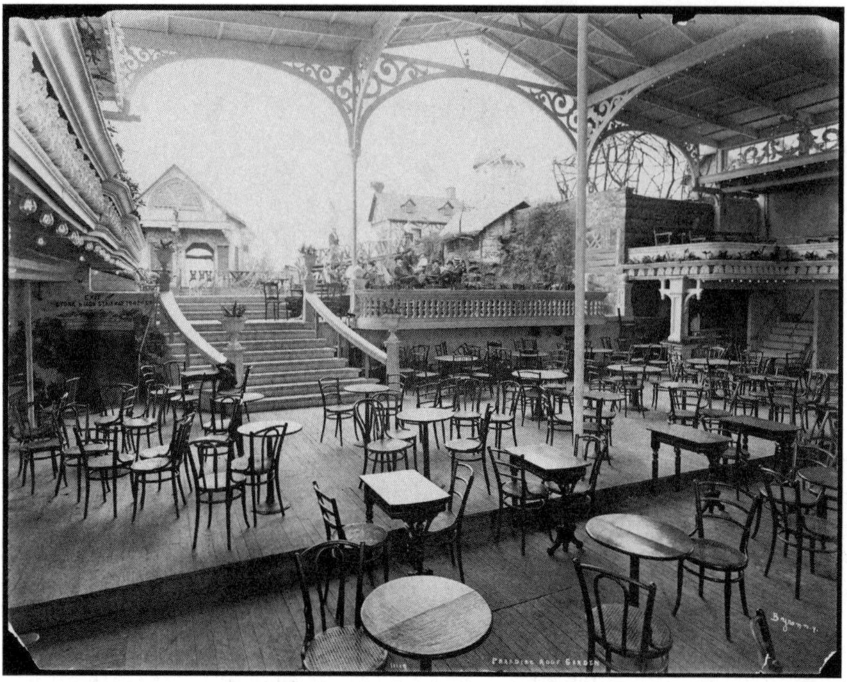

FIGURE 3.1. Paradise Roof Garden atop Hammerstein's Victoria Theatre, circa 1901. Byron Company / Museum of the City of New York. 93.1.1.10855.

She worked long hours, especially in summertime; choruses rehearsed twice a day and shows ran into the early morning. The Hoffmanns lived in a boarding house Gertrude calls Mrs. Deshure's, though the proprietor's name was Dougherty.[6] It was in a convenient location on Forty-Second Street between Seventh and Eighth Avenues, a block from Hammerstein's theater. In her diary, Hoffmann lists the theatrical stars who also stayed there, including Charlie Chaplin.[7] They later resided at the Royal Arms hotel where they befriended the future musical comedy star Charlotte Greenwood, daughter of the housekeeper.

Like many working women, Gertrude depended on female family members to help with childcare. Gertrude's sister Margaret seems to have been Max Jr.'s primary caregiver: in the 1905 New York census, she is listed in the same residence as the Hoffmanns, with the occupation of "home."[8] Because she balanced theater with family, Hoffmann felt a particular sympathy for working mothers in her troupe. One dancer in *Punch, Judy, and Co.* missed several morning rehearsals because she was wheeling her sick baby around the park to give the child much-needed fresh air. Hoffmann was so moved by her story that she rehired the woman and collected money for her baby.[9]

At the age of three, Max Jr. took the long trip west by train to stay with Gertrude's mother Catherine Hayes in San Francisco. Once Junior was left with his grandmother, he got into so much trouble that it made the newspaper: "Baby Steals Buggy and Tries Auto."[10] According to the story, Max Jr. slipped away from his grandmother and nurse, boarded an unattended buggy, and drove it several blocks. "He said he proposed to ride out to the beach and give the horse a chance to get his feet wet," according to the story.[11] No one was hurt, and Max befriended the horse and the policemen who caught up with them.

Gertrude Hoffmann's backstage work was pathbreaking. She was the first woman to be credited for her dance direction in a Broadway show.[12] "Now It's a Woman Stage Manager," marveled a headline in the *New York World*.[13] In that article, Hoffmann suggests that there is "a field of employment for young women in the staging of musical comedies and operatic attractions, not to speak of stock companies, provided, of course, they are fitted by special training to undertake the work."[14] It is unclear what is meant by "special training": perhaps Hoffmann dreamed of opening a school for women stage managers. Her special training took place on the road, and she never lost the resourcefulness of the stock company performer.

Her next show was *The Jersey Lily*, a Blanche Ring vehicle on the main Victoria Theatre stage. Hoffmann "staged and danced special novelty numbers" in the show.[15] She undoubtedly performed in "On a Chinese Honeymoon," a second-act song written by her husband. While Gertrude arranged and danced in *The Jersey Lily*, Max continued his working relationship with the Rogers Brothers. Gus and Max Rogers performed in eight farce comedies together from 1899 to 1907; Max Hoffmann wrote the music for the last four and served as musical director for three of them. This was a steady job, but it also took Max away from Gertrude for long stretches of time. Rogers Brothers shows toured the United States between New York City engagements and after they closed there. Max and Gertrude worked together when they could, whether on the Wells circuit (now the Wells–Dunne–Harlan circuit) or in New York City. One of the numbers Gertrude staged for their act was a "radium dance," which likely used radium as a medium for dress and set designs that would glow in the dark.[16] Over the Christmas holidays of 1904, they worked on *Me, Him, and I*, a burlesque starring the comic trio of Bickel, Watson, and Wrothe.[17] Gertrude took on a dual role, directing twenty-four dancers and playing the soubrette "Seattle Sal." The Hoffmanns were hired as a package in the summer of 1905 for the Wistaria Grove Roof: Max was music director; Gertrude was dance director. There they worked on the New York debut of Elsie Janis, a charming young celebrity impersonator. As a child performer, Janis had crossed paths with Max in Chicago.[18] Max Hoffmann's name was familiar to many performers, whether from his time in Chicago or his songwriting. But he denied any hint of nepotism: "'Give Gerty every bit of the credit; she did it all,' he said, not once but a score of times."[19]

A neighborhood grew up around the theaters and restaurants Hoffmann first saw in 1901. In the years when she began to work in the new theater district, the *New York Times* moved its headquarters from Park Row to Midtown, and the New York City subway opened. She saw these changes take place from up close: "Excavation was terrific, seemed to be about 200 ft. deep—all rock," Gertrude writes.[20] She sees the first wave of what the architectural historian Max Page terms the "creative destruction of Manhattan," a changing paradigm of development whereby the loss of the city's past is a necessary precondition for its improvement.[21] The changing neighborhood influenced Gertrude's sense of herself as a modern woman, as well as her rapid-fire revue style. It also galvanized her loyalty to the Hammerstein family, along with the other pioneers of Times Square.

Hoffmann worked primarily as a choreographer of female dance chorus numbers, known as "girl acts." In the next three years, she staged the dance numbers in more than a dozen shows. The modern American girl act developed from two British sources: Lydia Thompson and her British Blondes, who arrived in New York City in 1868, and "the original English Pony Ballet," trained at the John Tiller School, who performed in the 1883 New York show *The Casino Girl*. Thompson managed a burlesque troupe whose performances were spoofs of mythical stories with women in tights playing the male roles. Tiller's group of eight petite dancers (a larger number than was typical at the time) performed their moves in precise synchronization.[22] These two poles—the comedic ribaldry of the British Blondes and the dance precision of the Pony Ballet—defined the continuum along which the all-girl popular dance troupe was understood.

Hoffmann leveraged her experience as a performer and a producer when directing dancers. "I think I get better results with the girls than most men," she said in a 1905 interview, "because I can show them just what is wanted. I rehearse with them as well as rehearse them."[23] She never asked them to do something she could not do herself, which created a more equal relationship between director and chorus. Plus, her understanding of the chorus girl's experience keeps them on their best behavior. She observed, "They all try hard to please me; they know that I know their tricks, that I have been through just what they are going through, and for this reason they are willing to work when a man would only succeed in making them sulk."[24] In the shows, this also has a positive effect on the men, who felt equally motivated when they saw the women giving their all.

Because of her emotional intelligence and ability to relate to the chorus, Hoffmann considered herself to be a far better dance director than her regular collaborator Ned Wayburn. "These Wayburns were more policemen than directors," she observes cheekily.[25] She also thought herself more of an artist: "Wayburn knew about 3 steps, 3 dancing steps."[26] This criticism came after working with him for years: he was the music director for Mathew and Bulger's *Sad Sea Waves* in 1898, dance director for many Florenz Ziegfeld acts, and often composed songs that Max Hoffmann arranged. Around 1905, they held equivalent positions in the New York theatrical world. It is no surprise that Hoffmann felt this need to distinguish herself.

Both Hoffmann and Wayburn staged performances by a female dance chorus with occasional songs and solo dances. Ned Wayburn was an old pro at arranging "girl acts," and Gertrude Hoffmann was a fresh face. But critics in *Variety* saw them as practicing the same tired routine. A monologue placed in the mouth of "Corks," a drunken small-time burlesque producer, says as much:

> I don't know where Ned got his ideas in the first place, but they are all about the same, and the rest follow along until you get the idea that someone hired a whole orphan asylum and taught all the girls at once. There's the same stamping, the same hand-clapping and all that, and except for the name and the costumes, one act is the same as the other whether Weyburn [*sic*] or Gertie Hoffman or some one else put 'em on. They can't pay the girls a fair salary and make a profit out of 'em because a manager won't pay enough, and so they do the best they can, and the best they can is rotten.[27]

Corks dismisses these modern girl acts in part out of nostalgia: compared to the two-girl "sister acts" he remembers, these performers are skinny and unattractive, with interchangeable routines. But readers of this monologue are meant to take it less than seriously, since it is being spoken by a "human corkscrew" who staged a disreputable Adam and Eve act and spent time in a Mexican jail.

"Gertie" also dabbles in the world of burlesque, though she would never produce acts as seedy as those of Corks. She staged work for the comedian Alexander Carr, as well as for Rose Sydell and the Brooklyn Belles.[28] The early twentieth century was a transitional era when burlesque shows featured leggy girls and dialect comedians but were not yet fully associated with the striptease.[29] In this era the line between burlesque and musical comedy could be blurry. It was a definite step down in terms of prestige and audience: roof garden shows played to urban sophisticates and tourists, both men and women. Burlesque shows appealed to a "lunch bucket crowd," chiefly blue-collar men.[30]

By 1906, her services were much in demand. An agent named George Homans engaged her to develop a girl act.[31] A news item in *Variety* announced that Mark Luescher and Louis Werba would be presenting a new act called "The Pullman Girls," staged by Gertrude Hoffmann with music by Max. "The setting will be a Pullman sleeper," the story reads, "the whole side of which will be exposed to the audience, displaying the berths in various stages of undress."[32] "The Pullman Girls" sounds similar to the girl acts staged by Busby Berkeley more than twenty-five years later, from the setting of "Shuffle

Off to Buffalo" to the spatial arrangement and suggestion of nudity in "Pettin' in the Park."

Though "The Pullman Girls" does not seem to have made it to a stage, Gertrude's next act did. In March 1906, she collaborated with Max and the songwriter Harry Williams on an act called "In the Swim." The cast includes "six chorus men and six pretty girls and also a tramp juggler who works closely after the fashion of W. C. Fields."[33] After some comedy juggling, singing, and dancing, the show concluded with the chorus creating "an original fan effect" onstage while "a series of flags of all nations" are unfurled from the balcony.[34] Still in her early twenties, Gertrude was beginning to develop her style as a stage manager and director. She used the whole company to create abstract images, and she preferred to use the whole auditorium as a stage.

From 1901 to 1906 Hoffmann laid the groundwork for her later career as an auteur and impresario, both theatrical terms with masculine connotations. She could work as a woman stage manager and dance director in part because she worked in lower-stakes venues. Hoffmann went through a training process similar to those of later Hollywood directors who started their careers making B movies. She learned how to make what she wanted quickly and cheaply, with an eye toward a mass audience. Gertrude Hoffmann's behind-the-scenes work began to shape American culture. The girl act, as Hoffmann helped to develop it, is foundational to modern American popular performance. Stage musicals, nightclub revues, and movie musicals would feel underpopulated without them. She helped determine the course of the chorus.

Hoffmann performed while she was developing this movement idiom, but her solo style and stage presence were not as novel as those of her dancers. That was soon to change. During the 1906 summer tour on the usual Wells–Dunne–Harlan circuit, Hoffmann would find the act that highlighted her skills onstage. Her keen eye, which had been focused on stage pictures, was turned to the performers themselves. Hoffmann broke through as a star when she embraced her knack as an imitator.

Part II

✦

Solo Imitations, 1906–1909

Chapter 4

Imitative Caricatures

Gertrude Hoffmann developed into a full-fledged star in the 1906–1907 theatrical season by caricaturing the biggest stars on Broadway. First she supported Anna Held in *A Parisian Model*, and then she played the juvenile lead in the George M. Cohan show *The Honeymooners*. By fall 1907, Hoffmann was headlining New York City vaudeville bills as a solo act, performing what were dubbed "Imitative Caricatures." These early successes as an imitator shaped the critical reception of her work for the next decade: she was seen as a clever interpreter, but seldom as an innovator.

Hoffmann began performing imitations on the Wells–Dunne–Harlan summer circuit that she and Max had toured for years. In the summer of 1906, Gertrude Hoffmann and Her Manhattan Girls shared the bill with Max playing piano, the clown Frank "Slivers" Oakley, and the Hungarian twins Jenny and Rosie Dolly, who would later become the toast of Jazz Age New York and Paris. Charlotte Greenwood went on the tour as well, perhaps as one of the Manhattan Girls. Greenwood mused in her memoir, "As children the Dollys couldn't dance for sour apples, but they were so attractive that audiences never bothered about the missteps."[1] Gertrude agreed with her young friend Lottie's assessment: "They looked cute," she writes, "but had nothing else to offer."[2] For at least part of the tour, they performed the "In the Swim" number that played on the Hammerstein roof. The show ended with a sketch composed by Gertrude and Max, called "Everybody Works but Father."

Gertrude was hesitant to perform her imitations because Max found them ineffective. This changed in Petersburg, Virginia. Max was called to New York City to collaborate with Harry B. Smith on a new show, which would become *A Parisian Model*. Gertrude took this opportunity to try out a new version of her specialty, showing him before he left that she could be a success. She writes:

> I decided to go to it sat. Mat. [Saturday matinee] & show him he was wrong and that I could do the imitations. Also I realized that my costume was wrong—switched costumes. On Sat. AM took Lottie [Charlotte Greenwood] with me to toy shop and other shops. Bought toy hat, gloves, little umbrella, other props needed. Then I rehearsed

> Lottie to stand offstage in entrance and hand me props. Went on, did everything, cartwheel off—audience cheered & all women and children seen beaming in through upper windows. That did it—they would not let me off. On one of my bows I stopped dead & told Max that now you can go to N.Y.[3]

Gertrude used humor in her act before, since soubrette parts demanded a flirtatious and witty actress. With this act, though, the undersized props and acrobatic physicality moved her performance into the realm of clowning. She won over the crowd (and Max) with her imitations.

The props she used were likely for her caricature of Eddie Foy in drag as Sister Anne, the role he played in *Mr. Bluebeard*. In some promotional photos he wears a conical hat; in others, he poses with a paper umbrella, his hair piled on top of his head in a ludicrous ponytail. Figure 4.1 shows Hoffmann's interpretation of the character.[4] Hoffmann imitated George M. Cohan in this act as well. Both of these comic bits were based in part on her firsthand observation of the performers: Hoffmann had played in the chorus of a Foy show in San Francisco and had seen the Four Cohans on their western tours. She also called upon the publicity Foy received for his bravery in the wake of the Iroquois Theatre Fire, which broke out in Chicago in December 1903. Foy and Cohan were well loved across the country, so imitations of them reinforced the audience's sense of belonging in a shared theatrical community.

Hoffmann's summer tour made an impression on the critics back in New York City. One wrote that she was "hypnotizing" audiences in the southeast and leaving them "dazzled." [5] When she and Max returned to New York, Gertrude was ready to perform as a solo act. In her notebooks, Hoffmann says that the actress Grace George, who was married to the Broadway producer William A. Brady, offered her a booking at the Wistaria Grove, "where Elsie Janis had starred the summer before + by the way I staged the show."[6] Instead, she chose the Metropolis Roof, at Third Avenue and 142nd Street in the Bronx. This might be seen as the equivalent of trying her act "out of town"; since Hoffmann knew what the Times Square roof garden audiences were like, perhaps she wanted to start in front of a different type of crowd.

Her solo act included singing, dancing, and impersonations. She liked to break the fourth wall in inventive ways. This act had "ringers" in theater boxes who interacted with her during the first song.[7] By the second week, she was down to one assistant but still succeeded onstage due to her charisma.[8] Her mimicry of Florenz Ziegfeld's wife Anna Held was judged the best of her impersonations.[9] Max began working on the music direction for a new Ziegfeld-produced Held vehicle, *A Parisian Model*. Anna and Flo had worked together since the late 1890s, but five years had passed since their last hit, *The Little Duchess*.[10] Ziegfeld wanted to ensure success, and Max Hoffmann had written the music for the last three Rogers Brothers shows, so he was brought

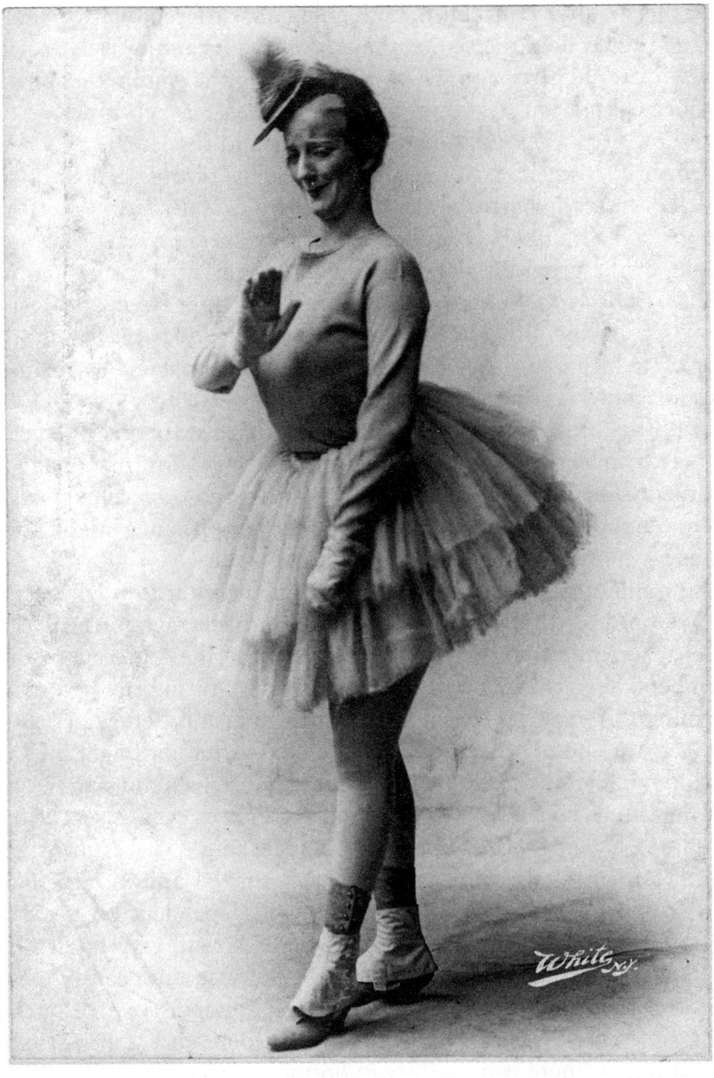

FIGURE 4.1. Gertrude Hoffmann imitating Eddie Foy Sr. in his role as Sister Anne in *Mr. Bluebeard*. Gertrude Hoffmann Collection—Brooklyn Public Library—Brooklyn Collection.

on. At first, no position could be found for Gertrude. Max "tried every avenue to get [her] into the show," while Gertrude looked for bookings elsewhere.[11]

This led to a minor crisis in their marriage. Though Gertrude wanted to continue to work with Max, she also intuited that she was about to hit it big: "I knew or felt that I expected to make good in my act this week + that

I thought this would be our finish, both going our different ways."[12] Gertrude went to the United Booking Office, the centralized location for vaudeville performers who wished to sign a contract to tour the major theaters of the Keith–Albee circuit. She asked for a generous long-term contract—$150 per week, with a forty-week guarantee—and was told that if she was a success at a tryout in Providence, she would have it. This tryout seems not to have materialized. Instead, Gertrude was brought on to *A Parisian Model* to help stage some of the numbers and perform a dance specialty.[13]

Looking at the program alone, one might assume that Hoffmann made a hit in *A Parisian Model* due to her dancing. She appears in the cast list as "Colombe, a dancing girl."[14] The numbers she receives credit for are the first act's "La Mattchiche," a scandalous tango-like dance that she performed with Anna Held, and a second-act solo dance. "La Mattchiche" saw Hoffmann dressed in drag: in her journals, she says the dance was too "naughty to be danced here by male + female—so Ziegf[eld] had his tailor [in] Chicago make me [a] tuxedo—he attended all fittings."[15] Hoffmann's dance experience got her cast in the show, but the best reviews of her performance talked about her imitations far more than they did her dancing.

Cast in a minor part, Hoffmann was elevated to stardom with a story of discovery so perfect that it could come from a backstage musical. She was performing her imitations of Foy and Cohan for the amusement of other cast members. She also imitated Anna Held, caricaturing the petite and coy Frenchwoman so perfectly that it was seen as an insult. "They all wanted me out," Hoffmann's notebook reads. "Anna—No—After mat[inee] she came on stage—told me, she wanted the imitation in but that I should sing her first act song 'Delightful to Be Married' which I did."[16] Press coverage set the incident on a train to Chicago tryouts of the show. According to the *Chicago Sunday Tribune*, Hoffmann was called upon to perform the imitation of Held the same night, which seems unlikely in a show so dependent on the women's costumes. Held's biographer Eve Golden has reservations about the story, noting that after Hoffmann left the show "she was replaced by Madalyn Summers—who was, if the papers are to be believed, discovered by Anna in the exact same way."[17] Though Hoffmann was sometimes guilty of believing her own publicity, there is no reason to doubt her account.

The anecdote conveys something of Anna Held's good humor, but it also shows a woman managing her own celebrity reputation. Asking Hoffmann to sing a different song suggests that Held was thinking about the caricature's impact in the show. Held was accustomed to Ziegfeld's publicity blitzes, including the decadent rumor that she bathed in milk to maintain her glowing skin.[18] Even stories that included critical details about her behavior added to her fame. Like newspaper stories, vaudeville imitations of female actresses were a sign of popularity and, in a certain sense, of respect. Famous actresses accepted the practice and even checked up on vaudeville mimics imitating them.[19] Held performed the same due diligence as Sarah Bernhardt and Ethel

Barrymore, though it was even more important since Held and Hoffmann were appearing in the same show.

Imitations were good for business.[20] They both assumed and built familiarity with the original stage performers.[21] It is possible that Held understood the power of Hoffmann's imitation as a signifier and amplifier of her originality. We can understand Hoffmann's freshness and cleverness working in tandem with Held's established fame to reinforce the celebrity of each. They were partners onstage; as in "La Mattchiche," Hoffmann's job in her imitations was to show off Held to her advantage.

This show kicked off a long friendship between the two performers.[22] After the show closed, Held gave an interview that dealt with the newest scandal in her life, the revelation of her adolescent daughter from a previous marriage. Late in that conversation, she talked about her own personality and stage celebrity with an admirable candor: "Mr. Ziegfeld, my husband, has several times said: 'Do you not think you are a little broad?' 'Do you not think you could modify some things a little bit?' I always reply: 'When I do things they are chic—they are different—they are—Anna Held! If I modify myself what will I be? Nobody! The same as hundreds of others.'"[23] Held understood the constraints of her stage persona and her obligation to maintain it. She was responsible for her own reproduction, and modification was not a possibility.

Held's career offers a vivid example of the ways that turn-of-the-century fame played out through the segmenting, doubling, and abstracting of the celebrity image. After she earned fame for her eyes, every show required an "eye song": one, "The Maiden with the Dreamy Eyes," was written by Bob Cole and James Weldon Johnson.[24] Ziegfeld erected an electric sign with a pair of rolling eyes above the marquee of *A Parisian Model*, though it was taken down after it repeatedly shorted and made the eyes look crossed.[25] Long after Held's initial career ended, her eyes served as a representation of her celebrity status, the part of her that stood in for the whole of her charms. Doubling of the female lead takes place in romantic ballets such as *Giselle* and *Swan Lake*, as Rhonda Garelick notes in her analysis of Loie Fuller's deconstruction of them.[26] Held appeared not as a doll or a double, but as a painted reproduction of herself. As the titular model, she is painted by her boyfriend; when a jealous rival steals the painting, she has to stand in for it to impress a wealthy art collector.[27]

Later in the show's run, Hoffmann's star ascended. Her billing changed by the time of the April 15, 1907, program. Instead of being listed as performing a dance specialty, she is listed as performing a "Dance and Caricatures of Famous Artists."[28] Though it is from Hoffmann's 1910 revue, figure 4.2 conveys Held's style circa 1907. Hoffmann wears a pale gown covered with intricate patterns of sequins. Her waist is narrow, her eyes wide; her dark pompadour and enormous, feathered headpiece encircle a small, exquisitely made-up face. Hoffmann's caricature was perceived as self-aware and original, thus commenting on Held's celebrity image.[29] Even though Hoffmann's

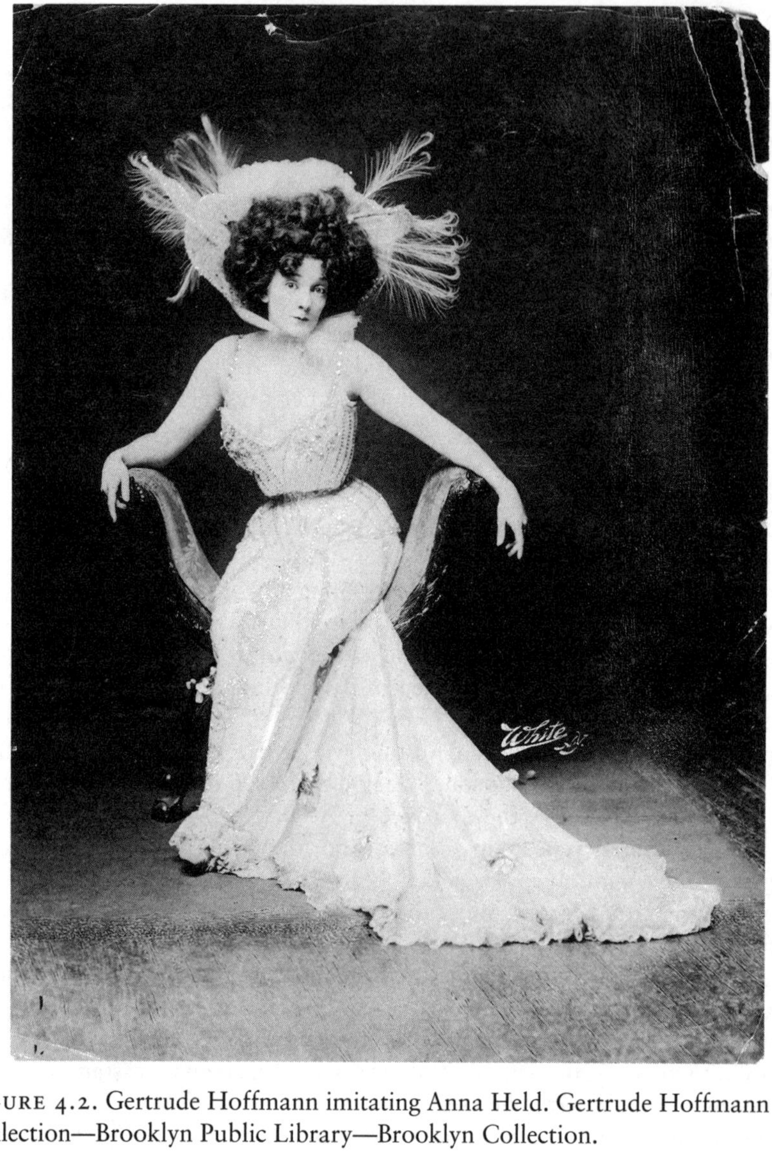

FIGURE 4.2. Gertrude Hoffmann imitating Anna Held. Gertrude Hoffmann Collection—Brooklyn Public Library—Brooklyn Collection.

caricature of Held was judged to be the most cutting in her repertoire, she appeared on the bill just before the butt of her joke. Anna Held follows Hoffmann performing her two hits of the show, "I Just Can't Make My Eyes Behave" and the newly interpolated "Won't You Be My Teddy Bear."[30] This billing suggests that Hoffmann's imitation is a kind of warm-up Anna, preparing the audience for the real thing. To have the imitation appear just before the original differs from a later version of the same tactic, commonly used by Ned Wayburn, which Barbara Cohen-Stratyner has called "instant debunking." In this form of celebrity caricature and doubling, a specialty act performed straight would be immediately followed by a routine burlesquing it.[31] Here too, the performers in question are aware of and consenting to the imitation. The rhythm differs: a move from imitation to original builds up the celebrity, while a move from original to imitation deflates her.

Once *A Parisian Model* was established as a hit, Ziegfeld moved on to planning the first of his eponymous *Follies*. Up-and-coming female performers approached Hoffmann, since she was a star with access to the producer. She says that "out of a clear sky they picked on me to show Z. their photos."[32] If Hoffmann's diary is accurate, a few of the women who asked her to put in a good word were cast, including Nora Bayes and Grace La Rue. Hoffmann herself waited in vain to be asked to join the *Follies*: "I expected he would want me—but he did not."[33] Hoffmann grew to understand why Ziegfeld kept her in *A Parisian Model*. She writes that she was "the applause hit of the show" and that if she had left to join the *Follies*, her "absence would have been noticed & commented upon—as it actually was."[34] Hoffmann was a vital supporting figure, one whose variety and versatility could serve as a complement to Anna Held's consistent performance of herself.

Late in the run of *A Parisian Model*, Ziegfeld devised a new way to showcase Hoffmann. *The Belle of Mayfair* was a British import that competed with his show but closed at the end of March. A month later, Hoffmann's second-act caricature scene introduced a travesty on Valeska Suratt's song from that show, "Why Do They Call Me a Gibson Girl?" Hoffmann wore a knockoff of Suratt's dress from the show, a sleeveless black velvet gown with hips comically padded to exaggerate the original star's hourglass figure.

This imitation takes on more importance in Hoffmann's career because it caricatures what had become an entire branch of popular culture. Charles Dana Gibson's first etchings of the Gibson Girl appeared in American mass magazines in the 1890s. A composite of older models of white womanhood and the features of contemporary friends and female celebrities, the Gibson Girl was both seen as an aspirational ideal and as a typical (white, middle-class) modern young woman. She was tall and active, with a curvaceous figure and a mass of hair piled on top of her head. By the middle of the first decade of the twentieth century, she was everywhere: on china, calendars, scarves, and wallpaper, and in every newspaper and magazine.[35]

Why was Hoffmann so successful in this role? The Gibson Girl by definition has an imposing physical silhouette; "The Weaker Sex," one of the most popular of Gibson's images, shows three giantesses examining the modern man through a magnifying glass. Hoffmann's performance accepted and refused the "Gibson Girl" moniker, bringing a vulnerability to the imitations that is wholly absent from the original image. The audience would have experienced the pleasure of recognizing a caricature of Suratt's performance coupled with a comparison of Hoffmann's appearance to that of the Gibson Girl from print culture.[36] Hoffmann's performance is both a comedic act and an act of representation, recreating an original image familiar to everyone in the audience. Her work should be grouped with other referential performances by women the period such as tableaux vivants, statue posing, and pageants.[37] Hoffmann's mimesis is more lateral in its references. Instead of pointing back toward a shared or imagined past, she gestures toward other contemporary stage performances and print publications.

Hoffmann emphasizes in her journal that the imitation (and the padding) were Ziegfeld's idea and that "he superintended all."[38] He did not get much of a return on his investment; Hoffmann left *A Parisian Model* soon after. Her departure from the show is mentioned in a *New York Times* article, which notes "that differences between Mr. Ziegfeld and Mr. Hoffman have come to a head since Mrs. Hoffman, owing to disagreement as to the advisability of certain stage business, left the company a few weeks ago."[39] Hoffmann began rehearsals with George M. Cohan for his summer show *The Honeymooners*, in which she would go on to perform the routine to much acclaim.

Though there does not appear to be a definitive explanation for Gertrude Hoffmann's departure, it seems important to note its proximity to the Gibson Girl debut. Perhaps "a certain stage business" performed during the routine led to Hoffmann's upstaging Anna Held? A more likely explanation was Hoffmann's continued desire to be part of Ziegfeld's upcoming *Follies*. She made an impact in a supporting part but knew she could be a leading lady. Max Hoffmann struggled with Ziegfeld as well. He signed a contract to serve as music director for the run of the show, but in late April he had been told that his services were not needed over the summer.[40] To make a point, Max took a risk that few in the theater business would.

Max had written the score for *A Parisian Model* before he was hired to conduct it. He argued that his contract as composer was signed with the production team Klaw and Erlanger, so the score was not Ziegfeld's to use.[41] If they fired him as music director, he argued, they lost his services as composer of the score as well. According to Gertrude, their lawyer, Nathan Burkan, recommended that Max "take out orchestrations on [the] quiet."[42] He asked the orchestra drummer Johnnie O'Neil to gather the sheet music and take it to the stage door; from there, Max took it home by cab.[43] The *New York Times* gives a different account, saying that the Hoffmanns took the score and then dined at the Hotel Metropole.[44]

Ziegfeld was furious. He met the Hoffmanns at Nathan Burkan's brownstone on 145th Street, where the lawyer tried to mediate a solution. There seems to have been more argument than negotiation.[45] The following morning Max Hoffmann was arraigned in the Jefferson Market court.[46] Gertrude sat six rows back, watching the action. Max was "pale as a sheet," listening to the charges against him from behind a wire screen.[47] No one contested that

Max had written the music. Instead, the charge was comically technical: larceny of the paper on which the score was printed.[48]

Gertrude was overwhelmed by Max's actions and their consequences. "I knew Max did a terrible unheard of thing," she writes, "taking away the music orchestrations of the biggest show in town + owned by the 2 biggest men in the theatre world."[49] The vaudeville producer Abe Erlanger attended the trial in his capacity as director of the Interstate Amusement Company, the plaintiff in the suit. He brought a claque of "yes-men" and Henry J. Goldsmith, the powerful lawyer. Nathan Burkan defended Max along with three "not too well dressed men," one of whom carried law books with him to the hearing.[50] Gertrude was already frightened, and this seemed to seal Max's fate: "I thought what kind of lawyers are they—they cannot be very good if they must carry law books to court—more shivering on my part."[51] Ziegfeld added to her anxiety, insisting that Max would serve a long prison term.

The court first decided in favor of the plaintiff. The decision was quickly reversed, though, since it was decided that Max did not display "criminal intent" when he took the score.[52] Max brought a countersuit for breach of contract, trying to prevent production of *A Parisian Model* without him.[53] The suit was settled, and Max returned to work for Ziegfeld as musical director for the *Follies of 1907*. The Hoffmanns played hardball with some of the most powerful theatrical producers in the country, and they won.

Gertrude's move from *A Parisian Model* to *The Honeymooners* was in one sense a step down: Ziegfeld shows were seen as sophisticated and urbane, while Cohan shows were decidedly corny. *The Honeymooners* cast Hoffmann as a vivacious co-ed in love with George M. Cohan's football-playing college boy. The play was a revival and revision of an earlier comedy for the Four Cohans, a 1903 show called *Running for Office*. The plot remained the same: John Tiger is running for mayor of a small town in Vermont, called Tigersville in the first version and Hazelnut in the second. Tiger is a widower who has remarried the former Mrs. Wright. The titular honeymooners avoid discussion of their previous marriages and college-age children. "Why don't you know that a man who has children can't be elected?" John reminds his daughter.[54] Those children, Madeline Tiger and Augustus Wright, attend the same college. They have fallen in love, unaware that their parents have married each other. The characters collide in Hazelnut where Augustus is due to play his football game, with farcical results.

Madeline Tiger's character and role in the show demonstrate the clear connection in this era between modern femininity and stage performance. In *Running for Office*, Madeline longed to go to "Paree," but in *The Honeymooners* she longs to "run away and go on the stage."[55] In the first act, she sings about being a "Musical Comedy Maid" in a show where "The audience will yell / At the sight of Anna Held."[56] Romantic and familial complications are resolved by the third act, with plenty of time for Madeline to perform in the public square. Hoffmann performed three imitations, which replaced the previous act 3 spectacle of a torchlight political parade.[57] Instead of presenting all three of her imitations in sequence, Hoffmann exited and the action continued while she changed costumes. This staging led Cohan to feud with some of the first-night crowd who liked Hoffmann's performances so much that they talked over the intervening dialogue, cheering for her to come back.[58]

As Hoffmann's star rose, her imitations made up a major part of the publicity for *The Honeymooners*. Her caricatures were caricatured in print. Over the month of June 1907, she was drawn several times—always in triplicate as Held, Suratt, and Foy. The Canadian American Boardman Robinson, who would later contribute to *The Masses*, drew her for the *Telegraph*.[59] Marius de Zayas, the Mexican American artist who would exhibit with Alfred Stieglitz and write for *291* magazine, drew the set in the *New York World*.[60] Robinson ties his three figures together with shading in the background. They all lean to the right and stand around the same height. De Zayas has cleaner lines and a more abstracting style. His figures are discrete, with one facing forward, the next in right profile, and the third in left profile. The faces are drawn so differently that they might not be the same person. And yet both sets of illustrations capture the poses and attitudes that define each bit of mimicry: for Held, her shoulders hunched up near the ears; for Suratt, a placid face and bent back; and for Foy, a clownish expression and awkward tutu. Their illustrations are second-order interpretations, ones that need to highlight both the performance choices of the mimic and the salient features of the original star.

When the summer season ended, *The Honeymooners* closed. Hoffmann had built up enough of a reputation as a performer that she could book engagements as a solo act in vaudeville. Unusually for the era, Hoffmann did not ally herself with one vaudeville manager in this period. She played at Hammerstein's Paradise Roof Garden theater in August 1907, then toured the Keith & Proctor circuit through the fall. Her act developed and changed over time, though the first successful "imitative caricatures"—Held, Suratt, and Foy—stayed in the mix. She came up with a novel solution to the costume-change delays of *The Honeymooners*. "It is the fashion nowadays for actors to reveal the secrets of their make-up and the arcana of their dressing rooms," says Robert Speare in a *New York Telegraph* review of her Hammerstein show, "So Miss Hoffmann had a dressing room in full view of her audience."[61] With two maids helping her, Hoffmann changed her outfits, shoes, wig, and makeup, all while giving the crowd a quick glimpse of the real performer beneath the trappings. Hoffmann moved her act to the Keith & Proctor circuit, with a new gimmick: a curtained opening in the back where she retreated, changed, and reappeared in a new costume. One reviewer finds this change even more suggestive: "The former frank display is now absent, and all the audience gets is a flash of lace from time to time to keep their interest on tip-toe of expectancy."[62] As Hoffmann's vaudeville act evolved over the course of the season, she continued to foreground the artificiality and titillation of her own imitations.[63]

Throughout these early seasons, Hoffmann's act showed how the work of caricature gets done.

The highest degree of difficulty took place not during the act of mimicry itself but while moving from one imitation to the next. The theater critic Caroline Caffin gives a backhanded compliment to the imitators who use costumes as part of their acts. Compared to the work of rubber-faced and many-voiced mimics, she says, the success of costumed imitators "belongs in great part to the wig-maker."[64] Even though the successful imitations do not arise from the skilled work of the body, she does admire the "economy of movement" that's necessary to transform from one famous personage to another. Hoffmann participated in this kind of performative efficiency with her maids (and even earlier in her summer act where Charlotte Greenwood handed her props offstage). These acts demanded forethought in terms of sequencing and coordinating props, and even required a kind of practical choreography.

Because of these quick changes between celebrity images, at least one reviewer thought that Hoffmann's show was a kind of human highlight reel. Her show offered famous people at bargain prices: "When she enables you to see Anna Held, Elfie Fay, George Cohan, Eddie Foy and Vesta Victoria better than they are themselves for one price of admission, what's the use of paying five prices to see the originals separately?"[65] It is worth interrogating why "imitative caricatures" of celebrities might be thought of as "better than they are themselves." When a mimic like Hoffmann presents a caricature, she performs not just the highlights of an act but the highlights of an identity, the recognizable quirks that make one celebrity image different from another. Seeing George M. Cohan in *The Honeymooners* might be a more thorough introduction to his style as an actor, but there are parts of that show in which Cohan was not "doing" George M. Cohan to the degree that Hoffmann would in her imitation. To perform a celebrity caricature onstage is to wittily reimagine that celebrity as a platonic ideal. Performative caricatures imitate and often critique, but they always condense.

Audiences enjoyed watching an actor make a quick transformation from one celebrity to another, in part because it showed just how quickly a celebrity's identity can be sketched. One review performs this speedy delivery in textual form, saying that Hoffmann "acted and sang like a foolish Eddifoy and an audacious Annaheld to perfection."[66] With portmanteaux that anticipate E. E. Cummings or John Dos Passos, the reviewer points out something important about celebrity culture: caricature work like Hoffmann's extends the understanding of individuality by emphasizing that it needs to come at you all at once instead of building up over time.

Caroline Caffin captures something of this strategy when she says of another mimic that he "could give us an admirable snapshot but could not elaborate a finished picture."[67] The performance of a caricature plays with the tension between the temporality of photography and that of theater. Hoffmann's audience recognized her imitations in a flash, but then waited to see how their expectations would be thwarted by the comedic direction of the piece. By all accounts, Hoffmann looked similar to Anna Held. The humor lies in how close to the original she began, and how far away from the original she diverged. "She seemed to have borrowed Anna's eyes for the Held imitation," says one reviewer of her performance in *The Honeymooners*; she also borrowed her coy voice, "which was gradually exaggerated until it ended in a scream."[68] The structure of Hoffmann's act reverses the logic of the celebrity caricature: we see the familiar image first, followed by a performance that undermines it.

When Hoffmann performed at the Maryland Theater in October 1907, she ended the act with "an imitation of herself as she appeared in 'A Parisian Model.'"[69] This period in Hoffmann's career illustrates several important things about the role of mimicry within American popular performance. She shows how the imitation of other stars serves as a vehicle for developing one's own star persona.[70] Her repeated performances of Eddie Foy, Anna Held, and the Gibson Girl show just how portable imitations were in an era before the integrated musical. The prevalence and acceptance of celebrity caricatures in this period demonstrate how they helped perpetuate celebrity culture.

This season was the beginning of her career as an imitator, and she remained faithful to the celebrities from this period long after she had gained more fame as a dancer and producer. "Do you know that I suffer from the fact that there are no people to imitate at the present time?" she asks the theater critic Alan Dale in 1913.[71] Dale admits that "the old subjects" (including Eddie Foy and Anna Held) are "a bit played out" but that "nobody has arisen to take their places."[72] Though it was an absurd remark to make at a time when Al Jolson's star was on the rise, Hoffmann communicated a kind of mournful nostalgia over vaudeville's loss of big personalities. Her imitations index a particular moment in celebrity culture, and they suggest that perhaps these stars of the popular stage circa 1907 became famous and stayed famous because they were easy to imitate.

After a successful move from supporting roles in musical comedies to commanding the vaudeville stage, Gertrude took a break. She and Max sailed for London in December 1907 aboard the *Oceanic* on the White Star Line.[73] It was Gertrude's first time in Europe; after working for so much of her young life, it is possible this was her first time taking "a pleasure trip."[74] When the Hoffmanns landed at home in January, they went back to work: Max mended fences with Flo Ziegfeld and again took up his baton for *A Parisian Model*. Gertrude prepared for her return to vaudeville. She rehearsed an act that skewered Eva Tanguay, the star known for her wild costumes and manic energy.[75] Tanguay's signature song "I Don't Care" gives a clear sense of her gleeful nihilism; the music critic Jody Rosen has called her a vaudeville "rock star."[76] Another addition to Hoffmann's arsenal was a send-up of the operetta *The*

Merry Widow. Her ambition as a mimic was increasing. Her vaudeville turn depended on contrasts for its effect, and there was no sharper contrast than one between Tanguay's jittery act and *The Merry Widow*'s elegant waltz. Both were wildly popular in the winter of 1908 and her imitations of both got Gertrude into a lot of trouble.

Chapter 5

Women's Rivalry and Copyright

Ideas about imitation and originality underwent a paradigm shift in the early twentieth century. Whereas copying was once associated with primitive minds and lesser forms of creativity, artists and social theorists alike were articulating new ideas about the inventiveness of imitation.[1] American popular theater was inundated with mimic acts, in both vaudeville and musical comedy. The otherwise unremarkable show *The Girl Question* featured a hit song calling this theatrical fad "The Imitation Craze."[2] The trend was dominated by female performers like Gertrude Hoffmann.[3] The summer that she played opposite George M. Cohan in *The Honeymooners*, one review called her "the girl mimic that seems to be deemed essential to a summer roof-garden show."[4] But with the dominance of women imitators came an increased interest in the rivalry among them. The *Honeymooners* article ranked Hoffmann in relation to her fellow mimics—"a follower of Cissy Loftus, a long way behind, but nearly alongside of Elsie Janis."[5] During a brief stretch of her career in the spring and summer of 1908, Gertrude Hoffmann was embroiled in several conflicts related to her imitations. She argued in the entertainment press and the judicial system for her right to imitate other people's acts. Though her claims were successful, they were seldom taken seriously. Women's debates over intellectual property were seen as a kind of catfight, or comic relief. The coverage of women mimics diminished the power of these transgressive performing women and rendered them more palatable.[6]

Hoffmann was supposed to return to vaudeville in winter 1908 as part of a powerhouse double bill. She and Eva Tanguay were booked to appear at Keith and Proctor's Harlem theater on 125th Street. Tanguay had previously challenged the British music hall performer Vesta Victoria to share the stage with her; this bill was seen as a follow-up, a way to take on another competitor. "Miss Tanguay will sing and dance," reads the *New York Tribune* listing, "and Miss Hoffman will give her amusing imitations of well-known players."[7] Hoffmann would play her imitation of Tanguay on the same stage as the star herself, just as she had done with her caricatures of Anna Held and George M. Cohan the year before. With Tanguay, though, her imitations competed with the originals.

Tanguay tried to prevent Hoffmann from imitating her, and the performers sparred over their position on the bill. An account from Hoffmann's future manager Morris Gest details the aftermath in colorful terms: "[She] wasn't Kitty Hayes and Irish for nothing. The fur flew. 'You think I'll let that spoiled brat dictate to me? We'll see!' And with that she ordered her trunks and properties out of the theatre, leaving Tanguay in lonely glory on the bill."[8] Hoffmann left the bill for that week. An advertisement suggests that she performed instead at Young's Pier Theatre in Atlantic City.[9]

The vaudeville stars continued their feud in the newspapers. Spectators, as Susan Glenn has theorized, enjoyed "watching women symbolically slug it out."[10] On February 25, Hoffmann published an ad in the *New York Morning Telegraph* daring Tanguay to play her usual penultimate spot on the bill and let Hoffmann close the show. An article in a later edition included the subtitle "Eva Afraid of Gertrude?" and Max Hoffmann was quoted betting $5,000 that his wife would best Tanguay, with "a committee to give the decision."[11] Tanguay responded in the next day's paper, insisting that "Miss Hoffmann left the theatre not because I wouldn't play with her, but because she COULDN'T have my place on the bill. The FACT was the ORIGINATOR remained and that the IMITATOR QUIT." Hoffmann was tipped off to this response, so she paid for a final retort on the opposite page of the same issue: "I will follow you and wager any amount of money you can cover that I will receive as much genuine applause as you do. You might 'bluff' foreign artists, but your hand is called now."[12] The reference to "foreign artists" was a nod to Tanguay's recent booking with Vesta Victoria. These heightened acts of public speech articulate different visions of female stardom. For Hoffmann a star was defined by her skill, her humor, and her nerve. (Note the extended poker metaphor of bluffing and calling one's hand in her final ad.) For Tanguay originality was more important than any other talents. Tanguay translates into present-day terms of celebrity (as a "rock star") because of this emphasis on personality, authenticity, and uniqueness. Gertrude performed others, while Eva performed herself.

Their clash highlights the tendency among vaudevillians to view their own acts as property to be defended in the court of public opinion. Vernacular performers did not invoke copyright law.[13] Instead, they claimed ownership in newspapers and trade magazines.[14] The section of *Variety* called "Artist's Forum" featured letters from acrobats, comedians, and other vaudeville acts who felt their material was unjustly borrowed by fellow performers. "Editor *Variety*," one letter begins: "There is an act calling themselves the 'Cycling Bordwells.' We wish to say we were the first to use the word 'Cycling' [i.e., as an abbreviation for "bicycling"] and people who are using the same would greatly oblige us by dropping it."[15] This letter was signed by the "Cycling Carrolls." A mechanism for protecting material was later formalized in Protected Materials Departments where performers could register their acts by mailing in an envelope with a hard copy of the material. When a plagiarism charge was brought, these hard copies could be consulted to identify the performer with the earliest claim.[16]

Hoffmann returned to Harlem the following week to take up her argument again. She played at the Alhambra Theatre, just across 125th Street from Keith and Proctor's venue where Tanguay performed. The Tanguay imitation stayed in the act. Just as in Atlantic City, Hoffmann piled her hair in a frizzy mop atop her head and donned a white corset, with matching tights and shoes. There was one addition: "The crowning touch in the duel came when, instead of inserting Miss Tanguay's name in the slots at the side of the stage for her "I Don't Care!" number, Miss Hoffmann displayed only a big "?"[17] The press enjoyed Hoffmann's one-upmanship. *Variety* discusses Hoffmann's booking at the Alhambra as it highlights problems with the United Booking Office, a managerial issue. Yet they still end the story with this deadpan detail: "On Tuesday evening it is related Miss Tanguay declared she would add to her performance 'an imitation of how Gertrude Hoffmann intended to imitate me.' Through a strenuous effort Miss Tanguay was induced to rescind her declaration."[18] The imitation craze can only be taken so far before it becomes ridiculous, the story suggests.

Gertrude Hoffmann won the battle with Eva Tanguay in the papers, but she still faced the consequences for failing to appear on the same stage. Her Alhambra booking was another double bill. In an interview with Morris Gest's biographer she says she was booked with her fellow mimic Cissy Loftus "as a punishment" since Loftus "was considered the greatest imitator of the times."[19] Hoffmann was a comic imitator, the thinking seems to have gone, but not a truly gifted artist like Loftus. A *Variety* review suggests that putting these two women on the same bill makes clear the "divergent directions" of their work: "Miss Loftus imitates in voice, gestures and expression; Miss Hoffman impersonates by assuming all the character, including the dress, and adding a bit of travesty. Miss Loftus is the personification of the art of mimicry; Miss Hoffman likewise of impersonation."[20] Their imitations differ, but so do their techniques. Loftus represented her characters from the inside out through movements that came from her body. Hoffmann represented from the outside in, assuming a character the way one might assume a title or an office. The emphasis on the supplementary components—not just the character but the dress, a bit of travesty added on to spice up the performance—underscore the ways Hoffmann's performance lay in the external.

Gertrude Hoffmann was often portrayed by her critics as an example of bad imitation to highlight the good imitation of other popular performers with a more skilled and trained relationship to their bodies. Other female mimics were celebrated for their ability to channel their performers and characters without external trappings. Reviews of Elsie Janis and Cissy Loftus emphasized the childlike and playful qualities of these performances; notably, both began their careers as child performers. Their imitations can be understood using romantic models of virtuosity: Loftus and Janis "obscure the mechanics of creative production" by making their mimicry seem effortless.[21] Hoffmann's acts often pulled back the curtain—whether literal or metaphorical—in order to show the work that went into her performance. She was talented, but she showed her work.

Hoffmann never imitated with the air of spontaneity that is ascribed to Loftus and Janis. Instead, her work seemed more calculated and theatrical, more about the pleasures of excess and playing dress-up than those of virtuosity. She often played someone playing a part, like her imitation of Eddie Foy as Sister Anne. A caricature in *Frank Leslie's Weekly* shows three of her imitations from this period: the Scottish comedian Harry Lauder, Eddie Foy, and the *Merry Widow* waltz.[22] Although two of them are imitations of men, all three costumes include versions of a skirt: a kilt, an old-fashioned dress, and an ethnic costume. These costumes emphasize the idea that, no matter how grotesque her outfit might be, there is an attractive, American woman underneath. There's an interesting mark of consistency beneath Hoffmann's disparate acts.

Later in the *Variety* review, after a caveat that her mimicry of Eva Tanguay "may rank as a pure imitation with any comedy subject Miss Loftus offers," there is a discussion of her Adeline Genée imitation, which depends on physical mimicry and costuming, an imitation setting, a cinematic projection, and seven men on horseback to accompany her.[23] This is a kind of laughably excessive move to make for a scene that made up a small part of a twenty-two-minute act. It becomes a testament to Hoffmann's ability to see a show and replicate an important number in its totality. The ability to do so, the review suggests, "entitles Miss Hoffman to the distinction of being the only 'production impersonator.'"[24] The taste for extravagant stage settings developed in her youth in San Francisco continued throughout her career. In this case, the extravagance was played for laughs.

Hoffmann carried on another tradition that was born in San Francisco, that of volunteering for theatrical benefits. She made several appearances in the March social season, as a costume judge for a masked ball held by the White Rats labor union and as the co-marshal of the "grand march" at the Keith & Proctor's Employees ball. She seems to have been comically ill-matched with her cohost Harry Leonhardt. The "Mountainous" manager "was forced into a series of eccentric cake walk steps to keep pace with his capering partner, to the huge delight of his friends in the box."[25] These appearances may mark Hoffmann as someone interested in charity or merely as a team player. But it is easy to imagine every appearance at an elegant masked ball as a fulfillment of the Mardi Gras wish from her childhood in San Francisco—and as a rebuke to the journalist who made her sound low class in that long-ago interview.

Though Hoffmann's clash with Eva Tanguay was resolved, a tougher battle awaited: her "Merry Widow" burlesque from the same act ruffled the feathers of Colonel Henry W. Savage, the producer of the original show. To understand the phenomenal success of *The Merry Widow*, we need to backtrack a bit. Franz Lehár's operetta *Die lustige Witwe* opened in Vienna in December 1905. Its English adaptation produced by George Edwardes opened in London in June of 1907. The show was wildly popular, both with the British and with Americans traveling abroad. When Savage's production opened in October 1907, a review notes, "The fame of this 'widow' had preceded her, and very many persons in the audience had seen her in Europe and wished to know if she had lost any of her gayety in crossing the ocean."[26] This review personifies the operetta as a woman and engages in light, witty banter similar to the tone of the show. Charming and sophisticated, with a hummable score and romantic dances, *The Merry Widow* dominated Broadway in the fall of 1907, earning over a million dollars in its first three months. The show's dominance was even more remarkable because it took place in the midst of an economic crisis.[27] With a stock market crash and runs on the banks, perhaps the public needed the theatrical escapism *The Merry Widow* provided.

The show inspired many homages, parodies, and competing productions. In an earlier era, if all parties were vaudeville performers, they might have fought out their case on the pages of *Variety*. Henry W. Savage made his intentions clear in an advertisement posted in the *New York Clipper* on December 28, 1907. "WARNING!! To all theatrical managers and operatic managers, agents and artists," it began:

> Take notice, that all rights of production, in all languages, of the operetta in three acts,
>
> "The Merry Widow"
>
> ("Die Lustige Witwe")
>
> by Victor Leon, Leo Stein, and Franz Lehàr, are vested solely for the United States and Canada in
>
> Henry W. Savage
>
> Messrs. Klaw & Erlanger, Booking Agents,
>
> and that the book and music have been duly copyrighted and fully protected; and that any person, persons or corporation making any production and presentation thereof, or of any part thereof, without license from the said Henry W. Savage, first had and obtained, will be prosecuted to the fullest extent of the law.[28]

Though the advertisement is a legal notice, it also engages in the conventions of theatrical promotion. The two names that are centered and bolded, in the largest fonts, are the title of the show and the name of the producer. The claim of rights "in all languages" warns any German-language theaters in New York against producing the original Lehár version, which several theaters in New York did. Most relevant to the Hoffmann case is his claim to the rights of "any part" of the play, which would preclude the parodic use of individual songs from the show.

Some critics and artists argued that Savage had a moral right to royalties even if his legal grounding was tenuous. Instead of working on a full-length *Merry Widow* burlesque, Edgar Smith, the regular librettist for Weber and Fields, left their company.[29] Smith felt any full-length parody of the show that included the original music would violate Savage's rights as a producer. "I have been with Mr. Weber more than ten years," Smith says, "but if it has come to the place where I have to do this sort of buccaneering I do not want to do it."[30] The language of piracy became common in discussions of theatrical borrowing. Participants in American performance culture use it to mark the violations of "informal norms" in the same way that Robert Spoo identifies in his discussion of the American publishing industry.[31] As Gertrude Hoffmann's career progressed, she was dogged by the claims that though her copying was not legally questionable it was morally questionable, in bad taste.

Weber and Fields did put on their performance, but they paid Savage royalties and credited him in all advertisements.[32] Their company was a mainstay of downtown theater and could thus afford the royalties. Smaller burlesque companies that traveled on the two established routes (or "wheels") were not so lucky. A *Variety* article in January 1908 announced that the law was on their side: "All proclamations to the contrary, the music is not copyrighted and anyone who cares to may produce an adaptation from the original in America."[33] It is unclear from a legal perspective how Savage obtained the rights and if they included the English translation, the Hungarian original, or both.[34]

Savage's copyright claims fueled debate in the theatrical community. *The Merry Widow* was involved in multiple charges of plagiarism, whether conscious or accidental. Less than a week after it opened, the *New York Evening Telegram* ran an article asking: "Did 'Mlle. Modiste' and 'The Merry Widow' Compare Notes?"[35] Victor Herbert, the composer of *Mlle. Modiste*, wrote back to defend himself, calling the accusation "irresponsible drivel."[36] This did not stop Joe Weber and Lew Fields from joking about their similarities: one song in their long-running burlesque switching back and forth between Lehár's "The Women" and Herbert's "Mascot of the Troop."[37] The playwright and drama critic Frederick F. Schrader took credit as the first to have noted the similarity between *The Merry Widow* and Henri Meilhac's play *L'attaché d'ambassade*, first produced in Paris in 1861.[38] *Munsey's Magazine* also noted these parallels in its March 1908 column, "The Merry Widow Travestied."[39] The *Washington Times* ran an article the same month with the headline: "Is the Merry Widow Waltz a Child of Mendelssohn's Brain?"[40] Because the show's music was so present in American culture, critics interrogated its sources and parallels.

The show's influence spread to vaudeville as well. From January through March, there were more than a dozen "Merry Widow" burlesques onstage, usually send-ups of the waltz. Performers danced with each other, with dressmakers' dummies, and with volunteers from the audience.[41] Shapiro Music Publisher plugged a song titled "I'm Looking for the Man Who Wrote the

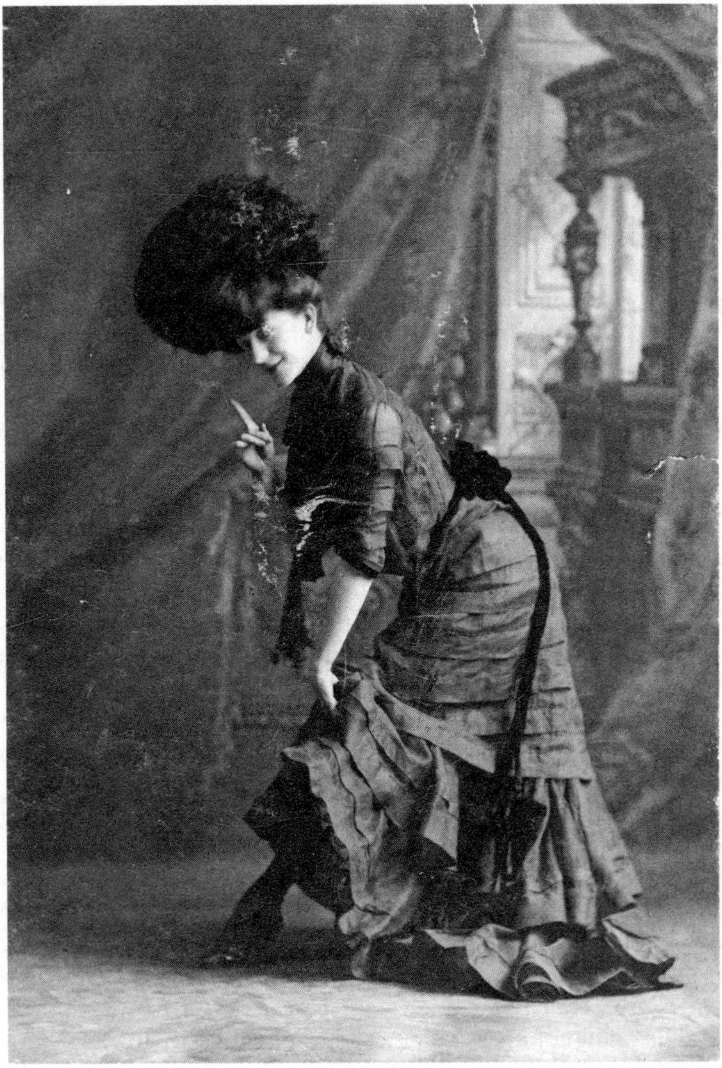

FIGURE 5.1. Gertrude Hoffmann as Sonia in *The Merry Widow*. Max and Gertrude Hoffmann Photograph Collection, Special Collections and University Archives, Wake Forest University, Winston-Salem, N.C.

Merry Widow Waltz," with a chorus that threatened: "And if I chance to find him he'll need more than smelling salts."[42] At this point, performers were burlesquing the cultural phenomenon more than the show itself. Once *The Merry Widow* crossed the ocean in 1907, she was impossible to avoid.

Gertrude Hoffmann entered the fray. Promotional pictures (see figure 5.1) show her dressed in a dark gown with a black sash at the waist and an enormous black hat, the picture of fashionable mourning. The hat became the signature accessory from the London production, and a "Merry Widow hat" giveaway at a June 1908 matinee of the show caused a riot.[43] Hoffmann bends at the wait, holding her skirt hem with her left hand to expose her ankle and pointed foot. Her right hand shakes a finger in a saucy gesture of warning. Hoffmann understood the risqué quality in the show, with its European air of sophistication and its tumultuous dances.

Her "Merry Widow" act is said to have lasted "from eight to ten minutes."[44] Both Hoffmann and her male dance partner were costumed as the principal actors are in *The Merry Widow*. The male performer sang Prince Danilo's song "Maxim's," then Gertrude Hoffmann entered, and they danced to the song that closed the operetta's first act. Up to this point, the act condensed the show, reproducing the high points of bachelor extravagance and romantic union. Then Hoffmann and her male assistant repeated the "Merry Widow Waltz" three times. They first danced to the song separately. Then they danced together in a recognizable imitation of the show's lead performers, while Hoffmann sang the lyric "I love you so." (That phrase, sometimes given as the alternate title to "The Merry Widow Waltz," is an important lyric but by no means the only one.) The imitation concluded with "a burlesque of the waltz to rag time."[45] The burlesque of the waltz also calls to mind the Hoffmanns' earlier career on the Wells circuit, where they would update old theatrical chestnuts by adding ragtime songs.

The play-by-play recounting of her act appeared not in *Variety* or the *New York Clipper* but in a judicial opinion for the case of *Savage v. Hoffmann*. Hoffmann did not seek permission for her burlesque, and so on April 1, 1908, Savage's lawyers the Fromme brothers filed a restraining order. Savage wished to stop her from performing the parody while the court made its decision regarding his copyright claim. The full demand was that "the defendant be restrained from imitating the postures of Barbanell [*sic*] and Brian [the *Merry Widow* stars Lina Abarbanell and Donald Brian], from singing the song called 'Maxim's,' and from using the orchestration of 'The Merry Widow.'"[46] The imitation of Abarbanell and Brian was the easiest for the judge to dismiss outright. His opinion puts aside any claims of similarity to Augustin Daly's copyright claim, where he asserted the rights to the first melodramatic scene in which a hero was tied to the railroad tracks. This case, *Daly v. Palmer*, established that dramatic incident could be copyrighted.[47] The judge found it obvious that a producer did not hold any commercial rights related to the two performers' physicality. If anyone had the right to complain about these imitations, the opinion states, it would be the performers themselves.[48] But their dance moves, poses, and other forms of presence were all held to be so idiosyncratic that they could not be associated with a literary property.

Choreography was protected in countries that signed on to the Berne Convention for the Protection of Literary and Artistic Works, but in 1908 the United States was not among those signatories. Dance choreography was not fully protected by copyright in the United States until 1976.[49] Earlier pantomimes and dances could be protected by common-law copyright if they were seen to possess "sufficient dramatic content."[50] Ruth St. Denis registered two transcribed versions of her dances, *Egypta* and *Radha*, as playscripts.[51] As dance scholars have observed, the early twentieth-century American legal system was sympathetic to narrative copyright claims but dismissed those having to do with extranarrative elements that were "merely" physical or aesthetic, such as dance. These legal protections, Anthea Kraut observes, were highly influenced by ideas about class and race.[52] Narrative art was perceived as more highbrow, white, and masculine while the vernacular performance arts—vaudeville, tap, burlesque, and the like—were more likely to be made by immigrants, African Americans, and women. But in the case of *Savage v. Hoffmann*, the lack of copyright protection for dances and postures worked in the vernacular performer's favor. She was seen to be imitating the idiosyncrasies of the performers, and not infringing upon the copyright of the performance itself.

Savage had no right to stop Hoffmann and her partner from dancing in the style of his lead actors. Nor did he present sufficient evidence for a preliminary injunction against her act for using the *Merry Widow* music or the lyrics to one song, "Maxim's." Instead, the judge allowed that when there was doubt about the complainant's rights to the material, the defendant's performance could continue. The Hoffmanns took advantage of the public's shared sentiment that *The Merry Widow* needed a dressing down. On the same day that this opinion was released, their lawyer entered affidavits and nine exhibits in opposition to the motion to continue.[53] This was Nathan Burkan, the same lawyer who had defended Max Hoffmann against Ziegfeld when he took the *Parisian Model* score. Though no records of these exhibits survive, their contents were discussed in the press, which advanced the argument that Savage could not claim exclusive ownership of *The Merry Widow* rights because that show's story and score were themselves borrowed from earlier sources. The press took up Frederick Schrader's claims about the similarities between Lehár's operetta and Meilhac's earlier play. They also added to the list of possible sources, claiming that the melody of the waltz could be found in *Le paradis de Mahomet*, a 1906 operetta, and that the tune of "Maxim's" was identical to a French folksong.[54] The case offered a piquant surprise: a vaudeville performer familiar with nineteenth-century French drama, pointing out that everyone borrows.

New York papers followed the case of *Savage v. Hoffmann* because *The Merry Widow* was the biggest moneymaker in an otherwise lackluster Broadway season. The sole voice defending the producer seems to have come from the *New York Press*, in an article that ascribed "moral rights" to Savage.[55] It argues that the Hungarian composer and American producer were responsible for creating *The Merry Widow* as a popular phenomenon: "If the composer and the producer had not applied the score to their uses, and if they had not invested a large amount of money in advertising it as a part of a comic opera, nobody would now be asserting the right to enjoy a share of its popularity."[56] This argument shifts the copyright from being something possessed by the creators to being something earned through publicity and marketing. The right to earn money on an artistic product is not inalienable, it is a return on investment.

The majority of theatrical and mainstream journalists took great pleasure in siding with Gertrude Hoffmann. *Savage v. Hoffmann* was a David and Goliath story: Savage was a wealthy real estate developer, while Hoffmann was a young, popular, and talented performer. Sharing the decision allowed writers to engage in the witty, though often sexist, banter that characterized reviews of the show itself. Stories about the court case expressed mock horror at the widow's age and her history.[57] The logic of female rivalry suggests that Hoffmann took the place of the widow because she was younger and prettier. One essay extends this language to Savage himself, suggesting that his aggressive pursuit of copycats was akin to the "jealousy of an amorous husband."[58] The pleasure that came from seeing female performers squabble with one another extended into this copyright debate, even if one of the women was fictional.

Hoffmann may have been perceived as a particular threat to the popularity of *The Merry Widow* because she performed in the "polite vaudeville" style that bridged high and low culture. The same was true of the operetta, which brought together conventions from opera and musical comedy. Weber and Fields produced a burlesque that played to a working-class, mostly male audience, but the same was not true of Hoffmann. Hoffmann's case, then, marked a new development in the discourse surrounding the rights of performers and producers. The owners of intellectual property asserted their rights more aggressively, but at the same time performers, parodists, and cultural critics insisted upon the value of mimicry.

Savage made strong copyright claims, but his case against Hoffmann failed, both because of the understanding that claims could not be made against parodies and because, at this point in the twentieth century, dance, posture, and other ineffable components of performance could not be copyrighted.[59]After the preliminary injunction was denied, the case fizzled out. On May 4, Savage's lawyers filed the replication, their response to the claims brought forth by the defendant.[60] In February, a note of issue was filed, meaning that discovery was complete and the case could be put on the calendar for trial. At the end of July 1909, the plaintiff's lawyers filed to discontinue the case. Hoffmann moved on, and Savage was making plenty of money with his Broadway, Chicago, and touring shows. What she moved on to would be the defining act of her career.

Chapter 6

A Vision of Salome

In the spring of 1908, word of Gertrude Hoffmann's court case spread from the daily newspapers to the weekly and monthly magazines. At the same time, the *New York Evening World* touted a "Mysterious American Dancing Girl in Poses That Captivated Europe."[1] She was Maud Allan, the Canadian-born and San Francisco-raised performer whose "The Vision of Salome" was captivating audiences at the Palace Theatre in London.[2] Hoffmann's imitation of Maud Allan brought her nationwide success and scandal.

"Salomania," the theatrical press noted, "is not a new craze."[3] Oscar Wilde wrote *Salomé* in French in 1891, imagining Sarah Bernhardt in the lead role.[4] Its production was prohibited in England; the questionable rationale given by the Lord Chamberlain was that it was illegal to depict biblical characters onstage.[5] The play was published in an English translation in 1894, with illustrations by Aubrey Beardsley. His languid, androgynous Salome, drawn with thick black lines and swirling organic shapes, epitomized decadent womanhood. (Twenty years later, Gertrude Hoffmann and Charlotte Greenwood were still said to strike Aubrey Beardsley poses onstage.)[6] Richard Strauss's operatic adaptation of Wilde was performed at the Metropolitan Opera House in late January of 1907. Olive Fremstad sang the role, while Bianca Froelich, a ballerina at the Met, performed the "Dance of the Seven Veils." [7] The final dress rehearsal was open to the opera house's board members, all important figures in New York society. They were shocked by the suggestiveness of Froelich's dance and by Fremstad's fondling and kissing of John the Baptist's severed head. The opera was canceled due to their complaints; it did not return to the Met until 1934.[8]

New York theaters presented scattered burlesques of the Met's abortive production, showing "a gradual unfolding of interest in the dancing girl."[9] The most prominent took place in *Ziegfeld Follies of 1907*, the first entry in the storied annual revue. The final scene of the *Follies* featured Emma Carus as "Salome, the one who sings" and Mlle. Dazie as "Salome, the one who dances."[10] Dazie's costume included "a low-slung gauzy skirt, a circle of pearls over each breast, an aigrette on her forehead."[11] The act mocks the Met production's ostensible indecency. Dazie's dance of the seven veils came to a climax and then was interrupted by a mock raid; policemen entered through the audience, but once onstage, they joined Dazie in a cancan for the finale.[12]

After the success of *The Merry Widow*, the transatlantic pursuit of European stars and scripts became a serious business on Broadway.[13] Rivalry between managers intensified the competition. The producer William Morris traveled to London, seeking to sign Maud Allan to an American contract as he did with the Scottish music-hall star Harry Lauder. Willie Hammerstein wanted to best William Morris, so he sought a performer to copy Allan's routine and perform it on the Paradise Roof in summer 1908. Morris Gest suggested Hoffmann for the job.[14] As a mimic and a dancer, she was especially qualified to observe Maud Allan. Her experience as a stage manager was useful as well, since Allan's skimpy costume, spare setting, and grotesque prop head all played a part in making her dance a sensation. Hoffmann reportedly asked for a thousand dollars per week in salary; when Hammerstein refused she counteroffered: "Twelve hundred and fifty! You should have heard me the first time!"[15] (By June of 1908, she was quoting $1,250 as her weekly price, refusing to play a Harlem vaudeville house for less.)[16] The hardball tactics worked. Gertrude and Max Hoffmann had spent their Christmas holidays in Europe, but by late April they left again, "silently," for London.[17]

Gertrude Hoffmann went abroad for twenty-one days in the spring of 1908.[18] During her trip, she saw Maud Allan perform "about fourteen times" at the Palace Theatre.[19] Hoffmann paid close attention to Allan's act, and especially her "Vision of Salome" dance, but she did so from a distance. "I never saw her any nearer than the back of the orchestra," Hoffmann said.[20] Hoffmann tried to take note of every detail of Allan's choreography, costume, lighting, and set. Imitation did not mean replicating the physical and verbal tics of a performer; it meant replicating the whole mood of their performance. Once she grasped the choreography, what might she have noticed during her sixth viewing of the dance, or the twelfth? The repetitions, one assumes, gave her a sense of the dance's core—which elements changed from night to night and which were central.

In this era, vaudeville audiences in America were introduced to foreign performers through their imitators: as Marlis Schweitzer observes, "Audiences in Boston greeted singer Harry Lauder as an 'old favorite' during his first appearance in the city because vaudeville imitators with access to the singer's sheet-music songs and recordings had already introduced them to the charming Scot through their impersonations."[21] But imitations from sheet music and recordings are different from reconstructions of live performances. "Consciously positioned against a series of originals and copies," Mary Simonson argues, "Hoffmann's dance was simultaneously an imitation and a unique original itself."[22] The borrowed performance style clashed in fascinating ways with the onstage immediacy of a semi-naked, sexually avid woman. Out of her repeated viewing, Hoffmann developed her "Vision of Salome," which embraced reproducibility and its complications.[23]

Once she returned to the United States, Hoffmann began rehearsing "A Vision of Salome." When she opened on Hammerstein's roof the week of July 4, though, she performed her act from the prior season. Morris Gest's autobiography suggests that Oscar Hammerstein got wind of Hoffmann's planned Salome dance and put a stop to it, concerned that it would diminish the perceived artistry of Mary Garden's upcoming performance at his Manhattan Opera House.[24] Hammerstein thought a copied Salome would decrease the value of his highbrow original, but Hoffmann knew that counterfeits made people crave the genuine article even more. Sometime during Hoffmann's first week as a headliner, Hammerstein changed his mind. Hoffmann suggests the reason for his reversal in light verse: "We talked to Oscar Hammerstein / He said it was the bunk / But he needed the dough very badly / So I sent around my trunk."[25]

Once the decision to perform "A Vision of Salome" was made, the Hammerstein publicity machine shifted into high gear. Newspaper articles hinted at the shocking nature of Hoffmann's upcoming dance. One story noted that she nearly lost her costume in a streetcar fire; she fled the burning car and left her purse onboard, with the flimsy outfit inside.[26] Another told of the night watchman at the Victoria Theatre who fainted from fright at the sight of her prop John the Baptist head.[27] Hoffmann's dance promised to be a sensation.

She first performed "A Vision of Salome" on July 13, 1908. A curtain opened, and Hoffmann descended marble stairs into a garden flanked by pillars. The lighting was weird and evocative: some reviews mention bluish light, others red. As the dance began, Hoffmann performed a series of sinuous steps and gestures suggestive of "the Orient" to audiences of the day. Her rippling arm movements during this section sound as if they were especially close to Maud Allan's.[28] She then discovered the head of John the Baptist, covered with a thin cloth or veil.[29] Hoffmann danced around the head with a series of actions that suggest alternating attraction and repulsion. She writhed in ecstasy and reached for the head while pulling herself away from it. After collapsing to the floor, she "snaked herself along the stage until she and the object were face to face."[30] She kissed the head and ended in a swoon.

The reception of "A Vision of Salome" was good, though tinged with uncertainty. Critics agreed that the performance's mise-en-scène was exquisite. A review in the next day's edition of the *New York World* called it "a model of stage manager's art" with "wondrous scenic investiture, dreamy, sensuous music composed by her husband and magnificent stage management."[31] There was serious disagreement about Hoffmann's presentation of Salome as a character. Was the interpretation meant to be funny or serious, artistic or provocative?

As with her earlier "production impersonation" of Adeline Genée's ballet, Hoffmann's "A Vision of Salome" humbles itself before an original while showily proclaiming its own skill. Hoffmann's act was billed as "an exact imitation" and "a life-like impersonation" of Maud Allan's work.[32] Unlike the viewing conditions for her imitations of current Broadway stars, most audience members would not have seen Allan's original dance. They would have seen still images and read tabloid stories as points of comparison. Hoffmann thus becomes the producer of these dances in the United States, the one whose first performances establish their essential character. Her reproduction of the stage settings and lighting places her in the same category as the drama critic and theater producer Kenneth Macgowan, whose books *The Theatre of Tomorrow* (1921) and *Continental Stagecraft* (with Robert Edmond Jones, 1922) introduced American theater scholars and practitioners to the techniques of the European theatrical avant-garde. Hoffmann's performance transmitted and arguably improved upon Allan's stripped-down stagecraft and choreography.

The ambiguity of imitation extends from set design to interpretation of character. Because she worked most recently in a comic vein, audience members were predisposed to find humor in Hoffmann's dance. "The rounders regarded her as Gertrude rather than Salome," said Franklin Fyles, "and they laughed when, after the dance was over and she had kissed the John's head, she sat down too hard on her overweight and turned heavily on her back."[33] Ending a serious, graceful dance with an awkward flop to the floor is just the kind of strategy Hoffmann might have used in her earlier imitations. The drunk first-nighters demonstrate their familiarity with Hoffmann's prior work and show how a star's earlier performances influence the reception of later ones, which Marvin Carlson has termed "ghosting." [34]

Though the "rounders" in the audience saw her as Gertrude, they may not have misread the act. The drama critic Ashton Stevens also understood the end of Hoffmann's performance as a send-up: "When she bore into the 'property' whiskers of the 'property' head and planted 'property' kisses therein, and fell into a grand 'property' swoon, you knew that the caricaturist and her secret [were] out!"[35] Stevens read Hoffmann's performance as one that began in imitation and ended in caricature. She crossed the line from homage into parody with gestures and actions that highlighted her awareness of the head as a prop. For Stevens, this self-awareness saved the dance from being a "nightmare" of overserious silliness.[36] It may also have saved Hoffmann from the critiques that plagued performers at the Met. The *Theatre Magazine* review says of her final kiss, "As a spectacle, it is repellent yet less objectionable than when done by Madame Fremstad at the Opera, because it is done with less art, and is therefore less convincing."[37] Here the reviews of the day disagree with Elizabeth Kendall's praise of "A Vision of Salome" for its creation of a mood that ran through the choreography, music, and set design.[38] Hoffmann's stage picture may have been a coherent one, but audience reaction and Hoffmann's interviews suggest the performance conveyed ideas in tension with one another. Whether it was a commentary on the original or a strategic hedging of her bets, the end of "A Vision of Salome" was performed in a style distinct from the rest.

Perhaps this discordance was an appropriate way of communicating Salome's dramatic movement between disparate emotions. Hoffmann insisted that her performance was not dance but "pantomimic acting."[39] Asked if she considered Salome from a psychological perspective, Hoffmann said, "Yes, indeed, I try to think I am really Salome and act the way Salome would."[40] In spite of this distance from the era, she says she could still evoke the necessary emotions to embody Salome, including "fleshly passionate love, revenge, fury, hatred, resentment, murder."[41] She loved pantomime and took every opportunity to practice her art.

The venue for Hoffmann's performance, though, made it seem less like serious artistry and more like a summer striptease. Marlis Schweitzer suggests that the intimate viewing space of roof gardens framed her dance in a context that "stymied" its serious intentions.[42] Audience expectations can be seen in descriptions of Hoffmann's costume. Her outfit included a headdress, two jeweled breast plates held together by strings of beads, further beadwork around her waist and draping to her hips, and an ankle-length, spangled black gauze skirt. She wore a flesh-colored bodysuit beneath her top and knee-length white trunks under her skirt. Her arms were braceleted, her legs and feet bare. "Her Salome Dress Fits the Weather," notes one headline; another story describes her "cool raiment."[43] Though roof gardens hosted underdressed chorus girls, their main acts were known for their sumptuous and elegant gowns. Hoffmann combined these two styles. A joke from the *Princeton Tiger* explains: One college man says, "I wonder where Gertrude Hoffman got her costume," and another replies, "At the jeweller's, I suppose."[44]

Blasé comments on Hoffmann's nudity belied the public's eagerness to see it up close. In vaudeville, the older male audience members in the first rows were called "baldheads." When they showed up for "A Vision of Salome," one critic dubbed them "Tenderloin Herods."[45] "Several rows of seats in the bald head division were torn out at Miss Hoffman's request, so that she might at least be decently aloof from the spectacle," said one review, "but every one brought his field glasses along, so it made no difference."[46] Susan Glenn sees Hoffmann commenting on the voyeurism of her audience: in interviews, she talks about revising Maud Allan's choreography to capture the attentions of the "Tired Business Man."[47] This critique spread: when Hoffmann toured with her Salome performance later that year, one newspaper cartoon showed an older woman refusing to hand over her opera glasses to her husband; another showed the audience full of leering men and grim-faced women.[48]

That tour came to pass with the help of Hoffmann's new manager, Morris Gest. After "A Vision of Salome" opened, Gest decided to make their collaboration official without asking permission. Hoffmann's act opened on a Monday night. By that Wednesday, "New Yorkers went to work blinking their eyes at huge posters from the Battery to the Bronx which shouted the town's newest sensation—GERTRUDE HOFFMAN—Under the Management of MORRIS GEST."[49] Hoffmann scolded him but moved on to the terms of his salary. They collaborated for the next six years, though the relationship did not end well. In Hoffmann's diary from the 1950s, she writes, "Morris Gest—He stole my credits and also my money."[50] Much of the resentment came from their work together on the Russian ballet and later revues, but Gest used questionable tactics with Hoffmann from the beginning of their partnership.

When it came to publicity, Morris Gest was indisputably a master. Two weeks after Hoffmann's debut, he was said to be planning a "matinee tour" that would take place once her stint at Hammerstein's was done.[51] He addressed Hoffmann's bare feet by placing an ad in the Sunday papers calling for a manicurist to treat them. Manicurists, pedicurists, chiropodists, quack doctors, and reportedly at least one blacksmith lined up at 9:00 A.M. to be interviewed for the stunt. A later cadre of more qualified practitioners returned at 4:00 P.M., when Hoffmann was present at the theater.[52]

After Gest's publicity barrage, New York City was overrun with "Dance of the Seven Veils" knockoffs performed by all kinds of Salomes.[53] The dances melded the sideshow orientalism of Little Egypt with the highbrow bombast of Strauss and Wilde, in differing proportions. Fanny Brice and Eva Tanguay performed comic takes on the dance; Julian Eltinge performed one in drag and blackface; Aida Overton Walker performed a refined version with no nudity to speak of.[54] Mlle. Dazie opened a "School for Salomes" in August 1908. She taught two-hour classes at the Jardin de Paris roof garden, where she had performed as Salome the year before in the *Follies*; at least 150 companies were supposed to leave New York for their fall tours, and Dazie hoped to provide each one with its Salome dancer.[55] It is useful to remember that the Salome craze was an outgrowth of vaudeville's broader imitation craze. Julian Eltinge and Gertrude Hoffmann both portrayed the Merry Widow in the prior season. Lotta Faust burlesqued a character from railroad advertisements—Phoebe Snow—in *The Mimic World* (1908) and performed her Salome dance in the same show until Hoffmann replaced her on tour.

Hoffmann posed for a series of Salome photos taken by Frank C. Bangs, an actor turned theatrical photographer.[56] These postcards did not display snapshots from the show so much as a kind of posed middle ground that was part re-creation and part imagination.[57] Figure 6.1 shows Hoffmann making her entrance. Her widespread arms and open stance suggest Salome as a *Follies* girl descending a staircase. In four later photos, she poses with the head of John the Baptist: two show her standing, one reclining, and one prone and approaching the head for a kiss. Two of the photos substitute John the Baptist's head with that of a lion, moving farther away from the narrative of Salome and toward a more general barbarism.

The series of seven Hoffmann images shot by Bangs circulated widely. A triptych of his photographs heads the August *Theatre Magazine* review of "Summer Shows at the Roof Gardens."[58] By September, they were being sold in the back of the magazine.[59] Hoffmann's postcard Salome images circulated

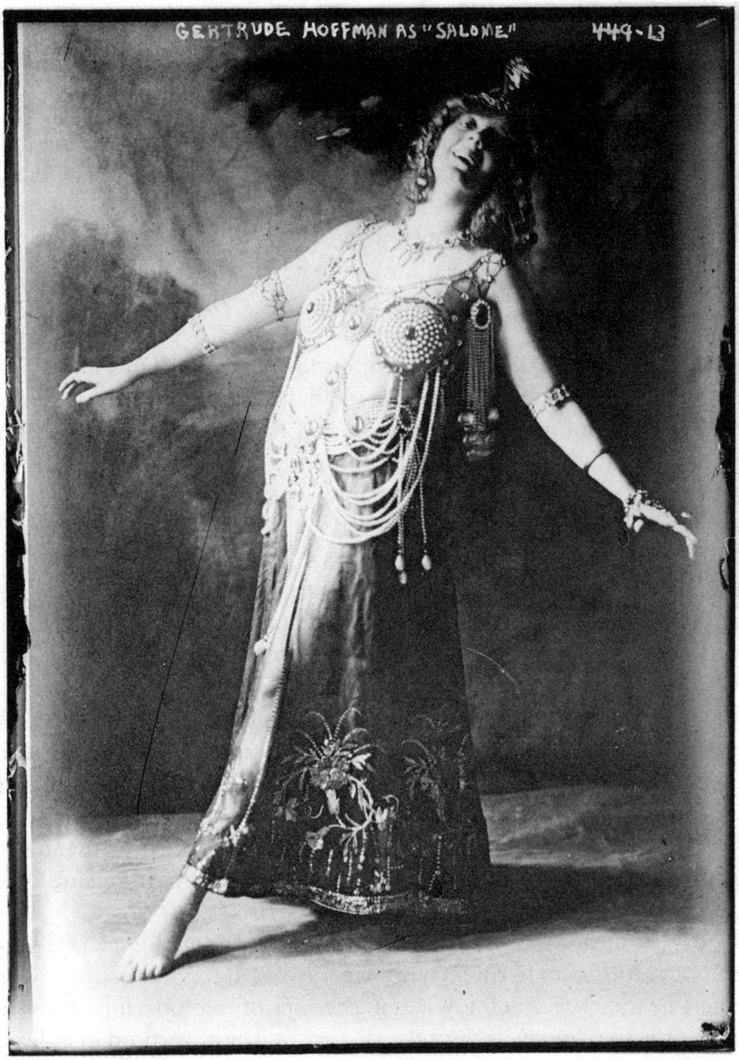

FIGURE 6.1. Gertrude Hoffmann as Salome. Photograph by Frank C. Bangs. Library of Congress, Prints and Photographs Division, LC-DIG-ggbain-02025.

as a promotion for and supplement to her act, fostering emotional connections in her fans. Penny Farfan suggests that postcard owners come into "physical contact with the star's being, and so in a relationship of distanced possession."[60] The possession could take on many forms: fetishism, identification, artistic appreciation. It seems likely that the postcard series shaped national anticipation for Hoffmann's tour.[61]

Her act was held over on Hammerstein's Roof until the end of September. Some newspaper stories suggest she wanted to leave because she was dissatisfied with their promotion of her act; others mention a commitment to play the Palace Theatre in London as a replacement for Allan.[62] When the conflicts were resolved, Morris Gest "loaned" her to the Shubert Organization for their touring production of *The Mimic World*, and she was to return to Hammerstein's the following summer. A musical comedy revue that burlesqued the previous season's Broadway plays, *The Mimic World* was a perfect fit for Hoffmann. The show was struggling, and she was a last-minute addition to the tour, one who would receive top billing. She claimed in a letter to Gest's biographer that they "pulled [the] show out of [the] hole."[63] Hoffmann introduced an additional dance, an imitation of Maud Allan's more pastoral "Spring Song." Loie Fuller originated the dance in Grecian draperies to the music of Mendelssohn; Isadora Duncan and Ruth St. Denis also performed versions.[64] This addition, plus her usual repertoire of imitations, made Hoffmann's act long enough to justify her name above the title. "Spring Song" also offered a more conventional aesthetic version of barefoot dancing to balance her more daring dance as Salome.

The Shubert Organization knew that Hoffmann would be the major draw for their show, but they disagreed on how to promote her. The theater manager Charles A. Bird and the publicity agent John Reynolds wanted to focus on "A Vision of Salome" as a highbrow attraction.[65] J. J. Shubert wished to promote Hoffmann's act as one might promote a circus, by blanketing a town with posters and playing up the spectacle.[66] A dismissive Chicago reviewer saw Hoffmann's onstage performance in circuslike terms as well, calling her partner for the "Spring Song" dance "a youth clad in a costume that would pass for classic Grecian in a Ringling Bros. pantomime."[67] Hoffmann's reception on tour paralleled that in New York: one could never be sure whether her dance would be taken as high art, comedy, or smut.

Whatever it meant, her image was everywhere. Reynolds placed multiple stories about Hoffmann to run in newspapers in advance of the show. He wrote to Shubert headquarters acknowledging receipt of two dozen pictures of her and asking for sixty more.[68] Her postcard series was advertised in at least one Chicago theater program.[69] A theater manager in Chicago complained about a prominent Hoffmann advertisement in his lobby.[70] Hoffmann's reproduction took another form in Kansas City. As Marlis Schweitzer has described, a conflict between newspapers and theater managers prevented Reynolds from his usual strategy of advertising in newspapers and supplementing with posters. Even after stories could be placed in newspapers again, Reynolds "papered the countryside, circulating posters and other advertising material within a 100-mile radius of Kansas City."[71] This was overkill: Hoffmann's image was too present, too far outside of the city. Kansas City residents led by the British evangelist Rodney "Gipsy" Smith petitioned for Hoffmann's dance to be stopped.[72] Their efforts succeeded, and Hoffmann performed her "Spring

Song" and imitations, but no Salome. During the same period, the Reverend Billy Sunday also protested Hoffmann's indecency in Springfield, Illinois.[73] This suggests that evangelists, some of whom borrowed performance techniques from vaudeville, saw themselves as competitors for the attention of the American public.[74]

Hoffmann continued her tour until April, when she returned to New York City. Because of her summer season engagement with the Hammersteins, she took her vacation a bit sooner than vaudevillians usually did. She left for Europe in April or May, accompanied by Max and Max Jr.[75] On June 1, 1909, Morris Gest married Reina Belasco, the oldest daughter of the famous theatrical producer David Belasco.[76] Their subsequent trip to Europe served two purposes: to celebrate their honeymoon and to retrieve Gest's star client.[77] The Gests and the Hoffmanns saw the seedier side of Paris together. After they were "ushered out" of the Moulin Rouge, they visited the Bal Tabarin, a cabaret full of "naked girls—cheapest girls with hanging busts—just awful."[78] Max and Morris wanted to stay in their box, so Gertrude and Reina went to the dance floor together.

Hoffmann returned to New York City and the Hammersteins' Roof. To welcome her back, Willie Hammerstein commissioned new scenery for Hoffmann's act.[79] She performed the "Spring Song" and "A Vision of Salome" dances as she had the prior summer. Ten days into her second run, she was arrested for indecency. A new police commissioner "inaugurated a new crusade against questionable theatrical productions in New York," and Hoffmann was his first defendant.[80] Hoffmann suspected that Morris Gest arranged her arrest as a publicity stunt.[81] Other Broadway regulars thought that Hammerstein himself might have been responsible.[82] In any case, her earlier tour made her an easy target for Commissioner Baker. "A Vision of Salome" traveled a circuitous route, gathering meaning along the way. When she began her performance in Times Square, it was understood in a transatlantic context as an imitation of Maud Allan. After performing it throughout Middle America, "A Vision of Salome" became a scandalous dance with its own history and associations.

The arguments against Hoffmann claimed that her costume was indecent not only in "A Vision of Salome" but also in "Spring Song." There was concern that her costume in the latter dance consisted of gauze and roses over her breasts. This was a major change from the initial reception of "Spring Song," which, even in *The Mimic World*, was understood by most critics as tasteful and even a bit old-fashioned. News stories tended to cast Hoffmann as a plucky heroine in her trial proceedings, following the same narrative as in the *Merry Widow* case. The arraigning judge asked if she wore trunks during "Spring Song." "False!" she defiantly replied, "I wear tights. I'll put 'em on now and show 'em to you."[83] Her trial was postponed to October 4, but the court decided that Hoffmann had to be overseen in the meantime by a "Mrs. McMahon of the Tenderloin Precinct." The police matron would ensure that Hoffmann wore full-length tights beneath both costumes.

Hoffmann's summer season continued before an audience of curious New Yorkers. While she gave repeat performances, she rehearsed a new imitation of *Radha* by Ruth St. Denis. St. Denis is an important, complex figure in the history of modern dance. Her quasi-eastern dances were influential in the early twentieth century, and her dance school Denishawn (cofounded with her then-husband Ted Shawn) fostered the talents of important choreographers including Martha Graham, Doris Humphrey, and Charles Weidman.[84] Her dancing itself tends to be considered mere exotica, indicative of the period's cultural imperialism.[85] St. Denis first performed *Radha* on a vaudeville bill in 1906.[86] She portrayed the Hindu goddess Radha, first in meditation and then in dances engaging with the five senses. St. Denis attracted the attention of a society matron, Mrs. Orlando Rowland; the dancer performed private matinees and "launched on the high art circuit."[87] Like "A Vision of Salome," *Radha* was a sensual, orientalist pastiche. St. Denis was unfamiliar with Indian dance at the time when she choreographed *Radha*, so she combined ballet, skirt dancing, and Delsarte poses with a generalized eastern air.[88] She used this performance as a stepping-stone from vaudeville sensation to cultural legitimacy, a transition that Hoffmann longed for.

Would *Radha* reframe Hoffmann's imitative talents as the work of a skilled producer and dancer? In short, no. A *New York World* headline may have blared, "Here's the New Dance to Bait Police Censors," but Hoffmann's *Radha* was far from indecent.[89] Instead, it was seen as too highbrow for her vaudeville audience's tastes. Hoffmann made her name in "A Vision of Salome" by uniting the Maud Allan imitation with her intrinsic ability to please a crowd. Elizabeth Kendall writes, "It took a clever and top-level vaudeville player to reveal Salome's dancing potential, and she did it by showmanship."[90] Her *Radha*, by contrast, was too faithful to the original. It lacked the broad smile, the wink to the audience seen in "A Vision of Salome." As the "Dance of the Seven Veils" floated free of Wilde and Strauss's dramatic narrative, Salome dances became their own act and not mere imitations of earlier performances. Their association with the "oriental" dances of Ruth St. Denis and the barefoot dancing of Isadora Duncan connected Salome dances to an alternative aesthetic tradition, one with more serious artistic associations.

Hoffmann's performance as Maud Allan embodied the tension between immediacy and copying, highlighting the ways that the copy points to the original and exceeds it. Her Salome is a version of what Elin Diamond has called "mimesis in syncopated time."[91] Diamond takes the idea of the theater as a space of "syncopated time" from Gertrude Stein, who was "troubled" by the clash between onstage action and audience reception: "The thing seen and the emotion did not go on together," Stein writes.[92] Hoffmann's mimesis can be similarly understood as an act taking place in syncopated time, and not just because her husband was known for his ragtime transcriptions. Hoffmann used her skills as a mimic to play the referential qualities of her dance against the unique ones. Hoffmann's performance was so fascinating because it drew on the ambiguities central to imitative performance.

By October 1909, Hoffmann ended her engagement with Salome: though she continued to perform the "Spring Song" in later revues, "A Vision of Salome" was removed from the repertoire. Her indecency charges were dropped: she was no longer performing the dances, and the lawyers and judge agreed that the public nuisance had abated.[93] When Maud Allan arrived in the United States and played Carnegie Hall in January 1910, Hoffmann again sat in the audience.[94] She added her comic touch to these proceedings, sending Allan a pot of orchids that, according to one account, ushers toted down the aisles of the concert hall and attempted to pass over the footlights like a bouquet.[95] Reviewers compared Allan to Hoffmann in unfavorable terms. Allan's choreography seemed a bit bloodless, more pretty than passionate, compared to their memory of "A Vision of Salome." Hoffmann's imitation Salome established the terms by which the putative original was read. It also inaugurated themes that became central to the rest of her career, including orientalism, the reproduction of the self, and the fine line between prurience and parody.

With her Salome dance, Gertrude Hoffmann blurred the line between producer and performer. She went to Europe in search of new talent just as the impresarios Charles Frohman, William Morris, and Oscar Hammerstein did. Unlike those producers, though, she reproduced the European act herself. As she prepared for *The Mimic World* and then returned to the Paradise Roof Garden, Hoffmann combined her Salome dance with other production numbers, thinking about how to balance an act and show off her talents to their best advantage. The staging and sequencing of her vaudeville turn became increasingly complex. Her ambitions as a producer sometimes clashed with her abilities as a performer and the expectations of her audiences. But in the years before World War I, no one had a clearer sense of how to combine modern dance performance and popular entertainment into a dazzling spectacle.

Part III

Producing Revues, 1910–1914

Chapter 7

Gertrude Hoffmann's Reviews

Beginning in 1910, Gertrude Hoffmann's vaudeville act resembled a whole vaudeville bill in miniature. Twelve distinct numbers were listed on the program and republished in several newspapers. She played a part in all of them, taking quick breaks and making costume changes when the focus shifted to her supporting players. This was a star-making turn, showcasing her wit and versatility. It also introduced vaudeville audiences to the review. "Whatever has previously been presented in vaudeville has been known as an act. This word can not apply to Miss Hoffmann's ambitious effort," one breathless account states; "'Review' would seem to be the only word, for it is a collection of bright burlesques on whatever is really worth while that Broadway has seen since last spring."[1] Gallicized as "revue," this form was a more sophisticated take on the theatrical burlesque, presenting the foibles of the current day and the current stage in a fast-moving, quick-witted way.[2] Sumptuous scenery and beautiful girls helped to smooth the transitions between bits. Ziegfeld's *Follies* was the best-known revue of the decade, and the Shuberts' *Passing Show* would soon enter the competition.

Gertrude Hoffmann brought the glamor of the revue to the middle-class audiences of the vaudeville theater at popular prices. As a woman who produced and starred in her own revue in the years of its development, she has vital insights on the form. Her musical numbers influenced the work of better-known producers and choreographers, including Florenz Ziegfeld and Busby Berkeley. They influenced modern drama as well: the famed set designer Robert Edmond Jones got his start designing Hoffmann's costumes. Though the shows sported different titles—*Gertrude Hoffmann's Review*, *Gertrude Hoffmann's Revue*, *Gertrude Hoffmann's New Revue*—she was always at the center. Gertrude Hoffmann's reviews shaped her career and American popular performance more broadly.

She returned to the stage on January 3, trying out her new act at Young's Pier in Atlantic City. Morris Gest hired Sri Lankan dancers and musicians to complement Hoffmann's newfound interest in Eastern exoticism. Billed as the "Royal Cingalese Troupe," they generated buzz in New Jersey that had "even [the] bell boys speculating."[3] Hoffmann and Gest sparred over whether the show should open in New York or go on a road tour booked through the United Booking Office.[4] They did not open at a Broadway theater. Instead, the Manhattan debut took place at Percy Williams's Alhambra Theatre in Harlem. Sam McKee noted that this booking was "completely reversing the usual theatrical routine."[5] Normally, theaters in residential neighborhoods would be visited by vaudeville stars long after their acts had run in Times Square. Perhaps as a compromise with Gest or as an acknowledgment of her popularity in the *Mimic World* tour, Hoffmann opened her show a bit off the beaten path.

In its first incarnation, Hoffmann's act ran for forty-eight minutes if every costume and set change went off without a hitch.[6] When changes were delayed, either by problems or applause, it could run more than an hour. "The entire act is fearfully hard work behind the scenes," Hoffmann notes in an interview.[7] She produced, directed, and starred, while Max Hoffmann conducted the orchestra. Along with two maids, Gertrude's brother George Hay helped with costume changes.[8] Hoffmann earned $2,500 a week for the act in the first half of 1910; her salary rose to $3,000 a week after June 1.[9]

She began the show on a nostalgic note, with a song called "It Isn't That Way Any More." As a part of this number, she mimicked the stage stars Eddie Foy, Ethel Barrymore, and George M. Cohan "as they were when they first attained popularity and as they are today."[10] Unlike the imitations she did in earlier acts, these were done without costume changes and so depended on Hoffmann's voice and physicality for their success. Her Barrymore sounds particularly wicked: Hoffmann showed her taking care of her new baby until she tired of it, then throwing it away so she could return to the stage. [11]

She followed this imitative montage with her Eva Tanguay—who merited a costume change into "white tights and a glittering bodice of silver"—and another attempt at Ruth St. Denis.[12] This time she imitated the St. Denis dance called *The Cobras* seen in figure 7.1. Hoffmann wore an emerald green jacket, a headdress, and rings that gleamed like snake eyes. The Cingalese performers drummed and danced. They were then joined by her "snake charmers"—the twelve chorus girls who also play "twelve nymphs" in an Isadora Duncan number. One critic was not sure where to look, noting that audience members "needed more eyes to observe at once that bunch of pretty, bare-footed snake charmers from Manhattan and the weird representatives of the Far East."[13] Hoffmann's revues would often return to this strategy of combining American chorus girls and foreign male performers.

The rest of the show alternated between Hoffmann's imitations and big numbers that used her dancers. She imitated the Scottish comedian Harry Lauder and the theatrical glamour girl Valeska Suratt. At the end of her Suratt scene, Hoffmann's scene partner Lee Chapin tore away her fashionable gown to reveal a swimsuit. She then performed a number called "You Splash Me and I'll Splash You" in imitation of the British music-hall singer Alice Lloyd. Her chorus members held pocket mirrors, reflecting light into the audience as Lloyd

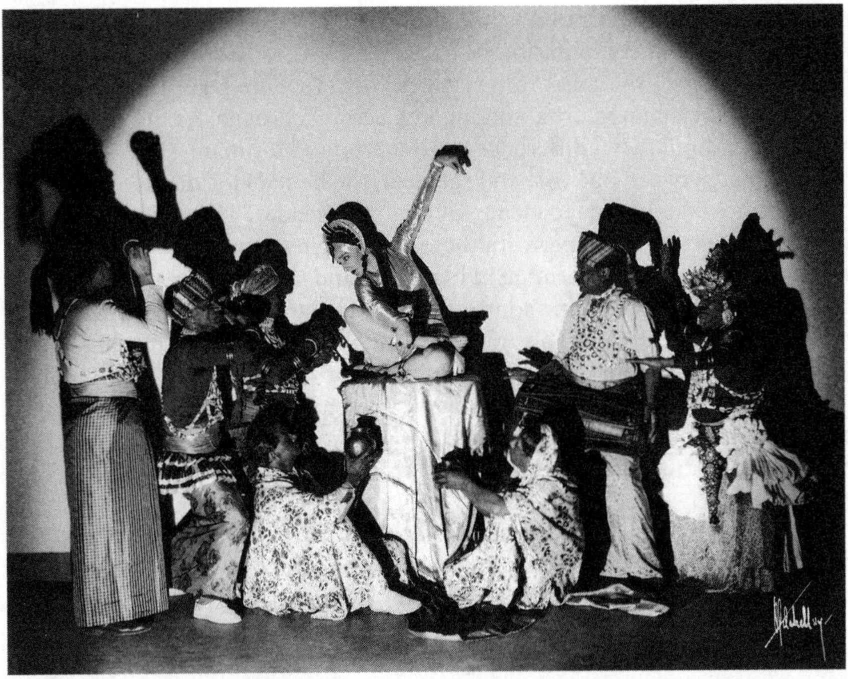

FIGURE 7.1. Gertrude Hoffmann performing Ruth St. Denis's dance *The Cobras*, surrounded by members of the Royal Cingalese Troupe. Max and Gertrude Hoffmann Photograph Collection, Special Collections and University Archives, Wake Forest University, Winston-Salem, N.C.

did in her number "Looking for the Lovelight in Your Eyes."[14] According to the program, they were dressed as "Twelve Brinkley Bathing Girls," after the fashionable illustrations of young women that the cartoonist Nell Brinkley published in newspapers.[15] Hoffmann then played the trombone like Harry Watson, a comedian she had worked with early in her career. The chorus performed "Just a Matter of Form," a number that "inspired [Mack] Sennett's bathing girls."[16] Then Hoffmann donned fake muscles to imitate Annette Kellerman, the swimming star who recently performed water ballets at the Hippodrome.[17] Suspended from wires, Hoffmann comically threatened to fall into an onstage water tank several times, then took the plunge. She ended the show with a solo number in blackface, singing "Booloo Eyes" as Eddie Leonard.[18]

Reviewing the act from beginning to end reveals how it functioned logistically and aesthetically. Her comic imitations were interspersed with serious dances; set pieces with a dozen chorus girls were followed by solo acts that Hoffmann could perform "in one," with the curtains closed so the set could be changed. The tone shifted from moment to moment as well: the familiarity of an Eva Tanguay imitation transitioned to the weirdness of East Indian music and dance; the pastoral prettiness of the "Blue Danube Waltz" was chased by Hoffmann in drag, singing in a Scottish brogue. As these examples show, gender and racial difference were central to Hoffmann's act. The wider the contrast between one role and the next, the better. Hoffmann's imitations demonstrate "the interdependency of race and gender" in vaudeville and the work that is necessary to perform these overlapping identities.[19] Jumping in a water tank and then performing in blackface and male drag to close the show seems like the most dramatic contrast of all: "It is very hard 'blacking up' after that soaking," she says.[20] This transition highlights the labor Hoffmann does throughout the whole revue. She conceals her whiteness and her femininity, and then she reveals their undeniable presence. Hoffmann "exploited the racial hierarchy of vaudeville," to use M. Alison Kibler's terms, showing how far she could stray from her own identity and how quickly she could return to the fold.[21]

The act played to packed houses in New York City and Philadelphia through May. The Ruth St. Denis and Isadora Duncan dances fit seamlessly within the larger program. Hoffmann struck a more successful balance between the exotic and the mainstream than she did in *Radha*. The Grecian beauty of Duncan dance offered a kind of palate cleanser between burlesques. This number was billed as an imitation as well, of Duncan's performance at the Metropolitan Opera House. One review describes Hoffmann's dance imitation as a kind of outreach to the masses who would not otherwise see something so highbrow.[22]

As Hoffmann was performing as Duncan in her revue, another dance act played the Metropolitan Opera House: the Russian ballet duo of Anna Pavlova and Mikhail Mordkin. The Met president Otto Kahn brought the dancers to America.[23] They made their debut at an inauspicious hour (11:00 P.M. on a Monday, after a full opera production) and thrilled the crowd.[24] The dance critic and modernist man-about-town Carl Van Vechten famously wrote about the pair's debut. In his first review of the performance, Van Vechten said Pavlova embodied the ideals of classical ballet.[25] In his second, he described some of her movements in painstaking detail and glossed over others with language that made her seem superhuman: "At times she seemed to defy the laws of gravitation."[26] Even the vaudeville trade papers took note, with a story in *Variety* observing that Pavlova was "a sensation."[27] The dancers appeared at social occasions and charity performances throughout the spring. They sailed for London on April 6, 1910, with a contract to return that fall.[28]

While the Russians were in town, Hoffmann turned her attention to Paris. The playwright Edmond Rostand, the author of *Cyrano de Bergerac*, premiered a new play called *Chantecler*. An allegorical critique of French society set in a barnyard, it would not seem to have the same cross-cultural appeal as Maud Allan's dances. Nevertheless, as the theatrical producer Charles Frohman signed the rights to bring the play to Broadway, Hoffmann added a *Chantecler* burlesque to her revue.[29] She wore a large and cumbersome rooster costume that appears to have been made of papier-mâché; her head peeked out of a hole in the rooster's neck, and her usually bare legs were covered in baggy tights that ended in oversized claws. Her twelve dancers were billed in this routine as "broilers," the slang term that applied both to chickens and to chorus girls. Publicity for the "Chantecler" number mentions the "most interesting part of the dance" will be a fight at its climax, between Hoffmann in her costume and a live rooster.[30]

Aside from its pure silliness, the coverage of this dance illustrates something important about Hoffmann's transatlantic ambitions and connections. A program for her Keith's Theatre shows in Philadelphia says that the "Chantecler" costumes "were obtained only by the diligent attendance upon the rehearsals of the play by one of the designers connected with the firms of Rich and Rich."[31] She paid enough attention to French theater to know that this play was important, and she had contacts abroad who were able to copy the costume while the show was still in dress rehearsal.

A string of newspaper articles emphasized Hoffmann's artistic side. She wanted to open her own theater, either on Long Island or in London; she frequented used bookshops and collected poetic quotations on the dance; she longed to play Camille.[32] Hoffmann's reputation as an entertainer inclined to crack jokes and show skin clashed with her highbrow ambitions. These articles showed one way that she (and perhaps Morris Gest, with his talent for publicity) tried to convert her image from that of a brassy vaudevillian to one of a dancer and patron of the arts.

At the same time, news coverage emphasized the exoticism of the Sri Lankan dancers and musicians in her company. One story claimed they would only accept payment in gold and threatened to return to Ceylon if the Hoffmanns continued to pay them by check.[33] A reporter found Max "in a facetious mood." When asked if it was true that the men did not speak a word of English, he said, "unless they think you are trying to get the better of them in money matters, and then they speak English both fluently and volubly."[34] That newspaper story lists the names of the troupe members, albeit with abbreviated first names and Anglicized surnames: K. Y. Kiva, R. D. Kiva, K. M. Saytowa, Runche Kiva, M. Suraya, K. D. Nida, and K. Addi.[35] Saytowa reportedly served as the troupe translator and prepared their food to follow religious and cultural customs.

During this stretch of the tour, she added several numbers to the revue. One called "The Bell Girls" was reminiscent of a number for *A Parisian Model*. In the former version, chorus girls played a melody with bells attached to their feet; the new bell number had them ring bells on their arms, feet, and heads.[36] The other new number, "Trapeze Sextette a la Charmion," presented six dancers performing a trapeze routine similar to that of the famed female bodybuilder. They were assisted by the Sri Lankan musicians, and some critics were troubled by their interaction.[37] One review late in the tour mentions a "Bacchanale," which may have been an imitation of Pavlova and Mordkin's *Autumn Bacchanale*.[38] She also added "Spring Song" back into the program. Hoffmann always looked for ways to breathe life into a show when it was on the road.

Hoffmann ended her tour in April 1911, after forty weeks of performance. During this time, she apparently never missed a show. A few articles discuss her recuperating at their summer home in Coney Island, where she planned to build a full-time residence.[39] She claimed that she was going to take the summer off from performing.[40] After a quick rest, she prepared for the most audacious imitation of her career.

Chapter 8

✦

Pirating the Ballets Russes

Debates about imitation continued to rage. Eddie Leonard, the "Booloo Eyes" singer whom Gertrude Hoffmann imitated to finish her act, placed an ad in *Variety* with the headline, "EDDIE LEONARD OBJECTS!"[1] Leonard called out the many singers who sang his songs or used his style without giving credit. Imitators who acknowledged their source material were not the subject of his ad; Hoffmann's name appears in the middle of the page along with other vaudevillians described in this way: "THESE PEOPLE ARE ARTISTS/NOT PIRATES."[2] According to the professional norms of the popular stage, mimicry that credited the original was still an acceptable form of imitation.

While Hoffmann was performing her celebrity imitations and modern dances, including her blackface imitation of Leonard, she prepared another project. Dubbed *La Saison des Ballets Russes*, this was her unauthorized reproduction of three Michel Fokine ballets. The choreography, costumes, and sets were borrowed wholesale from the Ballets Russes de Serge Diaghilev's 1909 and 1910 performances in Paris. Hoffmann took the title from a heading in the 1910 program of Diaghilev's company at the Théâtre National de l'Opéra, which is in her papers.[3] She mixed Russian ballet and revue style in a tour that traveled cross-country and lasted twenty-seven weeks.[4] *La Saison des Ballets Russes* engaged in imitative practices that today would be considered immoral, even illegal. Yet this tour marks an important moment in American dance. Aficionados saw Anna Pavlova and Mikhail Mordkin perform solos and pas de deux in the Russian style. Gertrude Hoffmann's *La Saison des Ballets Russes* then introduced a large audience to Russian ballet as a coherent aesthetic production. The Americanness of this Russian season interrupts and complicates narratives about modernist performance: when Diaghilev's ballet arrived in the United States in 1916, it was compared to the imitation.[5]

Hoffmann's pirated production is important to understand, both because it was influential and because it was legal. The United States did not sign on to the international author's rights protections of the Berne Convention until 1988, and it lacked bilateral copyright agreements with Russia. "Strictly speaking," wrote Gest's biographers circa 1935, "Gest and Miss Hoffmann had 'stolen' their repertory and their choreography from the parent company in Paris and Monte Carlo, for no copyright laws prevailed with Russia then any more than they do to this day."[6] Even if copyright agreements had been observed, choreography was not understood in this period as a product protected by copyright law.[7]

Robert Spoo's work restores important context to the discussion of pirated performances even though he discusses print and not performance culture. He observes that using the term "piracy" "gives a false aura of illegality to a practice that, though inconsistent with strict business morality . . . was a lawful form of cultural diffusion well into the twentieth century."[8] Gertrude Hoffmann was an artist and a pirate; her work in this period should be understood not as an embarrassing moral failing but as a strategy that made sense as an extension of the theatrical culture of the period, her career on the vaudeville stage, and her ambitions as a producer. Hoffmann's Russian Season serves as a useful illustration of how global theatrical culture made its way across the United States in the early twentieth century in a plagiarized, mediated form. Her piracy demonstrates how unauthorized cultural borrowing gives work a broader audience.

Hoffmann sought to bring important work from Europe through her pirated performances of the Ballets Russes in much the same way she did with her imitation of Maud Allan's Salome. Her fascination with the Ballets Russes began during her break from "A Vision of Salome" in May 1909. She then traveled to Paris and saw Serge Diaghilev's company perform the first season of Russian ballet at the Théâtre du Châtelet. She was enraptured by these dances, and concluded that it was her duty as an artist to bring them before American audiences. She went backstage to try to convince members of the company to tour with her. The choreographer Michel Fokine had signed on to work at the Coliseum in London after the Paris season. She had better luck with Theodore Kosloff, who committed to train her in the Russian style. Overwhelmed by the sheer beauty of the production and perhaps frustrated that she could not get the dancers to come directly to New York City, she noted that she "almost stole music off of rack, & costumes" because she was "so mad about it."[9] She told Morris Gest about the production, and they signed a contract forming the "Gertrude Hoffmann Corporation" to bring the dances to America.[10]

Hoffmann planned to return to Paris in May 1910 and then perform that summer on the Hammerstein Roof. By April she received an offer that complicated her itinerary and fulfilled a long-held ambition: Florenz Ziegfeld wanted her to star in his *Follies of 1910*. Trade papers buzzed with rumors; Willie Hammerstein threatened legal action for breach of contract.[11] The deal was kept from Eva Tanguay, the star of the *Follies of 1909*, who was still smarting from their earlier dispute. Also out of the loop was Morris Gest, who typically arranged her summer bookings.

Gertrude Hoffmann's Review was playing Philadelphia. Hoffmann and Gest seem to have argued about the Ziegfeld contract at a local restaurant. He asked if the rumors were true, and she admitted they were. Morris Gest's wife Reina burst into tears and left the conversation, perhaps to return to dine with her father. Reina Gest knew that without Hoffmann's financial support the plans to bring the Russian ballet to America were likely to fall through. Hoffmann thought about her previous agreement with Gest; she owned 51 percent of the shares in their joint venture, and she had not realized the responsibilities that entailed. "After much talking," she realized her heart was not in the Ziegfeld role. "Opening night he tore up [the] contract," she wrote.[12] Ziegfeld did pay Hoffmann the dubious compliment of imitating her act: a review of his *Follies of 1910* mentions "a bathing-girl scene which is almost a duplicate of one originated, and used by, Gertrude Hoffmann."[13]

The Hoffmanns sailed for France at the end of May 1910, with seven-year-old Max Jr. Gertrude Hoffmann's trip to Europe that summer received particular attention from the New York City newspapers, whose stories made note of her six-figure contracts for work that fall. One noted that she "crosses the water in search of material for an act which, it is promised, will be more magnificent and elaborate than her present offering, which has been generally accepted as the most pretentious in vaudeville."[14] (This use of "pretentious," which seems to have been peculiar to the vaudeville world, suggests ostentation and spectacle without judging it as excessive or unearned.)

Once they arrived in Paris, Hoffmann laid the groundwork for bringing the Russian ballet to New York. She met with Ida Rubinstein, the dancer in the Ballets Russes whose roles she planned to play.[15] Morris Gest's brother Sam translated between the two women.[16] Rubinstein was a wealthy Russian Jewish actress who, like Hoffmann, had performed as Salome. Since Rubinstein was not classically trained in dance from a young age as were most of the Diaghilev company, she worked with Michel Fokine. She had tremendous stage presence, pantomimic skill, and a willingness to appear onstage in various stages of undress.[17]

Rubinstein's entrance in *Cléopâtre* was just the kind of "pretentious" spectacle Hoffmann wanted to produce. The Egyptian queen was carried onstage inside a casket, first appearing as "a mummy swathed in veils."[18] Slaves unwound twelve scarves, each one vividly colored and richly decorated in designer Léon Bakst's signature style. Finally, Cleopatra revealed herself. With a blue-green wig and kohl-rimmed eyes, she embodied the femme fatale. For the rest of the dance, she lounged—observing and commanding the action but never engaging in it herself.

Cléopâtre was included in Hoffmann's ersatz Russian repertoire. So was the nonnarrative ballet with music by Chopin called *Les Sylphides*, which her first New York advertisement called a "romantic revelry."[19] Lincoln Kirstein's history of theatrical dance points out that this was a likely typo: Michel Fokine described the dance as a "romantic revery," and it is more dreamlike than lively and noisy.[20] Both of those dances were part of the Ballets Russes debut season. When Hoffmann saw the company again in 1910, they performed many new dances, including the now-canonical *Firebird*. The dance on that new program that most appealed to Hoffmann, though, was *Schéhérazade*. Based on *One Thousand and One Nights*, the ballet may have reminded Hoffmann of the pseudo-Arabian extravaganzas from her days in San Francisco. Unlike *Ali Baba, or Morgiana and the 40 Thieves*, this take on the Arabian nights was far more graphic in its sexuality and violence. Playing the role of Zobéide, Rubinstein struck poses of languorous beauty, passion, and terror. This role demanded the same skill set as Salome, against a larger backdrop.

Much of the work Hoffmann did that summer related to copying the costumes and signing the dancers. Morris Gest's biographers emphasized the secrecy of the planning: "To forestall rivals, all negotiations for personnel and repertory were conducted *sub rosa*—contracts and bonds for the dancers, who were responsible only to the Czar; arrangements for Marie Muelle to execute the costumes and scenery in Paris from the Léon Bakst designs, etc."[21] The published description elides the person making these arrangements. Hoffmann wrote that she met with Marie Muelle, the costumer who produced the openwork harem pants and fringed, beaded tops for *Schéhérazade*. She saw the plates with original designs that Bakst produced. She had contracts printed in English and French.[22]

Her notes betray a deep frustration with the division of labor between herself and Gest: "I told about Muel[le]—costumier—Pages + pages of directions," she writes, while he "was seeking a play for his father—Belasco."[23] She continued to study Russian dance technique with Theodore Kosloff, paying $60 an hour.[24] Kosloff was then producing and performing in London, at the Coliseum and the Hippodrome.[25] Hoffmann complained that Gest only saw the ballets in touring productions—either Milan or Monte Carlo—with "scenery of no consequence."[26] Later that year, touring with her revue, she received a telegram from Gest requesting $4,000. She sent the money and knew that now she was "in for it."[27] Unlike Gest's silent partner F. Ray Comstock, Hoffmann resented being treated merely as a source of funding.

For Gertrude Hoffmann, the decision to imitate the Ballets Russes served both pragmatic and idealistic purposes. She could not bring the originals, she was skilled as a mimic, and she had copied another European performance already. Along with Hoffmann's practical thinking, her desire to copy illustrates emotions of cross-cultural desire and identification.[28] "For two years," Hoffmann writes, "I studied patiently under foreign masters, not that I might dance with the Russians but that I might do my share of the work."[29] The unauthorized Ballets Russes production afforded her a long-term apprenticeship as an artist.

She and her family stayed in Europe until late July, with at least one outing with Anna Held and her daughter by the English Channel.[30] They returned to New York for what Gertrude Hoffmann claimed would be her last season in vaudeville. In a shipside interview, she said she had found "a splendid play by a French author" that would serve as her entry into the "legitimate drama."[31] Coverage of the trip gave Hoffmann the authority granted to Broadway producers, suggesting that she too had the money and the taste to find appropriate source material on the Continent.

A few details in this article suggest a certain anxiety about the transatlantic exchange of theatrical material. The "splendid play" was a feint, since her plan was to produce and star in dance-pantomime, not drama. The same article describes how Max Hoffmann remarks that he "had attended 'Hello, London' in London and had been surprised and gratified, but much more surprised than gratified, to note that the Londoners had appropriated one of his best songs and made it the basis of their play."[32] The borrowing at work in theatrical culture of the early twentieth century was bidirectional: that meant not only Europe but the United States could be visited, appropriated from, and imitated at a distance.

By September, Hoffmann was back on the road with her revue. Pavlova and Mordkin returned to the United States late in the month; they were due to perform their new program at the Metropolitan Opera House and on tour, beginning in mid-October.[33] That performance at the Met was hailed as another "triumph."[34] It revived *Giselle*, which had not played in New York since the early nineteenth century, and ended with a new ballet called *The Legend of Azyiade*, inspired by the success of *Schéhérazade* in Paris.[35] The Russian dancers crossed paths with Hoffmann in Indianapolis a week later: their one-night stand played at the Murat Theatre opposite her weeklong booking played at the Grand Theater.[36]

The New York theatergoing public was fascinated by Russian dancers that season, whether they were real or fake. The former Ballets Russes company members Lydia Lopokova and Alexander Volinine toured on the Orpheum circuit and performed in musicals.[37] Hoffmann knew Lopokova's work from vaudeville when she asked Morris Gest to book her for their Russian ballet tour.[38] These authentic Russian dancers competed with many ersatz performers. "Mlle. Bianci" presented a program of Russian dances; the reviewer pointed out that she bore a "remarkable resemblance" to Bianca Froelich, the ballerina who danced in the Metropolitan Opera's *Salome* and then performed in vaudeville.[39] The review for "Danses Classique Russe" at the American Theatre admitted the chorus was "home-made rather than from any 'Imperial Ballet.'"[40] After performing through the rise and fall of Salomania, Hoffmann may have seen this trend as proof that the American public would appreciate her production of the Ballets Russes. Perhaps she worried that the Russian dance bubble would burst before her production opened.

Theodore Kosloff trained the dancers to perform uncredited imitations of three Michel Fokine ballets: *Cléopâtre*, *Les Sylphides*, and *Schéhérazade*. The rehearsals were kept secret for a number of reasons. Clearly, they wanted to evade criticism about "borrowing" Fokine's choreography.[41] The secrecy also maintained an aura of exotic foreignness. In the wake of Pavlova and Mordkin's tour, the Russianness of the company's dancers was a benefit to trade upon: while some of them trained with the Imperial Ballet, the ranks were filled out with other Parisian dancers, Russians already touring in the United States, and, according to some sources, American dancers who took on Russian and French pseudonyms.[42] Ben Atwell and Max Rabinoff, the managers for Pavlova and Mordkin's summer tour, heard rumors about Morris Gest's planned Russian act and confronted him.[43] They attempted to come up with a publicity strategy that would foment interest in both tours instead of making them into competitors, but talks broke down.[44] Secret rehearsals also built up suspense. Hoffmann was a known quantity; she toured for forty weeks at a time, and she regularly appeared in trade magazines and newspapers. What would be her next move? *Variety* dropped hints in an article called "Gertie Hoffmann's Surprise," talking about the large cast (125 people) and orchestra (60 pieces), as well as the "large amount of money" that was "said to be represented in the production."[45] Whatever the content, readers knew that Hoffmann's new show would be extravagant.

Even more than the size, publicity for the ballet emphasized its European pedigree.[46] The Hoffmann production, this ad promised, was "The Introduction to the English-Speaking World of the New Cult in Art Which Has Enraptured and Enslaved the Pampered Parisians for Two Years."[47] These dances were pitched as acts of faithful transatlantic reproduction. They would be performed "exactly as done in Paris at the Chatelet Theater and at the Grand Opera House, and at La Scala in Milan."[48] Dancers and production designers in the ad were also tagged with their home theater and country of origin. No wonder so many contemporaneous descriptions of the show describe it as "imported."[49]

The copying extended to promotional materials. Consider the *Album Souvenir de "La Saison Russe,"* a keepsake booklet printed by the Gertrude Hoffmann Company in 1911. Its front and back cover and center spread are taken from a Parisian print source, without attribution to the journal or artist. The illustrations and page borders first appeared in a sixteen-page color supplement to the June 15, 1910, issue of *Comœdia Illustré*, a biweekly illustrated magazine that publicized the early performances of Diaghilev's troupe.[50] The front cover features "a brilliantly coloured design by Leon Bakst depicting the character of King Shahyrar from *Schéhérazade*"; this image was bordered by an "illustrated framework of Russian motifs" designed by Lucien Vogel.[51] The cover of the Hoffmann program seen in figure 8.1 features the same image, albeit in slightly less saturated colors. The Vogel border is reproduced, realigned so the bottom edge prints at the edge of the page. This cuts off the part of the *Comœdia Illustré* where the original artists' names appear: "Aquarelle originale de BAKST" printed in red is followed by "L. VoGeL" in gold.[52]

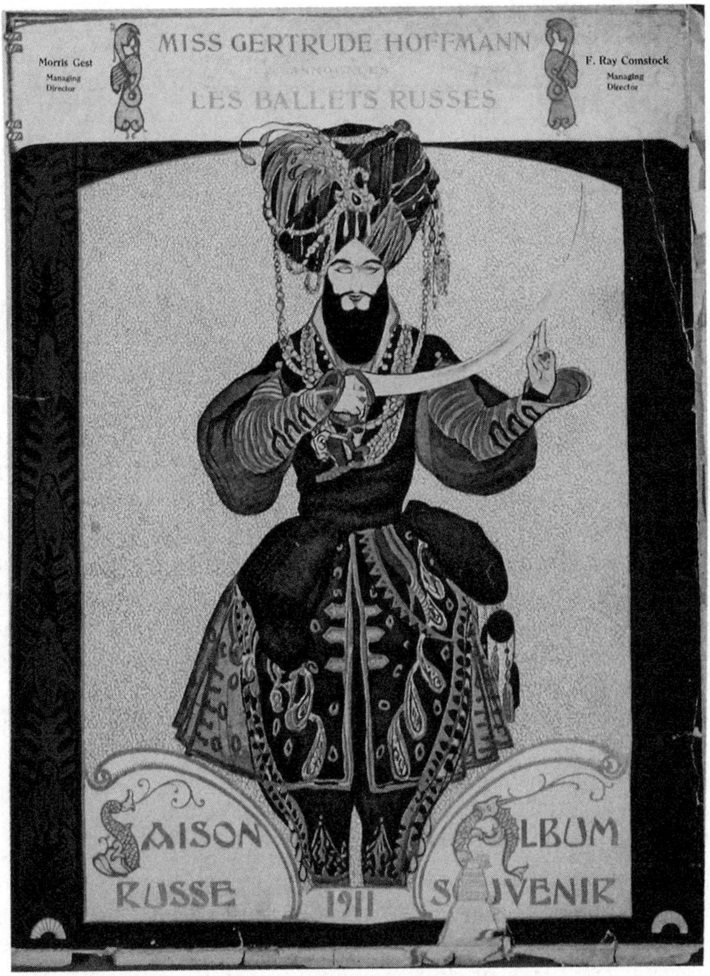

FIGURE 8.1. Cover of the souvenir program for *Saison Russe*, Gertrude Hoffmann Company, 1911. Collection of the author.

The central pages of this program display lavish illustrations of *Schéhérazade* costumes without any descriptive information: the reproduction has masked out the header crediting Bakst for the watercolor illustrations, two brief paragraphs describing the ballet and Bakst's career, and even the character names next to each sketch. These costume designs no longer have any clear relation to the ballets, and instead have become purely decorative in the same manner as the Lucien Vogel borders. Hoffmann's Russian Season is less interested in Russianness per se than it is in a decontextualized orientalist pantomime.

La Saison des Ballets Russes opened on June 14. The show began with *Cléopâtre*. Using a strategy similar to that of "A Vision of Salome," the setting was sketched out: heavy pillars suggested a temple, a distant strip of blue represented the Nile. The scene began with a high priest interrupting a rendezvous between lovers named Amoun and Ta-Hor, to announce the arrival of the queen and her court. Hoffmann's entrance as Cleopatra followed Ida Rubinstein's beat for beat: she was brought onstage inside a sarcophagus and unwound from a tangle of colorful scarves. Amoun showed his infatuation with Cleopatra; she agreed to spend the night with him if he would drink poison in the morning. Ta-Hor begged him to change his mind, but he accepts the queen's terms. The ballet ended with Ta-Hor discovering the dead Amoun.

The middle ballet was *Les Sylphides*. This selection of waltzes and mazurkas to the music of Chopin was less pantomime, more pure dance. Clad in white, the dancers provided a visual respite from the splendor of the first and last performances.

Schéhérazade concluded the program. This ballet was set in the harem of "Schah-riar, the king of India and China."[53] Lust and violence unfurled against a rich blue background, with blue and gold tapestries to complete the Persian aesthetic. Lynn Garafola summarizes the plot, which she notes now "seems the height of ballet camp. . . . A Shah, suspecting his favorite wife's infidelity, leaves home to test her; he returns to find the harem in the middle of an orgy and Zobéide in the arms of her Golden Slave. Scimitars flash, and the curtain falls on a stage full of corpses."[54] Hoffmann and Kosloff danced together in *Schéhérazade*, as seen in figure 8.2. She was Zobéide the sultan's favorite wife, while he was the "golden slave" famously played by Vaslav Nijinsky. One change was made to suit white American theatergoers' prejudices: in Hoffmann's production, the "golden slave" was renamed the "favorite Arab," to avoid associations with miscegenation and chattel slavery, one suspects.

First-night critics marveled at the show's decor, costumes, and music. The dance and pantomime were well-received, particularly that of Lopokova and Volinine in *Les Sylphides*. Hoffmann's performance was not. Charitable reviews noted that she did little dancing and looked beautiful; the less kind ones noted her clear lack of skill compared to the Russians.[55] George Jean Nathan who, along with H. L. Mencken, served as snarky doyen of American culture in the 1910s and 1920s, panned Hoffmann's performance in grandiose terms. He commands the reader:

> Picture to yourself a comic supplement cartoonist for the Hammerstein roof giving an exhibition of his craft in the Louvre. Picture to yourself a Casino show girl acting as a partner in the dance to a Rita Sacchetto. Picture to yourself a Keith and Proctor quartet tenor wrestling with "Aida." Picture to yourself any of these and you will gain a competent idea of the indecent bravado of Miss Gertrude Hoffmann, who injected her unclothed body and ante-vitagraph "art" into the sacred, definite, authentic and most exalted art of the most picturesque nation in the world.[56]

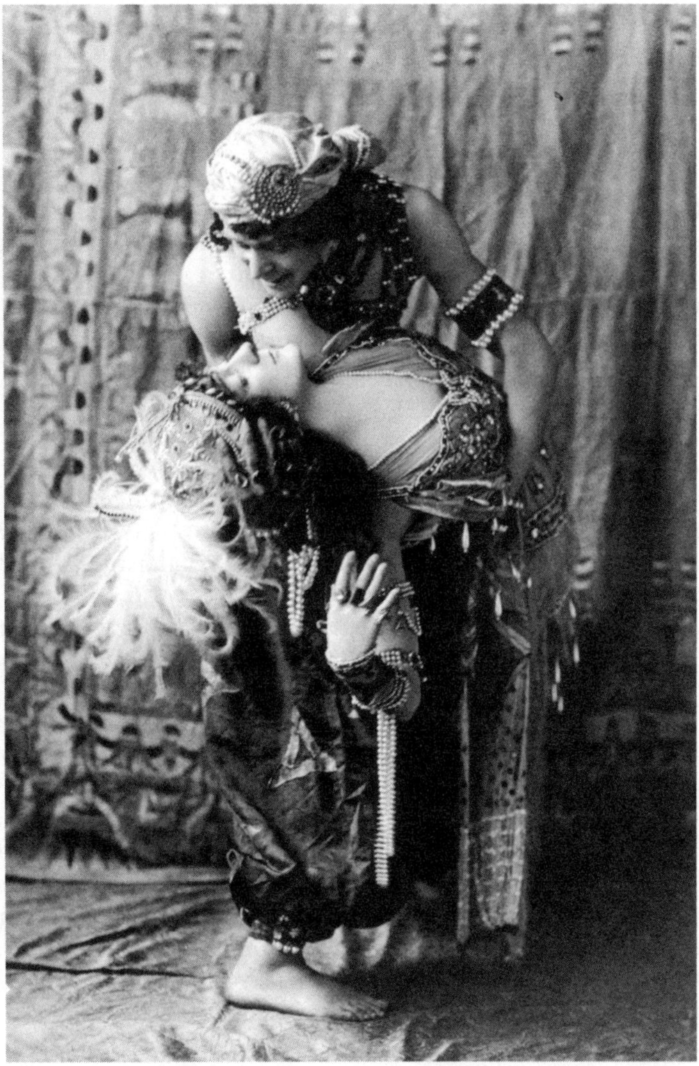

FIGURE 8.2. Gertrude Hoffmann and Theodore Kosloff in *Schéhérazade*. Photograph by Frank C. Bangs. Apeda Studios. Jerome Robbins Dance Division, the New York Public Library for the Performing Arts.

The indignation is palpable. Hoffmann is a popular entertainer daring to place herself among true artists. He asks the audience to picture any number of imaginary violations that might substitute for her own; like an act on a vaudeville bill, she can be swapped out. The other performers he gives as examples would never dare cross the same line: a tenor in a vaudeville quartet knows he is supposed to sing "Sweet Adeline," not opera. Hoffmann's indecency here is not a direct result of her nakedness. Instead, it's the "indecent bravado" of suggesting that she belongs on the same stage as classically trained Russian dancers. Her "art" can only be discussed in scare quotes, but their art is indisputable.

Nathan draws on relatively new ideas about the hierarchy among different parts of culture. Only around the turn of the twentieth century did critics begin to assert the division of "highbrow" from "lowbrow," and the location of the former in the concert hall and the latter on the popular stage.[57] This division was not an especially useful one when it came to dance. When Hoffmann began working in San Francisco, choruses of ballet girls were an expected element of operatic performance. Even the "Casino show girl" would have played a part in operettas, as well as Will Marion Cook and Paul Laurence Dunbar's *Clorindy: or the Origin of the Cake Walk*.[58] Gertrude Hoffmann posed a problem for critics of the era who were invested in this distinction because she is so clearly interested in dance with both avant-garde and mass appeal. As a San Francisco critic wrote of the *Saison des Ballets Russes* when it arrived on tour, "She has a punch in both hands—one for the highbrows and one for the roughnecks."[59]

The *Saison des Ballets Russes* played at the Shubert brothers' Winter Garden Theatre. The venue opened to great acclaim.[60] It was a large venue with a wide, shallow stage.[61] The interior was decorated in the style of a roof garden, and it promised to maintain a consistent indoor temperature, even in summertime.[62] This should have been an ideal venue to introduce the masses to Russian ballet performed by a full company, outfitted with the same costumes, sets, and music as in Paris. "But Gest and Miss Hoffmann had still another competitor on which they hadn't counted," wrote Oliver M. Sayler and Marjorie Barkentin, "the Weather!"[63] Though the critics lauded the performance, their praise could not convince people to sit through a long program inside a theater during a heat wave.[64] Another "indecency" controversy arose, but even the protests of the New York mayor William Gaynor failed to rouse the audience to attend.[65] The show closed on July 8, 1911. They tried to reopen it at the Winter Garden in August, with little success.

Hoffmann and Gest were losing thousands of dollars a week. That huge cast and orchestra translated to an extravagant payroll. Even on a tour that helped them recoup their investment, the large and ornate sets made it impractical to book one-night stands. Morris Gest convinced the passenger agent of the Lehigh Valley Railroad to transport the cast, crew, and sets to Chicago for free.[66] The *Saison des Ballets Russes* opened the fall season at Chicago's Lyric Theatre.[67] Even in the town where Max Hoffmann's career began, the show did not do as well as they hoped.

As the majority owner of their production company, Gertrude Hoffmann was on the hook for most of the expense. She came up with a solution inspired by her recent work in the revue format: interpolating her own imitations and dances between the Russian ballets. In Minneapolis, she added the highlights of her 1910–1911 vaudeville tour; she appeared third in the evening, after *Cléopâtre* and *Les Sylphides*, but before *Schéhérazade*.[68] Hoffmann's Cleopatra and Zobéide were placed in the same pantheon as modern divas Anna Held, Eva Tanguay, and Valeska Suratt. Even more daringly, she performed two straight dances among her imitations, *The Cobras* and "Spring Song."

Gest worried that this would spoil the integrity of the artistic program, to which Hoffmann replied "Wait and see!"[69] Her additions earned the second half of the tour far more money—and press coverage—than the first half. But the benefits of Hoffmann's revue came with a cost. Lopokova and Volinine left the company, objecting to the ways a revue cheapened the dances that shared the program.[70] While Hoffmann dealt with the aftermath of the Russian dancers' departure, Gest traveled to San Francisco to set up the last bookings in her western tour.[71]

There was one more hurdle to overcome before the tour could be proclaimed a success. Max Rabinoff and Ben Atwell, the producers of the Pavlova and Mordkin tour, undertook a smear campaign.[72] A poster with a dire proclamation appeared in the theater districts of cities across the western states: "Warning Against Pirates," it read across the top, the words underlined and flanked by skulls and crossbones. It suggested that any Russian dancers appearing in the weeks to come were mere "free-booters" and "buccaneers" trying to pass themselves off as true Russian dancers like Pavlova and Mordkin. The poster warned that "only two legitimate troups [*sic*] of imperial Russian dancers are coming to America," the Pavlova and Mordkin company and the Diaghilev company. The poster ominously concludes: "Several companies of disguised song and dance 'artists' from the ten, twenty and thirty cent vaudeville circuit, and supporting casts from cloak, clothing, boot and shoe, and suspender factories are in process of organization to sweep over the land NOW, making use of these illustrious names to deceive. Beware of the Pirates."[73] This language repeats the indignation expressed by George Jean Nathan, imagining that vaudevillians in disguise are setting out to take over the ballet stage. The cultural elitism and classism jump off the page, especially in the scare quotes around the word artist and the idea of a corps de ballet made up of factory workers. Valleri J. Hohman reads the classism as anti-Semitic as well, since it characterizes the "supporting cast" as "Russian Jewish immigrants rather than as Russian nationals."[74] The arguments separating highbrow culture from lowbrow could have a nasty tone.

The "Warning Against Pirates" poster depressed audience turnout in the Pacific Northwest until Morris Gest called in a favor. J. J. Shubert met with Ben Atwell and threatened him with jail time.[75] This was the end of their accusatory ad campaign. Atwell and Rabinoff had their own problems: Pavlova left, and Mordkin came down with appendicitis. Lopokova and Volinine took over Pavlova and Mordkin's dates.[76]

When her Russian ballet tour arrived in San Francisco in mid-October 1911, Hoffmann was hailed as a returning hero.[77] In a city that had lost so much during the recent earthquake, she served as a reminder of the fabled theatrical past. Reviewers loved to reminisce about her previous identity as Kitty Hayes the chorus girl. The show was also celebrated in Los Angeles, where reviewers embraced her "western" identity as a self-made success.[78] California reviewers shaped the reception of her ballet on its return tour: as the production moved back east, the reviews emphasized Hoffmann's skill, even her artistry, as an imitator.

Because Hoffmann spent so much of her career on the road, her reputation developed in national terms. New York critics first recognized her skill as a manager and producer during the run of her 1910 *Review*. It was critics outside of New York, though, who first proclaimed Gertrude Hoffmann to be an artist. The San Francisco critic Ralph E. Renaud anticipated the response to this claim: "'What!' you say, "Gertrude Hoffmann, the vaudeville headliner, a great artist!' I can only repeat it as my sober opinion. She is one of the most eloquent mimetic figures I have ever seen upon the stage. Outside of her versatility, which is dazzling, her work in 'Cleopatre' alone would place her in the front rank of graphic artistes."[79] For the reviewers on the western half of the tour, Hoffmann's work as an imitator stood up to that of the Russian dancers in their "mimodramas." Comparing her work to that of Theodore Kosloff and Alexandra Baldina, a Los Angeles critic said, "They represent classic dance; she represents, in its fullest and finest flower, the dance of pantomimic expression."[80] These reviews should be taken with a grain of salt. The critics were invested in Hoffmann as an icon of California dance, and perhaps they wanted to proclaim her the next Isadora Duncan. Western critics' ideas were echoed by more disinterested observers on the return tour, though.[81] As the ballet returned to Chicago in December, Ashton Stevens compared Hoffmann's mimicry to another new art that broke down boundaries between high and low, the art of the poster.[82] Hoffmann's mimetic prowess, already at a high level, must have improved as she continued to work with the Russian dancers. When she watched and copied high-quality artists, her imitations flourished.

Hoffmann's blend of highbrow and lowbrow art troubled critics who thought she should develop one part of her performance instead of insisting on variety. In the *Boston Transcript* review of the Russian Season, the dance critic H. T. Parker laments:

> What might she have been had life and work ordered themselves differently for her; had she sloughed her clowning and mimicking self and become the Hoffmann of these dancing episodes, beautifully imagined and beautifully achieved. Restless, temperamental, never quite escaping the bonds that bind her to the cheaper and the commoner side of her

> "reviews," yet seemingly ever struggling with them, she is one of the strangest paradoxes of our stage.[83]

This is the paradox of Gertrude Hoffmann in a nutshell: throughout her career, her "clowning and mimicking" coexisted with her dancing. Her work as an artist and as a producer was restless and temperamental, forever seeking the newest style of performance and then challenging herself to copy it. She continued to channel European modernism in her next act, though not in the ways she anticipated.

Chapter 9

Mainstream Modernism

Gertrude Hoffmann was not alone in bringing modern European performance to American audiences. While she was on the last leg of her *Saison des Ballets Russes* tour, a pantomime called *Sumurun* took New York City by storm. The German director Max Reinhardt fashioned a spectacle in the "Arabian nights" vein of *Schéhérazade*, with even more experimental lighting and set design than the ballet. Lee Shubert assisted Reinhardt in funding the American production, and when the show toured the United States it played at Shubert theaters.

Sumurun introduced the runway to the American stage, bringing the full cast in from the back of the auditorium and through the audience. This theatrical element, it was thought, disrupted the audience's sense of separation from the cast and broke through realism's fourth wall. The Shubert Organization co-opted Reinhardt's staging for its own revues, beginning with *The Whirl of Society* (1912). The drama critic Archie Bell notes dejectedly, "All theaters which play Winter Garden attractions have an electric-lighted runway into the audience, whereupon Tootsie Coughdrop and Mamie Gumshoe cavort and warble ragtime syncopations."[1] The aesthetic intent of the runway has been lost; instead, it is merely a vehicle that brings attractive chorus girls singing popular songs into closer contact with the audience. "If ever a big idea was thrown to the dust by someone who appropriated it," Bell continues, "this seems to be the case. But many of Reinhardt's ideas seem to have reached America in similar fashion. We think we are not ready for him, but we are ready enough for his imitators."[2] Clearly Gertrude Hoffmann fit the bill. She signed a two-year contract with the Shuberts that summer.[3]

On the surface, Hoffmann and the Shuberts seem an ideal match. They could both be said to follow the "Shubert house policy" of being "a canny copycat rather than an innovator."[4] But Hoffmann nursed a desire to be an innovator herself, or at least an innovative importer of European acts. As she renewed her relationship with the Shubert Organization, she felt torn between her desires to experiment and to popularize. She split the difference between the two in this period by presenting herself as a popular modernist who borrowed and mocked European avant-garde trends.

In what was becoming a habit, Gertrude Hoffmann followed up her Russian ballet tour with another trip to Europe. The Hoffmanns sailed on the RMS *Cedric* ocean liner on March 28.[5] This was another trip in search of a European act, which she planned to produce at the Winter Garden that summer.[6] Evidence suggests that she was interested in a pantomime called "La Bête" (The Beast) that was then playing at the Moulin Rouge.[7] Written by the Grand Guignol playwright André de Lorde, it tells the "Murders in the Rue Morgue"–like story of a rampaging gorilla who escapes from a Parisian fair. The gorilla hides on the rooftops; his trainer nearly apprehends him, but then loses his footing and falls. The gorilla "dreams of its infancy, in the forest."[8] This fantasy is followed by the scene of a ball at the home of a refined woman. After the party concludes, she goes to her bedroom, where the gorilla strangles her. Her lover is accused of the crime, but he finds an imprint of the gorilla's paw on her pillow and is vindicated. The animal is shot and killed.[9]

Imagining this play through Hoffmann's eyes, it looks like a good sequel to the Ballets Russes. "La Bête" combines fantasy, elegance, and primitive violence in a compressed storyline. It heightens the aesthetic and emotional abandon that Hoffmann loved in the Ballets Russes. (It may have heightened it too much: Grand Guignol plays were synonymous with excessive grisliness.) The *Variety* review of the act even calls it a "mimodrama," the word used in programs and reviews to describe the Russian narrative ballets.[10] Hoffmann returned to America on May 4, but she did not succeed in bringing "La Bête" to the American stage.[11] She may have been lucky in this respect; the eventual American production was poorly reviewed, and the Shuberts called it a "fiasco."[12]

The Shuberts were known for mixing high art with mass entertainment.[13] They paired *The Whirl of Society* with an operetta called *Sesostra* in the spring of 1912. They followed the same format for their summer show. The opening act was *The Ballet of 1830*, which played at London's Alhambra Theatre, choreographed by Hoffmann's Russian ballet partner Theodore Kosloff. But they followed this serious "mimo-dramatic ballet in 3 scenes" with something more playful.[14] The *Ziegfeld Follies* was postponed in spring 1912, so the Shubert brothers filled the gap with a new revue. They borrowed the title from an 1894 "topical extravaganza" produced by George Lederer that spoofed Broadway shows of the era.[15] The new version, called *The Passing Show of 1912*, claimed to be "a kaleidoscopic almanac in seven scenes, presenting the comic aspect of many important events, political, theatrical and otherwise."[16] Since she had brought one of the biggest European performances to America in the prior theatrical season, Gertrude Hoffmann was subject to parody in the *Passing Show*. Her "Spring Song" was mocked by the comedian Trixie Friganza.[17] Along with references to other Broadway hits of the day, *The Passing Show of 1912* included a harem scene from *Kismet* that also included nods to *Schéhérazade* as well as *Sumurun*.

Planning to headline a show at the Winter Garden in September 1912, Gertrude Hoffmann began rehearsals in late July; by the end of August it was clear that her new revue was in trouble.[18] The Shuberts hired a huge supporting cast and changed directors.[19] Meanwhile, *The Passing Show of 1912* was making serious money as each show played to capacity crowds.[20] Hoffmann's opening date was pushed back to October, and news reports suggested it would not appear at the Winter Garden at all.[21] Five months without appearing onstage must have seemed like an eternity.

To keep Hoffmann in the spotlight, Shubert press agents (or possibly Morris Gest) pushed a story about the costumes in Hoffmann's new show. She would wear outfits designed by the Ballets Russes visionary Léon Bakst, the stories claimed, as well as modern artistic designs invented by Bakst to stencil on her legs instead of stockings. These painted-on designs were the talk of the theater world, with responses ranging from scandal and disgust to amusement and celebration. Pictures of her painted legs as seen in figure 9.1 appeared in newspapers across the country in the first week of October 1912. Her shins display painted rabbits, "significant of the speed at which Miss Hoffmann dances," we are told.[22] Her initials appear below the rabbits; a diamond with four dots surrounding it appears as an additional part of the pattern on her right leg.

The Parisian actress Madame Polaire was shocked by Hoffmann's painted legs because they broke down the distinction between body and costume. She said, in her Gallic way:

> I cannot agree with Miss Gertrude Hoffmann in her idea of painting les jambes. I do not like that. It offends me. One should either be natural purely or don the embellishments to the natural. One would not paint a pearl or embroider fine lace. . . . One should either wear stockings or wear none. If they wear none, the ornamentation should be apart from the skin. Bracelets, jewels, bijous of various kinds can be placed upon it—but to paint it! I shudder![23]

Polaire's distinctions suggest that this is a period in which actresses can dress to emphasize either the natural or the decorative, but not both. To compare painting your legs to embroidering atop fine lace suggests that it breaks down the barrier between discrete types of decoration. In this way, this criticism anticipates the conflation of bareness and ornament in images of Josephine Baker.[24]

Some critics took Hoffmann's legs seriously, but the majority made jokes. A satirical magazine ran a column called "Watching Our Funny World Go By" where the author mentioned Hoffmann: "I don't like the rabbit on her ankle," he says. "I never did like to see hair on a girl's leg." [25] A play called *Birds of a Feather* includes a scene between a writer and an actress in which he asks her if she's got any "special stuff" for the "advertising man to talk

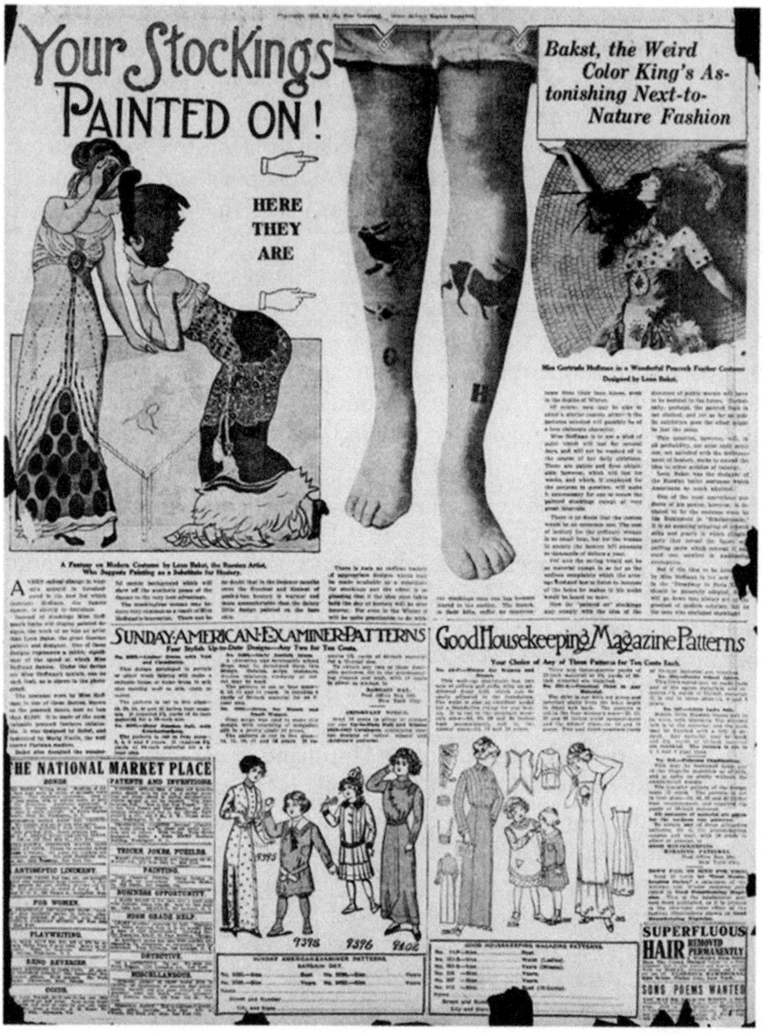

Your Stockings Painted On!

HERE THEY ARE

Bakst, the Weird Color King's Astonishing Next-to-Nature Fashion

SUNDAY AMERICAN-EXAMINER PATTERNS

Good Housekeeping Magazine Patterns

THE NATIONAL MARKET PLACE

SUPERFLUOUS HAIR REMOVED PERMANENTLY

SONG POEMS WANTED

FIGURE 9.1. Gertrude Hoffmann's legs at the center of a newspaper feature. *Chicago Examiner*, Sunday, September 29, 1912, 65. Chicago Public Library, Digital Collections.

about" like Gertrude Hoffmann's painted legs.[26] The actress replies sarcastically, "There'll be no room for the paint." She then notes, "Gee, look at the way that dame went up—why just a few years ago she was in the same chorus with me!"[27] Even if your legs are not much to look at on their own, the actress suggests, modern painting transforms them into a newsworthy spectacle.

Hoffmann's new show, titled *Broadway to Paris*, opened at the Winter Garden on November 20, 1912. She tried to make the show her own, which resulted in pushback from her producers at the beginning of their long, somewhat strained partnership. She gave the Shuberts a script, when they preferred their revues to be written in-house. Harold Atteridge, who Foster Hirsch dubs the "poet laureate of the Winter Garden," was hired to help craft the book.[28] She insisted on hiring her own stage manager; J. J. Shubert replaced him with Ned Wayburn.[29] It was the first of many times that year when Hoffmann would act more like a producer than a performer. The Shuberts reminded her "that there is a great difference between employee and employer."[30] Her artistic vision, and the money necessary to fulfill it, would often conflict with the producers' attention to the bottom line.

After planning her own revue in vaudeville, Hoffmann must have bridled at giving up control to the production team. With *Broadway to Paris*, she imagined a show with an even faster pace than her 1910 act: "In this revue," a *Variety* article optimistically states, "there will be thirty-three scenes, some not to hold the stage over a minute."[31] A letter in the Shubert archive nixed this rapid-fire, proto-futurist format. It told her that this structure was "absolutely impossible" and put her in touch with scenario writers who could work her scenes into a standard narrative arrangement.[32] Something of Hoffmann's original need for speed remained when *Broadway to Paris* opened: the critic Alan Dale said the show had "the pace that kills."[33] Hoffmann was constantly in motion—tumbling out of a hansom cab, riding around the stage on a bicycle, and performing her eponymous dance, the "Gertrude Hoffmann Glide."

The plot of *Broadway to Paris* is a conventional one, where the wealthy New Yorker Stuyvesant Van Cortlandt is engaged to the virtuous American debutante Isabelle Montclair, an heiress from New Jersey. Van Cortlandt becomes infatuated with the actress Anne Trelawney (played by Hoffmann) and follows her to Paris. Montclair and a pair of bumbling detectives follow after him. At a masquerade ball, Miss Montclair poses as Miss Trelawney and shows her fiancé the error of his ways.[34] After enjoying his adventures abroad, the hero ends up with the heroine from back home.

The show deals with Americans in Paris, both mocking their naïveté and championing their cultural superiority. The Greek deities Venus and Apollo serve as tour guides to Van Cortlandt when he arrives. He needs them as guides, Venus says, because "real Parisians know nothing of Paris. They ride underground in the Metro and never see anything."[35] The gods promise to show him the clichéd scenes he expects to see, but only if he pays them ten francs apiece. This artificial tour is necessary in the current economy: "You Americans have made restaurants so expensive in Paris that real students and grisettes cannot afford to go unless their expenses are paid," Apollo says.[36] This wisecrack leads into a Max Hoffmann–penned song, "Paree's a Branch of Broadway." The central conceit of the song is that Paris is underwhelming compared to cities in the United States including New York City,

Philadelphia, Boston, and even Yonkers. The lyrics suggest that Rector's restaurant is more exciting than the Moulin Rouge, that Parisian cafés are only exciting to hicks, and that even Parisian dress is outmatched by "outfits that are new" on "Old Fifth Avenue."[37] The show used its Parisian setting to the hilt, with scenes in a café, a casino, a theater, and a motordrome for bicycle racing.

As is the case in most musical comedies of this era, the characters and storyline provide the barest excuse for comic, patriotic, and glamorous production numbers. Hoffmann admitted as much in one version of the show's prologue: "If I was not down on the program as an actress," she says, "how could we stop the action of the play for ten minutes to give you my new 'Spring Song' or 'Garden of Girls,' for a dance of a fawn and a dryad, surrounded by a lot of nymphs, has certainly nothing to do with the plot."[38] Whether this was written by Hoffmann herself or by one of the many script doctors, it reveals the ways that audience expectations shape the possibilities of popular theater.

The show retains an amusing level of self-awareness throughout. One recurring joke is that Gertrude Hoffmann's fame is built on the fame of others. Anne Trelawney's name is based on a role Ethel Barrymore had recently played.[39] In *Broadway to Paris*, Anne Trelawney tries a publicity stunt made famous by Anna Held.[40] The "Gertrude Hoffmann Glide," with words and music by Max Hoffmann, demonstrates this borrowing most clearly. Performed in the first act with a reprise during the finale, the song mentions the "Gaby Glide" named after the current Shubert star Gaby Deslys, as well as George M. Cohan and Eva Tanguay.[41] The lyrics also give a mini-retrospective of her career with their injunctions to "try a little dash here of Salome," "add on the Spring Song," and "use the grace with which the Russians slide."[42] The song establishes Hoffmann's star persona in terms of what she does, not who she is.

Writing the song was just one way that Max helped craft his wife's reputation. An earlier newspaper article dubbed him "builder of Gertrude," and suggested (incorrectly) that he was the one who persuaded her to go by "Gertrude" instead of "Kitty."[43] That article also called Max "One Big Man" who served as a "Human Wall between Wife and World."[44] Gertrude Hoffmann wrote in her diaries of the ways she used Max to protect her from the threat of sexual harassment or assault. If a columnist or other bigwig asked to see her after a show, she would go—and Max would go with her.[45] He was over six feet tall, with an imposing physique and an aristocratic bearing. (At some point in his career, people began to address him as "Baron" even though he held no claim to a title.)

Max too was subject to criticism in the Shuberts' correspondence. One letter said that as the musical director for *Broadway to Paris*, Max "tries to do everything possible for the other people" in the show, but he "is not fulfilling his duties to them, as his whole interest is centered on" his wife.[46] He regularly visited the Shubert office with questions and concerns about Gertrude's career. One charming artifact is a note written in verse:

> Dear J. J.,
> By your request
> Per Morris Gest
> I called at seven thirty
> To figure out
> What punch and clout
> Is needed for our Gertie
> For hours I sat
> And watched the ladies
> Scrub your desk and tile and
> They tried to sweep
> Away my feet
> So back to Coney Island
> [signed]
> Max Hoffmann[47]

Max imbued his note with a Tin Pan Alley–style wit, including the rhyme of "tile and" with "Island." This is clearly a man who had written popular music for twenty years. His regular visits infuriated J. J., who insisted that Gertrude needed to address him directly instead of sending her husband as a messenger.[48] Max continued to advocate for his wife, eventually taking over for Morris Gest in the official role of her manager.

Broadway to Paris continued to play at the Winter Garden in December. On Sunday evenings, the venue often hosted "concerts," an excuse to get around laws prohibiting theatrical performances on the Sabbath. Hoffmann appeared on the bill at one such concert, and so did the British dancer Greville Moore. Earlier that summer Moore had performed in *The Ballet of 1830*, the show that played on the same bill as *The Passing Show of 1912*. Moore's mother was a noblewoman who wrote a pantomimic dance called "The Spirit of Opium," which her daughter was scheduled to perform. That plan was thwarted when Hoffmann "began to dismember the scenery, exclaiming, 'She shan't use it,'" and sitting on the pieces she had removed.[49] The matter was resolved by the stage manager, and after some delay, Moore performed her piece.

After all her other demands in the lead-up to the *Broadway to Paris* revue, this was the last straw. "I wish to state to you that I will not permit you to use any profane language or disrupt this organization," a Shubert letter to Hoffmann reads, "or air your personal affairs on the stage of the theatre or tear down scenery."[50] It continues, "Your action of last night was both uncalled for and unpardonable, and I trust that in the future, as long as you are a member of the 'Broadway to Paris' Company, that I, or the Stage Manager, who is in charge of the Company, will have no occasion to find any further fault."[51] Behind the legalistic language, the letter wants to put Hoffmann in her place, reminding her that the authority for the show was vested in the company's lieutenant, the stage manager.

It is unclear why Hoffmann felt so compelled to interrupt Moore's dance. She may have been jealous that another dancer got to perform the kinds of dances that she loved best. Moore appeared in the Alhambra Theatre production of *The Ballet of 1830* in London, thus working with Theodore Kosloff, Hoffmann's former *Saison Russe* collaborator. In *The Ballet of 1830*, Moore played the "Vampire Girl": this usage of "vampire," soon to be shortened to the more familiar "vamp," was a woman whose sexuality so overwhelmed her male lovers that she drained them of life. In *Broadway to Paris* Hoffmann undertook a "vampire dance" as well, which she called the "Dance Dracula." The set for that dance was visually striking and so expensive that the Shuberts made Hoffmann pay half the cost.[52] Perhaps the idea of this woman getting to perform another pantomime using sets she paid for was what sent her over the edge. There is no solid evidence for this opinion that Moore was stealing Hoffmann's thunder, but it makes sense in a period when Hoffmann was interested in making her mark on the "legitimate" stage. Moore and her "titled mama" epitomize the kind of aristocratic womanhood that was becoming more associated with modern dance.[53]

The Shuberts may have also been frustrated that Hoffmann's Russian ballet was such a success that it made touring with *The Ballet of 1830* impossible. The manager Gilman Haskell wrote to J. J. Shubert in late November, bemoaning the reception of the ballet in Boston. He noted that it "did not get a single hand," and later said, "I do not look for the show to do the business that the Hoffmann show did. I express this opinion after listening to all the conversation possible for me to over-hear. The concensus [*sic*] of opinion is 'Good but not as good as the other one.'"[54] Hoffmann's previous act poisoned the well for serious dances to come.

Broadway to Paris played at the Winter Garden through the new year, and then it set out on tour. At the same time, New York society was rocked by the International Exhibition of Modern Art. Better known as the Armory Show, this exhibition of modern painting and sculpture is often seen as a watershed moment for modernism in America.[55] The Association of American Painters and Sculptors brought the work of many European artists before the American public for the first time. Their work was shown with that of American experimenters who shared their techniques or attitudes. Marcel Duchamp's *Nude Descending a Staircase* was often referenced in the press about the show, with its abstracted time and motion study standing in for a full range of modern aesthetic experiments.

When the Hoffmann revue traveled to Chicago, it went head to head with the Armory Show, then remounted at the Art Institute of Chicago. Newspaper stories in Chicago teemed with advance publicity that promoted *Broadway to*

Paris by representing Hoffmann's body as the ideal medium for modern art. An article in the *Chicago Inter Ocean* on March 23, 1913, begins: "Although the first cubist gown was probably worn by the women of Noah's household in the ark, Gertrude Hoffmann lays claim, and justly too, to being among the leaders to introduce this new form of fashion to society." [56] After the strained cubits/cubist joke, this is a story about Hoffmann's trendiness. Once press agents recognized the vogue for cubist dresses, they claimed that Hoffmann anticipated them. "Many of the artists of the futurist school have studied the gown and pronounced it a perfect realization of their ideas," the story reads, "some of them even suggested that the actress allow it to be put on exhibition next week at the Art Institute, but Miss Hoffmann declares that she would sooner wear it in her new revue, 'Broadway to Paris,' in which she will be seen here the coming week." [57] It is difficult to make a claim about this dress as a costume, since there is no evidence that it existed or that she wore it. It is a publicity strategy that draws connections between risqué theater and avant-garde art, like the Shuberts' appropriation of Max Reinhardt's runway.

Critics in Chicago discuss Hoffmann's performance style using the same framework. Amy Leslie tried to represent Hoffmann's peculiarly modern quality using language borrowed from contemporary painting. "She is ethereal, but it is ether with phosphorescent edges trailing in ugly green and with sibilant hushes around her wraith. She is ghostly past impressionisty," Leslie says. She continues:

> Everything she does is well done. She is the cubist of the stage. If she dances she dances in perfect rhythm and exact figure; if she sings she sings in tune and pronounces her words excellently well. She never seems to breathe a normal breath, make a graceful move or sing a beautiful note be it ever so slight and genuine. She bathes in the weird, the morbid and degenerate of an art which she has entangled in unwholesome events.[58]

Hoffmann, like Picasso and Duchamp, was skilled at what she did. But as with the cubists of the canvas, Leslie cannot make sense of what Hoffmann was doing using previous aesthetic models. The decadence of Aubrey Beardsley is certainly in evidence, along with the color choices and distortions of the body that made Art Institute students dub Henri Matisse "Henry Hairmattress" and burn his paintings in effigy.[59] Peter Wollen points out the connections between the modern fashions of Paul Poiret, the costumes of Bakst, and the paintings of Matisse, noting that they shared a love of color, a similar aesthetic, and a similar relation to the body: "Each of them created a scenography of the Orient that enabled him to redefine the image of the body, especially, but not exclusively, the female body. All three of them were decorative artists."[60] But Hoffmann has, thus far, not been included in this history of decorative modernism. Juxtaposing her performance in *Broadway to Paris* with that of the Armory Show artists demonstrates that they shared aesthetic strategies including shocking colors, female nudity, and an emphasis on speed. Hoffmann's revue performances and press appearances, like the cubist dresses that did eventually appear in department store windows, filtered the avant-garde into the mainstream.[61]

Popular theater shows how European modernism was transmitted to the United States and how it was received by mass audiences.[62] Gertrude Hoffmann engaged in transatlantic and cross-cultural transmission. With her next act, though, she solidified her image as an all-American variety performer. Though she incorporated foreign influences, the shows she performed in and the acts she performed with only threw her national identity into sharper relief.

Chapter 10

All-American Artist

Broadway to Paris toured until the end of May, ending its run in Montreal. When the Hoffmanns returned to Brooklyn for the summer, Max Hoffmann submitted his petition for naturalization.[1] He had lived in the United States since 1879 and in New York City since 1901. He affirmed that he was neither an anarchist nor a polygamist and renounced allegiance to foreign governments and rulers. He declared his intention to naturalize five years earlier, when his hometown of Gniezno was ruled by Czar Nicholas II of Russia. Filing in 1913, he needed to renounce his allegiance to a different sovereign, Kaiser Wilhelm II. The paperwork for Max's petitions gives modern readers a sense of the territorial disputes in early twentieth-century Europe. It also anticipates the ways his wife's career would be tied up with the performance of national identity.

Gertrude Hoffmann received a big-ticket offer for the fall: the United Booking Office offered her a thirty-week contract for $90,000.[2] She took an offer with different terms—$10,000 in advance and a percentage of the profits.[3] She turned away from a conventional vaudeville booking in favor of an independent three-star tour, with each star a female performer whose work epitomized the character of her home country. "In a single evening's entertainment," audiences would be able to see: "Gertrude Hoffman, representing America; Lady Constance Stewart-Richardson, in the name of England; and Polaire, to wave the French tricolor."[4] The Three-Star Tour depended on the association of performance styles with national character. Stewart-Richardson was a British aristocrat whose act evoked both the natural world and the leisure to explore it afforded to a "titled dancer."[5] Madame Polaire was a French actress with a sixteen-inch corseted waist and a nose ring. She performed in intense, violent plays. Hoffmann dabbled in the same types of performance as Stewart-Richardson and Polaire, but her variety act was coded as distinctly American.

Hoffmann saw the contrast between herself and her costars even before she met them. She arrived at the train station to depart on the tour dressed for the long trip ahead, with a navy- blue peacoat and tam-o'-shanter over her street clothes. She wore her hair in kid leather curlers and carried a goldfish bowl.

Walking to the train she saw people on the platform: "Somehow I realized—not having seen them before—but from their outfits I knew—this was it."[6] Stewart-Richardson wore sandals, a turban, and a robe that was part toga, part kimono. Polaire wore a wine-colored negligee with a train, trimmed in sable. Their different worldviews were symbolized by their dress: "I was not at all awed by the get-ups of my co-stars, in fact I could have screamed laughing. To me, their outfits did not belong on a train bound for 18 wks of one nighters."[7] Hoffmann saw her costars as comically underprepared for life on the road. At the same time, she imagined how she looked through their eyes. "Taking a gander at G. H.," she writes, Stewart-Richardson and Polaire saw an outfit that "did not measure up to what a star was supposed to wear."[8] Though Hoffmann commanded attention when she was onstage, she did not always extend her star persona into her offstage life.

The program built from intimate to spectacular.[9] Stewart-Richardson performed solo in *Faun Dances*, and then Polaire starred in a one-act play called *The Visitor*. A glamorous actress returns from a party and discusses it with her maid. The actress hears a sound at the window; thinking it is her lover, she dismisses her maid and lets him in. When she discovers that he is a burglar in search of her jewels, she distracts him with her dance and stabs him in the back. Polaire's scene was dramatic, but it only involved three people. Hoffmann's act was titled *Gertrude Hoffmann's New Revue*. Her supporting cast of more than twenty-five people included chorus girls, comedians, and dancers. The rest of the act followed her recently established revue format, moving from imitations "in one" to lavish group numbers, and alternating between comic scenes and elegant ones. She performed an Argentine tango and imitated the Scottish comedian Harry Lauder and the French performer Gaby Deslys. Other numbers included a harem scene and one in which her dancers were dressed as geisha girls. *Gertrude Hoffmann's New Revue* had a kind of melting-pot flair.

Morris Gest hoped that fights among his stars would goose the show's publicity. Hoffmann was told in advance that "the papers" were going "to be full of rivalry, jealousy."[10] In order to bring that jealousy into being, Gest sowed the seeds of conflict.[11] Each woman was promised her choice of rooms on the train leaving for the tour, the finest suite in each hotel, the largest dressing room. Each star had her own press agent, so their stories competed for space in the newspapers. To play up nationalistic rivalries among audience members, each star's contract reportedly demanded twenty tickets per show be given to "her countrymen. . . . Polaire, of course, will give her seats to Parisians of the Boulevard type. Lady Richardson will distribute hers among monocled Englishmen, and Miss Hoffman will endeavor to find in every city a score of typical Broadway first nighters to be her guests."[12] This contract stipulation, whether true or not, suggests an increasing awareness in the 1910s of the self-identified ethnic and cultural groups and their influence in major American cities. It seems notable that "typical Broadway first nighters" might be found outside of New York City. Mass media distribution of news about Broadway and the circuits many Broadway shows traveled meant that not only "Paree" was a branch of Broadway, but Boston and Baltimore were too. Angry about the billing order, Stewart-Richardson accused Gest of placing Hoffmann in the headlining spot because she was his mistress. Max Hoffmann was sufficiently furious with Stewart-Richardson that he called his lawyer Nathan Burkan and demanded that he sue her for slander.[13] The disputes continued, and the tour broke up at the end of October. The alliance lasted for less than a month.

After the Three-Star Tour collapsed, Hoffmann continued touring with her revue. Max Hoffmann wrote to J. J. Shubert in February 1914, asking him to call off Claude Greneker, the Shuberts' press agent. Greneker threatened to sue Gertrude Hoffmann for her imitation of Deslys. Max explains, "The skit Gertie is doing is the old Suratt imitations with a few slight changes. She did it for you in Boston. It is the one in the course of which she bites Miss Chopin in the leg and hits her over the head with a shirt box."[14] She swapped at least one new imitation into an old sketch.

Another number satirized the social dance craze. In the 1910s, "dance madness" overtook New York City.[15] The scene demonstrating its effects began on a subway platform, where members of the Hoffmann company pretended to be mascots in station advertisements: one of her dancers was the Dutch girl in Old Dutch cleanser, and an Arab dancer doubled as the Cream of Wheat Man. After the advertisements came to life, commuters of every stripe began "indulging in the bunny hug and the turkey trot, and the tango, and what not."[16] This was the modern urban crowd as melting pot.[17] Though the chorus members engaged in different fashionable dances, they all followed the same tune.

On her tour, Hoffmann was supported by a bevy of performers from diverse ethnic backgrounds. These new performers may have served a purpose similar to Polaire's and Stewart-Richardson's, setting into sharp relief Hoffmann's all-American quality. She had shared her revue bill with foreign performers in 1910, the Sri Lankan musicians and dancers who filled out her Ruth St. Denis parody. These new performers were not just "part of the set design" as in her previous act.[18] They did their own turns. The Chinese magician Ching Ling Foo (Chee Ling Qua) performed internationally and inspired myriad imitators.[19] His troupe juggled and tumbled, and his daughter Chee Toy sang American ragtime songs.[20] Ching Ling Foo played on tropes of oriental mysticism, but he also challenged the indolent, feminized vision of Asia in the era.[21] The North African performers from Hoffmann's Ballets Russes–style dance now had their own spot on the bill as well, performing their acrobatic routine. They were "especially imported," according to the program, by manager Hassan Ben Ali.[22] Susan Nance discusses how Arab acrobats in this period were understood as representatives of American ideas about "success and self-improvement."[23] A later interview with Hoffmann confirmed that she shared the same perspective: "I find them much easier than Americans," she said, and "they are willing to learn; they don't 'know it all,' and I can make them do what I want."[24]

How did the experience of traveling and performing with these acts shape Hoffmann's dance practice? Maybe working with actual Moroccan and Algerian performers grounded her orientalist fantasias a bit more in reality. There are few artifacts of what Priya Srinivasan calls "kinesthetic contact" with the performers on this tour.[25] Gertrude Hoffmann eagerly absorbed whatever new performance style she encountered, though, so they doubtless left some trace. Like her Chinese and North African costars Hoffmann imitated and synthesized, even at moments when the work claimed to be most culturally authentic. She insisted, for instance, that "Zobeide's Dream" was performed "in the Russian manner," and yet included in this dance "at least one turn which never saw the snows of St. Petersburg," in which two groups of dancers circle in opposite directions. One characteristic of Hoffmann's dance direction is its integration of avant-garde movement with the choreography of the chorus line. Hoffmann's hybrid dance style showed that she could move between cultural spheres.

Variety theater offered a place where audience members saw the effects of immigration in action, not only in the stereotypical ethnic humor of the period, but in the ways that different ethnic groups share the stage.[26] In this era some types of foreign performance were seen as glamorous and exotic but others were perceived as threatening. Many factors came into play: the region of the country, the class of theater, the interaction between performers of different backgrounds. One review from this tour gives a sense of how some audiences were threatened by her multiracial cast. Her *New Revue* played a three-night stand in New Orleans on December 7, 8, and 9, 1913.[27] After viewing the first night of her show, a critic felt the need to intercede on behalf of white supremacy:

> Let us pause a moment for a word as to Gertrude Hoffmann and the management of her production. In the beginning, with a desire to assist rather than to knock: This is the South. The average Southerner has certain convictions and sentiments along racial lines. In making use of the Arab troupe in the strenuous scene, "Zobeide's Dream," along with the white girls, and in placing Arabs opposite white girls in a love song and dance the management doubtless did not look at it as did many who were in Sunday night's audience.[28]

The aside in this review shocks for a few reasons. The author suggests that Yankees such as Hoffmann and her management might not be familiar with the "convictions and sentiments" of the "average Southerner." (This although Hoffmann performed in the South for more than a decade, starting with her stock company experience on the Wells circuit.) The audience members did not suspend their disbelief and watch "Zobeide's Dream" as a dance taking place in an abstract harem. Instead, they saw brown-skinned performers dancing with white women. Some audience members may have missed the program note and assumed they were African Americans; others read the note and were still offended. Their pairing in a "love song and dance" suggested miscegenation and thus should be cut. He goes so far as to say later in the review that the Arab performers should be removed from the bill. The Arab acrobats kept their place in the revue through 1915, though, and many of them continued to perform with Hoffmann's troupe in her next project.

White southerners were reeling from the trial of Leo Frank, a Jewish factory superintendent convicted of murdering a thirteen-year–old employee Mary Phagan. Frank was awaiting an appeal of his case at the time this review was written; his sentence was commuted in 1915, and he was subsequently lynched.[29] The defense of white womanhood from swarthy men is a major issue in D. W. Griffith's *Birth of a Nation* (1915). It also occupies a central place in the ideology of the Ku Klux Klan. This review makes explicit many of the tacit assumptions that enabled the Klan's resurgence in the late 1910s and early 1920s.[30]

By February 1914, Hoffmann had parted ways with Ching Ling Foo. "The show made money when starting south after the union of the two features," said a *Variety* article, "but has barely broke even since coming back and playing week stands." [31] Both parties would make more money as vaudeville acts on preestablished circuits. Hoffmann also ended a longer partnership: she did not renew her contract with Morris Gest. Gest insisted that their parting was motivated by money. His complaints seem unfounded, though, since they appear in a story about Hoffmann selling out Chicago vaudeville shows.

Hoffmann regained a certain level of artistic freedom. She made sure that her audiences knew who they should credit for the eleven-scene revue: one program features the headline, "'GERTRUDE HOFFMANN in GERTRUDE HOFFMANN'S REVUE, Originated and Staged by Gertrude Hoffmann."[32] A critic remarked that her performance "is not a vaudeville act—it is a production."[33] She was the closest female competitor to a George M. Cohan (who wrote the book and songs for the shows in which he starred), or a Florenz Ziegfeld. In some ways her act resembles the *Ziegfeld Follies*, where African American, Irish, and Jewish performers spiced up the visual spectacle of modern white womanhood.[34] But Hoffmann's performance embodied both glamour and comedy. She imitated ethnic comedy and sang dialect songs, but she could also look as elegant as a Ziegfeld girl. Perhaps her act was meant to illustrate how a white woman performer could incorporate—or at least briefly embody—all different types of identity and performance.

Gertrude Hoffmann was popular and well paid. She signed a $105,000 contract for thirty weeks of touring, or $3,500 a week, though it should be noted that her salary paid her large supporting cast as well. [35] Hoffmann established herself as a headliner at the height of vaudeville's popularity.[36] She was a reliable show-woman whose act brought in crowds from coast to coast. She regularly played the Palace Theatre, the pinnacle of New York vaudeville success.[37] "What is Miss Gertrude Hoffmann to do?" a newspaper review asked. "Where is she to turn for new worlds to conquer?"[38] She returned to her favorite source, avant-garde European performance. But times changed, and she could no longer easily return to Europe to see a show firsthand. Max Hoffmann's citizenship application was approved by the Brooklyn Supreme Court on July 23, 1914. Less than a week later, Austria-Hungary declared war on Serbia. The Great War in Europe had begun.

Part IV

✦

New Directions, 1914–1923

Chapter 11

✦

Grecian Dance, Pantomime, and Silent Film

Gertrude Hoffmann still had "a hankering for the legitimate," so she set her sights on an old desire: marrying commercial success with artistic acclaim.[1] Hoffmann cultivated her reputation as a performer and producer. She sought another respected European production as a vehicle for her talents. She even pursued opportunities to break into the movies. The timing made sense. Since the turn of the twentieth century, vaudeville bookers had attempted to use certain kinds of female performers' acts as a way of elevating the audience's taste.[2] Hoffmann always mixed refined acts—her "Spring Song" and "Blue Danube" dances in particular—with more lowbrow comedy. By the mid-1910s, the attitude toward this "uplifting" culture had changed. American mass media covered the news from elite cultural circles. The coverage of the Armory Show in the American press meant that even everyday newspaper readers were familiar with the innovations in modern art.[3] Gertrude Stein became a popular celebrity, even when her writing was mocked.[4] Smart magazines began to engage in "art-and-commodity-blurring publishing practices" where advertisements looked like art and actual art was used to sell things.[5] Even if they did not understand its aesthetic aims, popular audiences understood the cultural capital associated with high culture. And Gertrude Hoffmann understood popular audiences.

First, she put forth a new image inspired by Isadora Duncan. Frank C. Bangs, her Salome photographer, took a new series of Hoffmann shots in 1913 and 1914. Some photos showed her posed in long grass with her hair up and one arm raised, looking like an ancient Greek statue. More active images showed Hoffmann with her hair loose, dancing in the tide. She is not as scantily clad as in her Salome photographs: in figure 11.1, her toga-like draperies cover her chest, and her bare feet are hidden by the water. The wet draperies do cling to her lower body, and her bare legs are exposed from knee to thigh. Where her Salome image was decadent and artificial, the new one tried to achieve a natural expressiveness.

Her long-standing love of the ocean was born in her San Francisco childhood and nurtured in this era when Gertrude, Max Sr., and Max Jr. lived in the Sea Gate neighborhood of Brooklyn, a gated community west of Coney

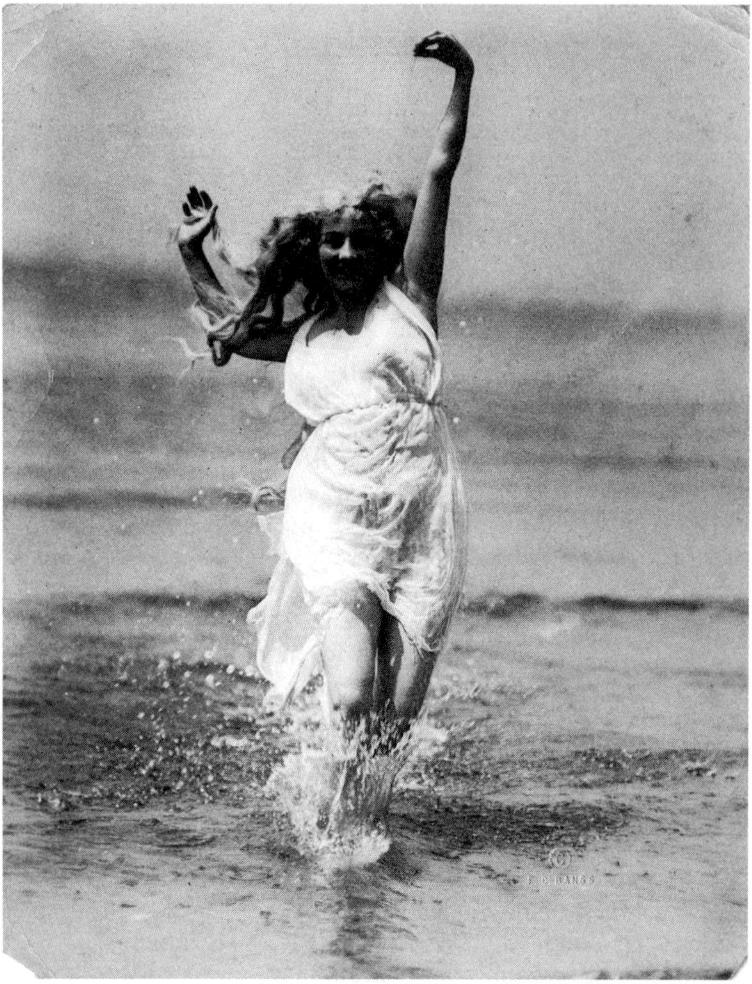

FIGURE 11.1. Gertrude Hoffmann in the water near her home in Sea Gate, Brooklyn, circa 1913. Photograph by Frank C. Bangs. Max and Gertrude Hoffmann Photograph Collection, Special Collections and University Archives, Wake Forest University, Winston-Salem, N.C.

Island on a peninsula that juts out into Gravesend Bay. This new image drew on modern dance and physical culture, in which a Hellenistic aesthetic prevailed. Isadora Duncan felt that Greek dance and sculpture epitomized the ideal of art in harmony with the natural world.[6] Grecian dress and imagery pervaded women's popular demonstrations in the 1910s, from historical pageants to suffrage protests.[7] All this work was inspired in part by the system of posing and emotional expression theorized by François Delsarte.[8]

These Grecian-style photos first appeared in an article about Hoffmann's exercise routine, "The Well-Watered Woman," written by Hoffmann herself.[9] This article was syndicated in American newspapers in 1913, serving as publicity for her Three-Star Tour. This means it was pitched by Morris Gest or Hoffmann's press agent Abe Levy.[10] She discusses her exercise and beauty routine: when she cannot run on the beach as in the pictures, she jogs in place in her bathtub with the shower spraying her "at full force."[11] (She notes that readers should place a rubber mat or towel in the bottom of the tub to prevent slipping.) She shot more beach photos with Frank C. Bangs, posing in the rigging of a shipwreck near the Sandy Hook peninsula in New Jersey. These were first published in the July 1914 issue of *Vanity Fair*, as illustrations to another Hoffmann-penned article.

Frank Crowninshield took over the editorial reins at the magazine in 1914.[12] Crowninshield, an enthusiastic supporter of modernism, collected modern paintings and served as the publicist for the Armory Show.[13] He championed modernism in *Vanity Fair* too, though within a broader cultural context. He told the publisher Condé Nast that the magazine should, in effect, provide information about the things people talk about at cocktail parties. This included art, theater, and literature, but also humor, sports, and celebrity gossip.[14] *Vanity Fair* appealed to moneyed elites from urban centers; as its influence spread, its audience encompassed not only people who already belonged to that group but also those who aspired to belong.[15] Gertrude Hoffmann appeared regularly in the pages of *Vanity Fair* over the next decade. She added visual interest to their layouts with her portraits—often gracing a full page—in exotic costumes.

Hoffmann helped the magazine communicate this message of sophistication in her 1914 essay, "Dancing, and the Magic of the Sea: The Ocean as an Inspiration and a Background for Outdoor Dancing."[16] The topic is the same as in the "Well-Watered Woman," but the approach is more upscale. Where the newspaper article describes her exercise routine to housewives and working women, the *Vanity Fair* article shares her artistic motivations with fellow lovers of nature and culture. She showed her readers how to appreciate one part of the natural environment—the ocean—in an educated way that involves the body as well as the mind. The essay begins with an epigraph from an Algernon Charles Swinburne poem.[17] Hoffmann revels in the beauty of Swinburne's language and then suggests that they would have been friends because of their shared love for the ocean. Her notorious nudity is here recast in wholesome terms: her swimsuit is "scanty as possible," as readers might expect, but this is merely because she loves "the smooth, salt feel of the ocean." Her description of swimming naked "until she is weary" and feeling the salt water as a "tonic" align her less with stage burlesque and more with the athleticism of the physical culture movement.

Hoffmann's tone is less than convincing. She writes, "The Greeks loved the sea and they loved dancing, and they were, as everyone knows, the most perfectly civilized people who ever lived."[18] Both "as everyone knows" and "perfectly civilized" seem more like Dorothy Parker jokes, cracks in the facade of a worldly woman's voice. This is the Hellenic ideal as secondhand gossip. She concludes the essay by noting that she saw "through her field glasses" a shipwreck three miles offshore. "I thought it would make a wonderful setting for a picture," she writes, "a far more beautiful scene than I could ever secure on the stage, so we sailed out there one afternoon and—here are the pictures."[19] The photos taken by Frank C. Bangs were obviously a collaboration and not the singular artistic vision she makes them out to be, but no matter—the stage manager has returned.

One photo from the Grecian series was mislabeled in a telling way, giving Hoffmann's tour a newsy hook by connecting it to the Great War raging in Europe. Hoffmann poses in long grass; she wears her Grecian draperies and holds her arms in a ballet style, with the right arm curved over her head and the left extended to her side. The photo is titled "Dancing on the Sand Dunes," and the caption below it claims that she is "lightly tripping an impromptu fantasy over the sand dunes of West Flanders, which are now being rudely plowed up by competing projectiles from hostile big caliber guns."[20] (Elsewhere, the photo was labeled "Gertrude Hoffmann in One of Her Graceful Dances.")[21] Germany began its occupation of Belgium in August 1914, and British troops shelled the Flanders coast through the early months of 1915. Perhaps Hoffmann's toga and delicate beauty communicated something of the editor's sentiments regarding "brave little Belgium." The dunes were not Flemish, though; they were part of either the Brooklyn or New Jersey shore.

The United States would remain neutral for several years to come, but American vaudeville performers were already shunning European tours because they feared submarines might attack the ship on their journey.[22] The London booking agent George Foster placed a full-page ad in *Variety* noting that "nothing could be more ridiculous than this attitude on the part of the Americans. The ocean is absolutely as safe as it ever was and there never was a time when American novelties were in so great demand as at this moment."[23] Foster's timing could not have been much worse. *Variety* published the ad on April 16, 1915; three weeks later, the *Lusitania* ocean liner was torpedoed by a German U-boat and sank. One night when Hoffmann was performing at the Palace, an audience member threatened her: "If you mention Gaby Deslys's name again you'll suffer the fate of the Lusitania. I won't let any one with a name like Hoffmann take Gaby's name in vain."[24] (It's unclear whether this confused outburst was anti-German or anti-Semitic.) Booking agents continued to recruit American vaudevillians throughout the war, to little effect.

Hoffmann finished her season at the Palace and took the usual summer break. When she launched her newest show in August 1915, it was a few miles down the shore from her home in Sea Gate. A *Brooklyn Eagle* reporter attended rehearsals at the New Brighton Theatre in the Brighton Beach neighborhood. Because the costumes had not yet arrived for Hoffmann's "seaside attraction," he noted, the actors and stagehands were all dressed in informal "beach garb": bathing suits for the women, rolled-up trousers and shirtsleeves for the men.[25] Sketches next to the article showed a woman with her hair tied back in a bandana and a "man with loose hands, feet and a shaggy head."[26] The gender ambiguity connects Hoffmann's cast to the bohemian figures of Greenwich Village, and these rehearsals take place the same summer that the Provincetown Players presented their first works in an oceanside setting.[27] Provincetown was establishing itself as an artist's colony at this time, but Brighton Beach was a beach neighborhood with a boardwalk, rides, and carnival attractions. Here Hoffmann ran her out-of-town tryout of *Sumurun*, the Max Reinhardt pantomime that dazzled New York City's theatergoers in 1912.

With *Sumurun*, Hoffmann worked within some limits that had not been imposed on her earlier European projects. The war in Europe discouraged the kind of transatlantic travel to which she was accustomed. *Sumurun* borrowed from an earlier American tour and depended on reconstruction from memory. Once again Hoffmann showed her strengths as a producer, identifying important modern performances and adapting them to the norms of popular theater. The Reinhardt production was adapted to vaudeville's constraints of time and attention, most likely by Hoffmann herself. There are two versions of *Sumurun* in her papers, one a summary of its eight scenes and another a draft script trying out different phrasings for the narration of each scene.[28] By shortening the pantomime to the length of half a vaudeville bill, Hoffmann follows a pattern established in the small-time performance venues of the Midwest, known as "tabloid" or "tab" shows. These shows boiled down Broadway musical comedies to their bare essence. They kept the musical numbers, with just enough plot and dialogue to string them together.[29] Reinhardt's *Sumurun* was the ideal source for a tab show. It had pantomimed action, stylized sets, and glamorous costumes; each character was associated with an orchestral motif. Hoffmann's vaudeville adaptation shows just how close the original show was to a musical melodrama to begin with.

Many commentators in 1915 noted the logic of reviving *Sumurun* in an era when audiences were accustomed to the pantomime of silent film.[30] The evolution took place on screen and in the audience. A history of pantomime from 1916 argues that film actors have moved beyond conventional expressions and poses, and that they are beginning to develop a more realistic mode of acting for the camera.[31] At the same time, audiences have "learned to understand the meaning of gesture and expression."[32] In the mid-1910s theater critics and academics were still thinking about pantomime and silent film as parallel media forms with shared audiences. The skills learned in the movie theater could be transferred to the vaudeville house.[33]

Hoffmann collaborated on *Sumurun* with Richard Ordynski, the Polish protégé of Max Reinhardt who directed the initial touring production. He coached the cast through the pantomime, while Hoffmann served as the dance director. Ordynski and Hoffmann also performed in the pantomime. He played the old hunchback and she played the enslaved dancer he loves and sells away, known in the program as the "Beautiful Slave of Fatal Enchantment." Ordynski initially worried that Hoffmann would ask him to compromise his vision, but he found their working relationship to be a good one.[34] Like Theodore Kosloff before him, Richard Ordynski engaged in a symbiotic relationship with Gertrude Hoffmann: her popularity boosted him, while his European avant-garde credentials legitimized her.

Putting on a costume of foreignness, whether through beads and veils or makeup, gave white women in vaudeville the license to be openly seductive. In *Sumurun*, Hoffmann enacted that performance through another example of racial masquerade. Earlier acts featured brief imitations in blackface. She took the practice further this time, performing the Beautiful Slave of Fatal Enchantment in full-body brown makeup, as seen in figure 11.2. Her brownface aligns her with the dancer Ruth St. Denis, who painted her arms, legs, and face at the beginning of early concert performances of Indian dance.[35] It also situates her in the vaudeville tradition of white women's acts of minstrelsy, which allowed them to take on a "childlike wildness" not otherwise granted onstage.[36] The onstage substitution is similar to that of the "Dance of the Seven Veils," in which a white woman takes on the role of a racialized other in order to gain more sexual freedom in her onstage performance than might otherwise be allowed.[37]

When the show opened, Hoffmann claimed that she was following the example of the original Reinhardt troupe's actress who dyed herself "in a solution of liquefied copper." "This was possible," Hoffmann said, "because a celebrated scientist at Mannheim had invented a solvent" to remove the dye from her skin.[38] Because the war impacted shipping from Europe to America, she ran out of solvent and remained, "even in private life, of a color somewhere between a Patagonian and an aboriginal Persian."[39] Without the scientific innovations from Europe, Hoffmann cannot take her racialized costume on and off as easily as she would like. She is forced to remain in a not-quite-white condition. This story was in some ways typical publicity: the link to the war makes it timely, and the topic is suggestive without being tawdry. It also tells us something important about Hoffmann's thought process when she engages in the primitivism and minstrelsy so central to modern performance. She performed in blackface when she imitated Eddie Leonard's songs and Bert Williams's poker routine. Though Leonard was white and Williams black, both were blackface comedians: she did their acts, imitating an imitation. She distanced herself from the orientalist performances of Salome, the Ballets Russes, and Max Reinhardt as well. The story about her copper dye stands out because it made her borrowing explicit, but it also acknowledged the ways it marked her physically. Her stereotypical "eastern" roles came secondhand from European sources, but they nevertheless left traces on her body.

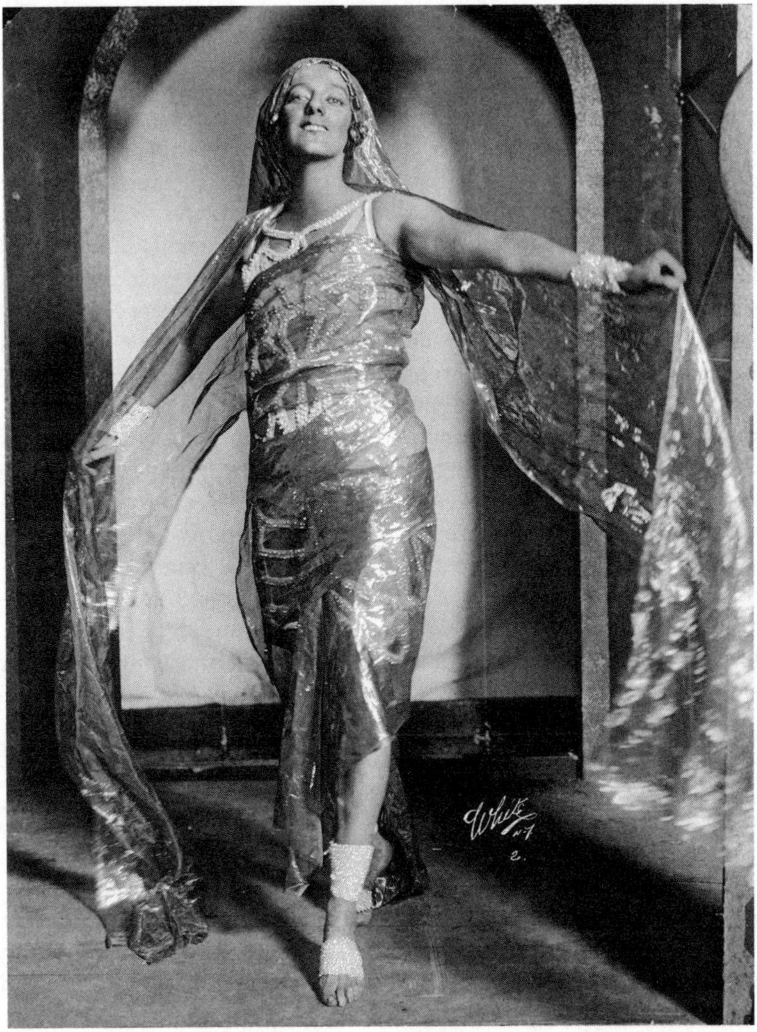

FIGURE 11.2. Gertrude Hoffmann as the Beautiful Slave of Fatal Enchantment in *Sumurun*. White Studio / Museum of the City of New York. 52.248.38 © the New York Public Library.

The *Sumurun* pantomime tells another *Arabian Nights*–inspired story of sex and death. The setting was evoked with stylized silhouettes and plain white turrets. The story begins in a marketplace where a slave dealer's shop and "little theatre" stand near the stall of the carpet merchant Nur-al-Din.[40] Members of the royal family circulate through the bazaar. The Sheik's son falls in love with the Beautiful Slave of Fatal Enchantment; Sumurun the

Sheik's favorite wife does the same with Nur-al-din. The Sheik enters the bazaar, sends Sumurun back to the palace, and buys the slave from the Hunchback for himself. The Hunchback "tries to kill himself for love of her" according to the scenario, "but the poison sticks in his throat and he only falls insensible."[41] Both the Hunchback and the eager lover Nur-al-Din are smuggled into the palace, where they sneak into the harem. The Beautiful Slave dances for the Sheik, who then rests beside her. The Sheik's son wakes the dancer, and they embrace; the Old Sheik discovers them and stabs his son. The jealous Hunchback kills the Beautiful Slave of Fatal Enchantment. While this takes place, Sumurun and Nur-al-Din are making love in the harem. The Sheik discovers Nur-al-Din and tries to kill him too. The Hunchback kills the Old Sheik before he can destroy another couple's happiness. "All the wicked die," the scenario concludes, "and the good walk over the Flowery Path to happiness."[42]

The "flowery path" was a runway: "Flowery path" is the literal translation of *hanamichi*, the Kabuki theater's runway that Reinhardt borrowed for his production. A runway now called to mind both the Reinhardt show and the many Shubert productions with parades of chorus girls. Columnists joked about its effectiveness as a theatrical device. At the Brighton Theatre, cast members who tried to enter by the runway were locked outside the theater in an alley, and at the Palace, where the pantomime appeared last on the vaudeville bill, the "harem ladies" and "eunnuchs" [*sic*] collided with audience members leaving for the night.[43] While a runway might be an evocative way to bring the actors close to the audience, it lacked practicality.

Sumurun opened to mixed reviews. The *Brooklyn Eagle* called it "magnificent" and said that Hoffmann had "come into her own" as an artist.[44] The *New York Tribune* drama critic Heywood Broun called it "one of the best things that has been done in vaudeville."[45] Ordynski was universally lauded for his miming abilities, while Hoffmann was praised by some critics and panned by others. *Variety* critics were dubious about a vaudeville *Sumurun*, finding it neither artistic enough to be legitimate theater nor entertaining enough to be vaudeville. Sime Silverman, the magazine's founder, deemed the Brighton Theatre production "not a wise choice for vaudeville, for vaudeville will not appreciate it even if it wants it."[46] When the show moved to the Palace, another review called it "semi-sensational, but not entertaining."[47] Mass audiences may have learned to appreciate pantomime from watching the movies, but critics were unsure about their reaction to the genuine article, or even a "vaudeville reproduction."[48] It is unclear whether this was true because the pantomime was ineffective or because they were still unwilling to see Hoffmann as an entertainer who could engage in serious mimicry.

A few weeks into the show's run at the Palace, Hoffmann upped the entertainment factor. She added a bathing scene in which several harem ladies swam in an onstage tank of "warmed and perfumed water."[49] The tank included a central fountain, akin to Esther Williams's aqua-ballet sets. Hoffmann added the scene in the third week, when her act moved from the headliner's spot to the less prestigious first-act closer. This addition ensured that the act felt fresh for audience members coming to see Fanny Brice and Eddie Leonard, the new headliners. The change bothered Frederick James Smith, the editor of the Vaudeville section of the *New York Daily Mirror*. He wrote, "Gertrude Hoffmann has, we fear, Flo Ziegfeld-ized the 'Sumurun' of Max Reinhardt. . . . The wordless drama is an appeal to the imagination, but there's nothing mental about a chorus girl in a one-piece bathing suit."[50] Critiques of Hoffmann often centered on her taking "mental" experiences of high art—the Russian ballet, the German pantomime—and reminding the audiences that those acts depended on women's bodies. When Ada Rubinstein was unwrapped at the beginning of Fokine's *Cleopatre*, audiences were thrilled. When Gertrude Hoffmann played the same role, her unwrapping was uncomfortably close to striptease. The same was true of *Sumurun*: Hoffmann's adaptations reminded reviewers invested in European high art that these performances—with their vivid colors, gorgeous costumes, and spectacular action—were most analogous to Broadway revues. The second scene of the pantomime, in which a snake charmer and puppet act precede the slave girl's dancing in the Hunchback's "little theater," also draws attention to the popular performance elements of the play.

Hoffmann's bathing scene created an intertextual spectacle, one that reminded audiences of the oriental drama *Kismet* (with similar swimming maidens), as well as the Australian swimmer Annette Kellerman (who performed in the same tank). In the matinee performance when the bathing scene debuted, Hoffmann even reenacted a scene from another revue—perhaps accidentally. While performing a "seductive dance," she fell into the pool; she was helped out of the water by the Sheik, but the wet stage caused her fellow dancers to skid into the footlights, "to the accompaniment of an uproarious response from the other side" (that is, the audience).[51] Hoffmann's accidental fall echoes a scene from *The Passing Show of 1912*. In that revue, the portly Trixie Friganza parodied Hoffmann's "Spring Song" dance and stumbled backward into a bathing pool "in the harem of the Sewerman."[52] Because her mistake so closely imitated the Friganza routine and took place when Hoffmann's act moved down the bill, it may have been an intentional way to ensure continued publicity.

The brief interpolation allowed Hoffmann to stay on the Palace bill for another week; *Sumurun* played around New York City for a few more weeks without the bathing scene. In November, the large *Sumurun* company went on the road. Advance publicity in California reported that she was touring with "sixty artists," though that number probably included musicians as well as cast members.[53] They made stops in the eastern venues of the Keith–Albee circuit through the fall, and the midwest and western venues of the Orpheum circuit through the winter and early spring.[54] *Sumurun* was a financial success on the road, though critics continued to be unsure about how audiences would react. The *Christian Science Monitor* claimed it was a "test of vaudeville patron's favor," and *Variety*'s Chicago correspondent noted that audience members laughed at the show in one local venue and maintained a respectful silence in another.[55] The company stayed in California for more than two months, playing San Francisco and Los Angeles.

The long California stint signaled Hoffmann's goal for her post-*Sumurun* career: she wanted to make the jump from vaudeville to film. Before *Sumurun* opened, she hinted that she might hire movie actors and actresses for pantomime parts, "believing their training in gesture and expression may be put to good advantage."[56] She cast Kenneth D. Harlan, "a former Biograph Company player" who had worked with D. W. Griffith, as the Sheik's son.[57] When the tour visited Boston, she told a reporter that she was interested in producing her version of *Sumurun* for the motion pictures.[58] One newspaper columnist stated that Hoffmann was planning to film her production of *Sumurun*, but this seems not to have come about.[59]

Sumurun opened at the Orpheum Theatre in Los Angeles on March 20, 1916. The show ran for two weeks; gossip circulated about Hoffmann and her harem girls making the rounds of the movie studios.[60] Perhaps she sought a film contract at Universal Pictures: while Hoffmann was in Los Angeles, she wanted to screen a film of the studio's called *The Dumb Girl of Portici*, which starred Anna Pavlova and was directed by Lois Weber.[61] As a famed dancer who moved into filmed pantomime, Pavlova provided a direct model for Hoffmann. So did Weber, a former stage actress who wrote, directed, and sometimes starred in her own films.[62]

Another candidate for Hoffmann's attention was D. W. Griffith. Griffith was fascinated by the artistic potential that stage pantomime and motion pictures shared.[63] Though its racial politics are reprehensible, *Birth of a Nation* (1915) is often mentioned as the first feature-length film to shift moviegoing patterns away from melodramatic or jokey one-reelers to extended, complex narratives.[64] Hoffmann had several connections to Griffith. While the cast was in Los Angeles they visited the set of a Douglas Fairbanks film at Fine Arts Studio, Griffith's studio on Sunset Boulevard.[65] Griffith had attended previous Hoffmann performances in Los Angeles and recruited two of Hoffmann's dancers, Blanche Sweet and Gertrude Bambrick.[66] Bambrick worked as a dancer and choreographer in his films, and Sweet rose to fame as an actress.[67] The theater and film scholar David Mayer suggests that Hoffmann influenced Griffith in important though indirect ways through her training of these two dancers.[68] Ruth St. Denis and Ted Shawn had a more direct influence, training the actors and dancers who worked in Griffith movies, as well as choreographing and performing in the Babylonian dance sequence in Griffith's epic *Intolerance* (1916).[69] Griffith and Hoffmann both attended a benefit for the Actor's Fund of America, but this seems to have been the extent of their contact.[70]

Sumurun ran in Los Angeles through early April. Then the tour headed back east, playing the Palace again in May 1916. A report appeared in the press that

Hoffmann had "signed a contract for a long period and an exceedingly large salary" with Lewis J. Selznick's production company.[71] That report did not pan out.

While Gertrude Hoffmann failed to gain a foothold in Hollywood, her influence reverberated throughout New York City and spread through further coverage in *Vanity Fair*. Along with Ruth St. Denis and Isadora Duncan, Hoffmann brought about a rage for barefoot dancing.[72] The illustrator Dorothy Ferriss sketched languid figures posing in arabesque and skipping with scarves draped around them. The tongue-in-cheek feature claimed in its subtitle that Grecian-style art dance was "Now Wrecking Cabaret Life, Studio Life, Music Hall Life, and Even Married Life."[73] If you were a sophisticated New Yorker, you could not go anywhere "without having a bevy of beautiful barefoot dancers come rushing at you, waving their gossamer veils, 'playing dead' on the floor, leaping after toy balloons, clashing cymbals, flinging their hair about, stamping on the ground, hurling property rosebuds at your head and otherwise behaving like ladies in a madhouse." Hoffmann and her fellow barefoot dancers inspired amateurs to engage in ridiculous behavior. This form of dance is at once too natural and too artificial, with animalistic and childlike imagery alongside the cacophony and props of bad theater.

The sophisticated public was losing interest in this style of dance. Hoffmann plotted her next move. Her new act, *Variety* reported in August 1916, would be Hawaiian.[74] The hula dancer Doraldina became a well-known figure in New York vaudeville circles, and Hoffmann sought to capitalize on that trend. As soon as these plans were announced, they fell apart.[75] The Hawaiian act was supposed to star Guarany Schriff (also spelled "Shiff" and "Shriff"), who played Sumurun's maid to substantial acclaim on tour. Hoffmann promised to place Schriff within the year in a $50 a week position for thirty weeks.[76] The Hawaiian act "didn't take."[77] Their relationship broke down, and Schriff sued Hoffmann for breach of contract.

A passport application from late November 1916 suggests that Gertrude Hoffmann planned to travel to London in December and perform the following year.[78] The contract was about eight years old, since it was signed when Hoffmann visited London to copy Maud Allan's Salome dance.[79] Though the passport application lists the departure date and ocean liner for her planned voyage, the trip seems not to have taken place. At the very least, the performances did not. Reasons for canceling this trip are unclear, but it is likely that they have to do with the ongoing war in Europe. H. B. Marinelli was well known as a manager of international vaudeville talent: his firm brought the Scottish comic Harry Lauder to the United States, and he was just as adept at booking American acts abroad.[80] According to Marinelli's obituary, the Great War "wrecked" his system of booking acts, "and it never recovered."[81] Hoffmann took the war effort as a point of inspiration for her revues, putting on patriotic dance numbers and holding charity drives. But it is fair to say that Hoffmann's transatlantic borrowing process never recovered either. *Sumurun* was her last European imitation.

Chapter 12

✦

Snake Acts and Other Wartime Spectacles

The fall vaudeville season began without any performances from Gertrude Hoffmann. She and Max went back to work for Florenz Ziegfeld: he served as music director for *The Century Girl*, which premiered on the main stage of the Century Theatre, and she staged a dance for the autumn roof garden show *The Midnight Frolic* that harked back to the "bell number" in Anna Held's *A Parisian Model.*[1] Eventually, she found a place in Ziegfeld's *Dance and Grow Thin*, which opened in January 1917. The show ran in the Cocoanut Grove Theatre, on the roof of the Century Theatre at Sixty-Second Street and Central Park West. The cabaret-style venue was reminiscent of the roof gardens of Hoffmann's earlier days. *Vanity Fair* notes that the club "has sprouted on the roof of the Century Theatre through the skillful horticultural efforts of those two notable gentleman-farmers, F. Ziegfeld Jr., of Chicago, and C. B. Dillingham, of Hartford."[2] Transplants they may have been, but Dillingham and Ziegfeld defined New York nightlife. They co-owned the Century and coproduced the upstairs show, which shared its DNA with Ziegfeld's *Midnight Frolic.* The show began at midnight and ran until nearly 2:00 A.M. Food was served during the intermission by Reisenweber's Cafe, whose Columbus Circle location was popular with theater types.[3] *Dance and Grow Thin* included mainstays of revues in the period, such as two-man comedy sketches, love duets, and songs in which white men praise the American South.[4] Perhaps the best-known act from this show is "Letter Boxes (Just Placed in New York)." Chorus girls wore mailbox costumes, and patrons at the front tables were given paper and pencil so they could slip a note to the girl of their choice. The chorus girl's proximity—circulating among the tables, and even sitting on customers' laps—was one of the main draws of the cabaret.[5]

Hoffmann took advantage of the intimate setting when staging her group numbers. During the "Blue Danube" dance, according to *Variety*, her "choristers mingled" in the audience.[6] Her "best and rawest effort" featured Hoffmann and four other girls undressing on trapezes.[7] A reviewer was disappointed, though, that the girls did not toss their clothes into the audience as the strongwoman Charmion had done a decade before.[8]

This new program shows a shift in Hoffmann's style. Although she still included modern dance influences, they are mitigated by performances that belong on the midway. Hoffmann began her Cocoanut Grove act with her longtime partner Enrico Muris. Unlike Vernon and Irene Castle's cool and upright version of the dance, Hoffmann and Muris danced a passionate tango.[9] Then she presented solo imitations: first Ruth St. Denis, then belly dancer Princess Rajah. Rajah was another performer who borrowed orientalist tropes; unlike the Salome dancers, she performed her act while fully clothed. An Edison kinetoscope from 1904 shows her doing a lively shimmying, hip-shaking dance and balancing a chair in her teeth.[10] For her interpretation of the death of Cleopatra, Princess Rajah partnered with a live snake.[11] So Hoffmann brought a snake into her act as well.

The snake, named "Black Baby," figures prominently in Hoffmann's journals from the era. She entered Ziegfeld's office full of "excitement and enthusiasm," to ask "guess what I have?" When she showed him the snake, he "nearly fell over with fright" and "yelled at [her] to get out with it quick."[12] She rehearsed with the snake in the Hoffmanns' pied-à-terre on West Fifty-Ninth Street. A few visitors watched her, including her older sister Margaret Hay and the Ziegfeld girl Marion Watson. The snake got loose and frightened them all; Max recaptured it while dressed in a nightshirt. On opening night, Hoffmann writes that Black Baby "got away from" her and slithered down the center aisle. The Vanderbilts sat at a nearby table, and they screamed.[13]

A snake was a prop of diva identity, one of the ways that oriental imagery helped vaudevillians and dramatic actresses claim a more complex and exotic performance style. Drama critic Archie Bell pinpointed this strategy in an otherwise complimentary article about Hoffmann titled "Can't Be Real 'Oriental,' You Know—on the Stage—Without Your 'Sarpints.'"[14] Dancers used snakes in much the same way that Salome acts worked a decade before, as part of their stereotypical evocation of generalized Middle Eastern culture, one filtered through World's Fair and dime museum performances. The snake substituted for the striptease as a signifier of exotic otherness.

Hoffmann may have been trying new things in her Cocoanut Grove act, but she did not stay in the show for long. Evidence suggests that she disliked this cabaret environment. Every night, she wrote, Ziegfeld and William Randolph Hearst sat at the center table. The Hearst columnist C. F. Zittel (known as "Zit") requested that Hoffmann visit the newspaper mogul.[15] As was her usual strategy when dealing with lascivious men, she brought Max with her. She preferred to maintain a distance between herself and her audience. *Vanity Fair* reports that Hoffmann "had to withdraw from that fascinating spot because, in such close and intimate relation with her audience, it frequently happened, early in the morning, that a guest thought the snake was his, and tried to kill him."[16] A patron might mistake a snake for his own if he had been drinking heavily; before drunks saw pink elephants, they saw snakes in their boots.[17] She was used to performing in front of tired businessmen, not inebriated ones.

The division between audience and performer was more clearly marked in vaudeville. Hoffmann also had more creative control with her own vaudeville act than she did in a cabaret show produced by someone else. She finally left *Dance and Grow Thin* because of a dispute about the lighting for her act: the management wanted to use blue lights during her "Blue Danube Waltz"; Hoffmann, less literal and more artistic, asked for amber lights and was denied.[18] She quit the show.

This early departure began a rough period. Hoffmann's dance partner, Enrico Muris, died of pneumonia. Muris was Italian, though he had reportedly come to New York by way of South America "with the first splash of the tango dancing craze." The Hoffmanns paid for his gravestone and funeral.[19]

Hoffmann threw together a vaudeville act that debuted in Brooklyn. She had lost a skillful and seasoned dance partner, someone who added a level of professionalism to her show. She received among the worst reviews of her career. *New York Clipper* critics said that the first performance looked more like a dress rehearsal than a big-time vaudeville act.[20] "To say the best for the newest Gertrude Hoffmann act," the *Variety* review begins, "is that she presented an unprepared production."[21] This was the most charitable comment. Silverman savaged the act as badly cast and rehearsed: the six girls performing on trapezes "made a thorough botch of the bit," and nearly half her cast was made up of "chorus girls, without singing or dancing ability."[22] Hoffmann liked to hire inexperienced chorus girls because of their freshness as performers, but this group seemed especially green.

Problems extended to Hoffmann herself. When she closed her act by taking requests for imitations, audience members called out "Milo"—presumably for the Venus de Milo—and "September Morn," for the Paul Émile Chabas painting that depicts a nude young woman standing in a lake. These were not imitations in Hoffmann's repertoire: they were roundabout ways of shouting "Take it off!" Critical dismissal may not have mattered if she was giving the audience what they wanted, but the audience "laughed loudly at the sallies" from these hecklers, suggesting that they too wanted a more titillating show.[23]

The newest addition to *Gertrude Hoffmann's Revue of 1917* was a striking spectacle called "Song of Nations." This was less a musical number than an international fashion show. Chorus members wearing the native costumes of different countries paraded down a black velvet-lined staircase.[24] They sang as they walked down the stairs, but according to Sime Silverman in *Variety*, their voices were too weak to reach the first balcony.[25] As the Great War raged, even fashion shows were politicized; "Song of Nations" shared nationalist costumes and fiery red light with Ziegfeld's recent *Midnight Frolic* number called "The Melting Pot."[26] The backdrop for "Song of Nations" was said to be "the largest flag in vaudeville."[27]

"Song of Nations" epitomized the fashion for nationalism in U.S. popular theater. The actress Hazel Dawn appeared on the cover of the January 1917 issue of *Theatre* magazine dressed as Columbia, the female personification of the spirit of America.[28] Dawn played the lead in *The Century Girl*, the show Max Hoffmann was conducting downstairs from the Cocoanut Grove. That show also included two patriotic songs: "When Uncle Sam Rules the Waves" and "Uncle Sam's Children." The former was an "undersea extravaganza," similar to the pantomime spectacles Hoffmann had danced in as a girl.[29] The latter was an imperialist number with actresses dressed as American territories: Alaska, Hawaii, the Philippines, and "Porto Rico."[30] The show also featured a Ned Wayburn–staged precision dance routine in which chorus girls marched, dressed as soldiers and sailors.[31] Popular entertainment in the lead-up to the U.S. declaration of war against Germany was patriotic and "increasingly militarized."[32] New York City vaudeville and musical comedy circa 1917 looked much like San Francisco theater at the time of the Spanish-American War.

The United States entered the Great War on April 6, 1917. Whereas President Wilson had declared the country "too proud to fight," he now felt that American participation was necessary so that the world could "be made safe for democracy."[33] Vaudeville performers contributed to the war by enlisting as soldiers or volunteering for relief efforts. The U.S. government encouraged Americans on the home front to economize.[34] Producers and performers tried to heed this call. The Selective Service Act was passed on May 18, 1917; theaters put on "chorus boy-less musicals" to account for the smaller pool of able-bodied men.[35] By 1918, theaters closed on Tuesday nights as part of a fuel conservation strategy.[36] The actress Blanche Ring "tabooed extravagance," learned how to knit, and canceled a tour so she could cook for her son while he was enlisted.[37] But this call to conserve resonated differently for acts like Hoffmann's, which were built on "flash" and extravagance.

Hoffmann's revues, like the fashion industry and the popular theater more broadly, depended on novelty and visual interest. These industries responded, as Marlis Schweitzer notes, by articulating "an even stronger link between consumption and patriotism."[38] Before the United States entered the Great War, women were told that they should forsake Paris fashions for clothes "Made in America."[39] Now that the nation joined the war effort, an essay in *Theatre* magazine titled "True Patriotism!" suggested that it was the obligation of American men and women to keep buying new clothes and attending cultural events in order to keep the economy strong.[40] A *Variety* review of Hoffmann's act at the Palace joked that the patriotism of vaudeville audiences would keep the "long-suffering tailors" and "upholsterers" in business, since those patrons stood whenever "the flag was shown" onstage or "something was played that even distantly resembled 'The Star Spangled Banner.'"[41] Apparently, patrons sometimes stood up when the "Song of Nations" began because the number featured "an American flag as big as the Palace proscenium."[42]

The beauty and glamor of the show was tied to the patriotism it evoked at a reflexive level.

Producers such as Florenz Ziegfeld and Gertrude Hoffmann reconciled the aesthetic pleasure of the revue format with the news from overseas. In her review of the *Ziegfeld Follies of 1918*, Dorothy Parker mused, "One sweetly solemn thought comes to me o'er and o'er, 'Can they ever produce a revue, when we get through with the war?' I brood over the thing practically without ceasing, but I can find no answer to it. I can see no future whatever for our musical entertainments once peace is declared."[43] Parker listed the clichés of wartime theater, from showgirls decked out in flags of the Allied powers to "property sandbags" used to represent the trenches.[44] As Parker describes it, "The audience staggers out of the New Amsterdam Theatre, all used up with patriotism, muscle-bound from applauding Dolores swathed in the stars and stripes, and Kay Laurell simply gowned in the French flag." During the Great War, fashionable women performed aesthetic and allegorical service. These women literally wrapped in a flag created a spectacle—as did the huge flag that Hoffmann flew from the proscenium—that allowed audience members to perform their citizenship in physical and emotional ways.

The chorus girls in Hoffmann's revue supported the war effort offstage as well. They participated in a recruitment campaign sponsored by the *New York American* newspaper. The press agent Walter Kingsley dressed them "to represent the Allies."[45] They seemed approachable in the same way as the young women of Howard Chandler Christy's illustrations. Christy's wartime recruitment poster shows a young woman dressed in a sailor's uniform; she hints, "Gee!! I wish I were a man. I'd join the Navy."[46] The Hoffmann girls may have been dressed as foreign countries, but their faces were recognizably young, attractive, and all-American.

After its run at the Palace in New York, *Gertrude Hoffmann's Revue of 1917* made its way west to Chicago. At least one critic there was unimpressed by the wartime aesthetic. Percy Hammond, a reviewer for the *Chicago Tribune*, said Hoffmann's show "cause[d] the American flag and the American anthem to be merchandised as the by-product of a gilded and voluptuous leg show."[47] An honest burlesque would be preferable, Hammond seems to suggest, compared to this commercial hybrid of nudity and nationalism.[48]

The revue played at Chicago's Majestic theater in late May, and its run was extended into June. After the show closed, Hoffmann made another appearance in the Chicago newspapers, endorsing a "malted food drink" called Askum.[49] The ad quotes "the most wonderful classic dancer of modern times": "I can't dance after a heavy meal. Askum supplies the necessary nourishment and satisfies my hunger."[50] Her signature is reproduced below the quote, with an oversized, looping G and extended Fs. An illustration of Hoffmann in a fringed dress and turban adjoins her testimonial, striking a vampish pose. Stage actresses such as Lillian Russell and Sarah Bernhardt had endorsed products in the past.[51] Now Hoffmann was on the leading edge of a resurgence of celebrity testimonials.[52] Before the decade ended, she would lend her name to chewing gum and motorcycle advertisements as well.

Along with her advertising contract, Hoffmann continued to seek one for motion pictures. That summer, her former dance partner Theodore Kosloff shot his first Cecil B. DeMille film, an Aztec costume drama called *The Woman God Forgot*.[53] The theatrical agent H. B. Marinelli pitched a three-picture deal for Hoffmann, with an asking price of $75,000.[54] No one took up the exorbitant offer. She may have been too old—at thirty, she was twice the age of Blanche Sweet and Gertrude Bambrick when D. W. Griffith hired them—or have asked for too much money. By September 1917, she gave up the quest for a film career and decided that she "prefers vaudeville."[55]

The *Gertrude Hoffmann Revue* played midwestern and southern venues through the end of 1917. Hoffmann participated in the "Smokes for Sammies" campaign, standing near barrels placed in theater lobbies to encourage the collection of cigarettes for soldiers at the front.[56] Audience members continued to make the same mistake as New Yorkers, rising and saluting the giant American flag when it was lowered onstage for the "Song of Nations."[57] "The error was all right, though," wrote the theater critic Giles P. Cain, "it is best to be patriotic at the wrong time than not to be patriotic at all.[58]

The war had other effects: Hoffmann's chorus boys kept enlisting or getting drafted.[59] She found a new partner who was too young for conscription in her teenage son. Max Jr. was enrolled at Bordentown Military Institute in New Jersey. He took a leave of absence to perform in the show, dancing with his mother in "Spring Song" and singing in the "Song of Nations" number.[60] This was his first professional engagement.

The relationship between mothers and sons was a fraught one in the wartime era. "I Didn't Raise My Boy to Be a Soldier" was a major hit in 1915, when the United States was still neutral.[61] In the ensuing years, American songs and films responded with images of good mothers eager to send their sons to war and bad mothers who pulled strings to keep their sons at home.[62] A charming fifteen-year-old trained at a military school may well have been eager to lie about his age and join the war effort. I suspect, though without any direct evidence, that the Hoffmanns put their son in the show to keep him from enlisting. Max Jr. often did impulsive things while his parents were away on tour.

Max Jr. supported his mother in a show that was dependent on spectacle. At this time, reviewers began to betray a suspicion that "flash" acts were passé. A write-up of the Chicago show compares the Hoffmann revue—with its dazzling scenery and costumes, its huge cast, and its own crew of technicians—to the act of the singer Miss Ray Samuels who preceded Hoffmann on the bill. "Miss Hoffman's efforts were rewarded by enthusiastic applause," the review says, "But Miss Samuels, all by her electric self, stopped the show for three minutes."[63] A critical consensus was taking shape that the magnetism of an individual performer was the best measure of vaudeville success. Caroline

Caffin begins her 1914 treatise on vaudeville with a chapter called "The Force of Personality." For her initial case studies, she presents vaudeville performers "whose appeal has that originality which for want of a better name we must call genius."[64] These are performers who convey their uniqueness in a vibrant and modern way. Hoffmann's act, by contrast, depended on what Caffin calls her "flexibility of style," a charitable way of saying that she's a good mimic but not an original.[65]

Hoffmann did have one singular quality as a performer: a predilection for dancing in a state of undress. While her nudity was an expected part of her act in the years after Salome, it stirred up more trouble in the fall of 1917. The Chicago Women's Church Federation denounced Hoffmann's act because she performed while "nude below the thighs."[66] She responded by asking if they expected her to "appear in an overcoat and golashes [*sic*]" when performing as "a Greek nymph."[67] Her audience did not need to be protected from her body, she slyly suggests, anymore than she needed to be protected from the rain.

The United States was going through a period of increased legal attention to the morals of its residents. Hoffmann could not overcome late Progressive Era policing with her wit alone. After two days of performing in St. Louis, she was arrested for public indecency. Some writers joked about the incident. In Illinois, a columnist suggested that Hoffmann had taken wartime thriftiness too far by conserving her clothing.[68] Back in New York, news of the arrest was received with skepticism; those in the know suspected it must have been a publicity stunt to drum up business.[69] The initial arrest took place in November. The Hoffmann tour traveled south for bookings in New Orleans, and then stopped off in St. Louis once again in December on the way to Des Moines, Iowa, performances. Gertrude requested that the charge against her be amended from "nudity" to "partial nudity"; she was acquitted even of the modified charge.[70]

New York theaters felt the aftershocks of Hoffmann's arrest. A warning circulated in December that all women in musical comedies should perform in full costumes, including tights and shoes.[71] Concerns about theatrical indecency had not been major news since 1913, when the "white slavery" play dominated Broadway.[72] These new calls for censorship would grow into the 1920s, leading to the passage of the Wales Padlock Law in 1927; under that New York State law, if a play was deemed obscene by the courts, its theater could be "padlocked for a year."[73] In the popular imagination, American culture became increasingly freewheeling from the 1910s to the 1920s: the moves toward theatrical censorship show that this was far from universal.[74]

Patriotism went hand in hand with prohibition: the war brought about food shortages, which in turn led many countries to outlaw distilling.[75] By the end of 1917, twenty-three states in the United States had banned the drinking of alcohol.[76] The government passed a few wartime restrictions on distillation and possession; they passed the Eighteenth Amendment on December 18, and sent it to state constitutional conventions for ratification.[77] The Hoffmanns ran afoul of another midwestern morals squad later that same month. On Christmas Eve their train car traveled through the "dry" state of Nebraska. The company celebrated the holiday with champagne. Their guests reportedly include the mayor of Omaha and the theatrical couple Mr. and Mrs. Sydney Drew.[78] Gertrude recorded what happened next: "noise—confusion outside—porter knocks—warns of prohibit[ion] officers 6 miles out town—tells us throw any liquor down toilet—me defiant—Max gave me a big boot—sent me on my way off train to Hotel. He says he allowed p.[olice] Officers to open snake basket. They ran."[79] While this description makes the raid sound like a screwball comedy, it had some serious consequences. Max and several members of the company (including a carpenter and one of the Cingalese dancers) were arrested.[80] The case was dismissed a few days later, with the judge ruling that the private train car was the Hoffmanns' home and therefore their possession of alcohol within it was not illegal. Although Gertrude was not arrested, the hearing was nevertheless used to generate some Ziegfeld-style publicity. Max submitted into evidence two telegrams from their New York City doctors, who explained why their alcohol consumption was medically necessary. The first telegram said that Gertrude was prescribed a glass of champagne after each meal "to counteract the fatigue caused by the tremendous strain on her heart by the conditions of the present act."[81] In later versions of this story, a reporter used the shorthand that Gertrude Hoffmann drank "champagne for the nerves," a decadent tonic for what was seen as a modern woman's condition.[82] She rejected the claim then, insisting that she never drank. Max's doctor made his case in less dramatic terms, asserting that he "prescribed martini" to help him sleep.[83]

Since the nineteenth century, American doctors had considered how the speed and strain of modern life could affect people's health.[84] Stress was thought to have an adverse effect on the heart.[85] Though the doctors' telegrams were sent to keep the Hoffmanns from being convicted, they also show them as a couple both made and unmade by modernity: while they produced the pleasures of the present—speedy, spectacular entertainment underscored by jazzy music—they also felt its negative effects in their bodies. The Hoffmanns disprove the cheerful progressivism of Vernon and Irene Castle's *Modern Dancing*, in which that couple insists "while we dance . . . we are warring against fat, against sickness, and against nervous troubles."[86] The Castles made it their business to associate partnered dance with clean, healthful living.[87] Gertrude Hoffmann's dancing was always associated with a certain degree of pathology, from the Salome "epidemic" to the dance craze.

The Hoffmann revue toured the Pacific Northwest to begin the new year, playing Orpheum houses in Canada and Washington State. The Spokane performance added six new showgirls to the "Song of Nations" act: Red Cross volunteers in their uniforms. According to a review, "The Spokane maids descended the staircase in the spotlight and tripped across to the wings," where they received a round of applause.[88] When the Hoffmann troupe arrived in California, a critic connected the dominance of revues to the "saloon closing" orders: "If the amusement-loving public cannot have wine, they are going to have plenty of 'woman and song.'"[89] They played the Bay Area and then turned back east, with stops in Denver, Colorado, and Lincoln, Nebraska, and a return to St. Louis where the tour closed in mid-May. The Hoffmann company toured for seven long, tumultuous months, and finally returned to New York City.

That summer, Hoffmann embodied the spirit of the West in print ads that appeared in mass-circulation magazines. Both *Life* and *Ladies Home Journal* ran advertisements for Adams California Fruit Gum; as in the Askum ads, a picture of Hoffmann in a dance pose appeared next to a testimonial about the product over her signature. In the ad seen in figure 12.1 Hoffmann wears a Grecian gown like her "Spring Song" costume. She poses with a cornucopia of semi-exotic produce: not just California oranges but grapes, a banana, a pineapple, and stone fruit. Hoffmann's rosy complexion and bounteous offering are reproduced in a lush four-color halftone photomechanical print. Although Askum was only sold in Chicago with her name attached, these ads ran nationally. In both ads Hoffmann's power as a spokeswoman arose from her authority as an energetic performer who brought Americans intense, spectacular entertainment in short bursts of time. The products she endorsed worked the same way. If you did not have time to sit down and eat a full lunch, you could still get the calories packed into a drugstore soda with Askum; if you did not have access to the fresh fruits of California and the Pacific, you could enjoy the next best thing by chewing California fruit gum. Even in a period of wartime economizing, Hoffmann's image seems to suggest, Americans could still treat themselves to something quick and delicious.

While her image circulated, Gertrude and Max sold their old Sea Gate home and built a new one. The labor shortage affected construction work as well as vaudeville, so Max "had to jump in" and help build the house.[90] He joined another labor pool as well. When the Selective Service Act was first instituted, American men ages twenty-one to thirty had to register for the draft. In August 1918, the age range was extended to include American men from eighteen to forty-five.[91] Max Sr. was just within the limits, at age forty-four when he registered for the draft in September.[92] Max Jr. was still too young.

For the first time in nearly a decade, Hoffmann overhauled her vaudeville turn. When she performed in the fall season, it was as a solo act. Long tours with large companies and complex sets helped her gain a following, but the expense and logistics needed to manage this type of act were unsustainable. The *Variety* review of her Palace performance noted as much, saying: "In these days of heavy rail tariffs, she is very wise to eliminate the factor of carrying a large supporting company."[93] It was a frugal decision with a brave message: "It says that it is 'Gertrude Hoffmann' after all—she doesn't need a 'troupe.'"[94] The gambit paid off, setting the bar for single acts that season.

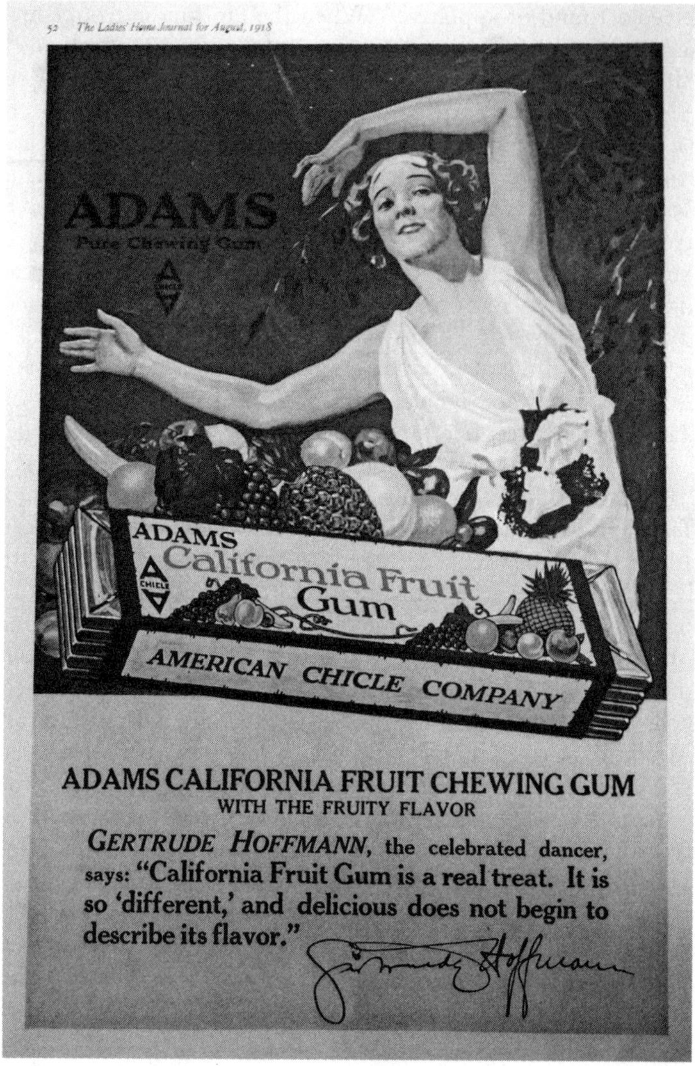

FIGURE 12.1. Gertrude Hoffmann in an advertisement for Adams California Fruit Chewing Gum. Collection of the author.

She began with several dances that demonstrated her continued love for vivid contrasting colors. For her Spanish dance, she wore a costume of "black satin, maize, and topaz."[95] "Dance of the Allies" was an allegorical pantomime of the present war, which she danced in "a wisp of red cheesecloth before hangings of deep blue."[96] Performed to a Sousa march, the dance sounds as if it fell into the no-man's-land between serious mimodrama and kitsch. This section was followed by imitations of newer stage stars, including Ann Pennington,

Bessie McCoy, and Fanny Brice. She ended the show with musical imitations, playing percussion instruments to suggest different activities on "A Trip to Coney Island." When she opened at the Palace, she was billed in advertisements as "Vaudeville's Greatest Versatile Genius."[97] The act seemed designed to rebut criticisms from the last tour, both that she was underprepared and that her act was all flash and no genius. This time, the spotlight was on Gertrude Hoffmann alone.

Hoffmann's return to success at the Palace was a small victory in a period when the nation was going through monumental struggles. Hoffmann and her fellow performers faced an enemy at home—the Spanish influenza pandemic.[98] October and November 1918 were the most devastating in terms of U.S. casualties. *Variety* published lists of entertainers felled by the virus.[99] Outside of New York City, many public places were closed to prevent further spread of the disease. A stock company actress recounts her experience: "People were wearing masks and gargling every hour. Often we'd get to a town to find the schools and churches—and theaters—had been closed that day. We'd sit in our hotel rooms gargling too, and the lists of the local dead filled up the front page columns."[100] To Americans at least, the pandemic was deadlier than the war itself.

Hoffmann was stricken with the flu in November.[101] She stayed at home to recover, canceling a week of shows. By mid-November, *Variety* claimed that the epidemic had ended.[102] Quarantines were lifted, and theaters began running their usual bills once again. The Great War ended as well, and Germany signed an armistice agreement on November 11.

Gertrude Hoffmann's act embodied the contradictions of U.S. culture during World War I. She brought together the hedonism of the cabaret and the patriotism of the pageant. She represented the timeless bounty of the harvest in one advertisement and the speed of the modern age in another. After the war, Hoffmann struggled to maintain her old routines. Even after recuperating from influenza, she kept her engagements close to home: she played the Orpheum and Bushwick theaters in Brooklyn, and then ventured to Boston in December. While performing her Ann Pennington imitation at the Alhambra Theatre's New Year's Eve show, she lost her footing: a *Variety* article was waggishly titled "Gertrude Hoffmann's Slip."[103] Sources disagree about her injuries: she may have dislocated her elbow or sprained her ankle, but in either case, she left the bill.[104] Hoffmann's virtuosity was taking its toll on her body and her self-image. Chapter 13 discusses her growing dissatisfaction with her career, echoed at a larger scale by the breakdown of the vaudeville system itself.

Chapter 13

✦

Just Drifting

Changes were afoot in the vaudeville industry. As early as 1910, twice as many New Yorkers went to the movies as attended a vaudeville show.[1] Profits for touring theatrical productions fell after 1915, a long and slow process called the "decline" (or sometimes the "death") of the road.[2] Small-time theatrical circuits like those owned by Marcus Loew challenged the dominance of the more expensive Keith–Albee circuit.[3] On a broader scale, the United States went through an economic recession after the end of the Great War. Max Hoffmann placed an ad in *Variety* selling "all scenery and equipment" for "Gertrude Hoffman's Revues and Sumurun Production."[4] This included an "illuminated steel run way" from *Sumurun* and the "five section steel diving tank" from Hoffmann's Annette Kellerman imitation.[5] The solo show with easily transported backdrops may have led the Hoffmanns to decide they would never reuse the complex and bulky scenery from earlier shows.

Newspapers reported that Gertrude Hoffmann disappeared for a few days in July. On the evening of July 23, Gertrude left Max Hoffmann's car to buy something in a midtown drugstore; what happened next is subject to dispute. Max reported that when his wife left the car, she never came back. He went into the drugstore himself, but did not find her.[6] In a newspaper report the following day, Max said that he had enlisted the services of a private detective.[7] According to at least one source, she was missing for three days but then "turned up . . . at the home of her sisters in Yonkers."[8] She and Max may have quarreled: he was quoted in the article as saying, "'Some differences of opinion had come up' but these 'had been adjusted.'"[9] The news columns in *Variety* were far calmer about the whole incident, claiming the event had been cooked up for publicity and that "during her reported absence" she was seen around the theater district.[10] Until a letter or other explanation comes to light, the occurrence remains a mystery.

A theatrical era ended that summer: Oscar Hammerstein died on August 1, 1919. Gertrude Hoffmann's diaries include an extended reminiscence on Hammerstein; the writing style makes it sound like notes for a public speech, either requested or imagined. She proclaims, "To me, Times Sq. began with The Great Oscar Hammerstein"; typical accounts of the area give more credit to the *New York Times* editor for moving his offices to Longacre Square and thus renaming it. Perhaps due to the early divorce of her parents, Hoffmann maintained a deep affection for the theatrical father figures of her youth. She continues, "To know him intimately was to know both a dreamer and a terrific action man. He had the confidence and courage of a lion."[11] Hammerstein had hired her as a dance director when she was a teenager; at the time of his passing, her career had moved into a new phase as well.

That summer and fall, Gertrude Hoffmann's influence could be felt throughout Midtown Manhattan. A *Vanity Fair* article, "Keeping on with the Dance," insisted that "the dance craze is still going strong. In fact, it's more violent than it ever was."[12] Three of the six types of dancing sent up by the article had been part of Hoffmann's acts. The elegant sketches done by "Fish" (the illustrator Anne Harriet Fish) include ersatz Ballets Russes dancers performing a scene from a fake dance called "The Golden Vodka," a "Spring Song"–inspired barefoot dance in Central Park titled "The Birth of the Crocus," and even a "Dance of Salome." Though it may have seemed decadent a decade earlier, the author says of the Salome dance, "Perhaps the secret of its appeal is the sweet, wholesome joyousness of it all."[13] Another Salome danced in the *Passing Show of 1919*, and newspapers marveled at how permissive society had become since Gertrude Hoffmann had toured with her Salome.[14] Hoffmann established the standard for vibrant, upscale women's dance culture. At the same time, her association with a particular place and time was used by cultural commentators to mark the ways society had progressed beyond that era.

One dancer who suggested potential new directions was Adolph Bolm. He moved easily between production and performance, and he drew on international dance traditions as well as American popular culture. Hoffmann saw Bolm perform in Paris in 1909 as part of the Ballets Russes. He was skilled at character dance and pantomime, as well as in powerful masculine roles.[15] Bolm was interested in staging ballets and performing in them, but at that time Diaghilev saw Vaslav Nijinsky as the star and had little time for anyone else in the company.[16] Bolm toured America with the Ballets Russes in 1917 but when he fractured vertebrae due to a stage accident, he was forced to remain in the hospital.[17] After his recovery, Bolm stayed in the United States, where he taught, choreographed, and danced.[18] Bolm worked in places that ranged from high (the Metropolitan Opera) to low (a musical revue called *Miss 1917*). His source material was equally eclectic: he choreographed and danced in ballets inspired by Oscar Wilde's fairy tale "The Birthday of the Infanta" and the George Herriman comic strip *Krazy Kat*. Bolm offered a model for the kind of work Hoffmann longed to do.

Hoffmann's work and interviews during this period suggest how closely she followed Bolm's career. His dance "The White Peacock" premiered in late June of 1919.[19] When Hoffmann opened her fall vaudeville season, Bolm's "The White Peacock" was the only addition to her routine. She may have learned the dance from Bolm himself. A 1963 letter from the dance critic John Dougherty reports that Beata Bolm told him that her husband had taught Hoffmann the dance himself.[20] Hoffmann's experience reinforces a story about American ballet that contemporary dance scholars have begun to tell in detail: the story of how, even before the 1933 arrival of George Balanchine in New York City, European ballet influenced and was influenced by practitioners of American popular dance forms.[21]

"The White Peacock" may have interested Hoffmann for other reasons. It seems to have been performed as part of a "movie prologue," a live dance performance with orchestral accompaniment that preceded motion pictures.[22] Using the "tone poem" composed by Charles T. Griffes and conducted by Hugo Riesenfeld, Bolm's "interpretative ballet" debuted at the Rivoli Theatre, a movie theater.[23] The dance performance served as an opening act for the film program, a Mack Sennett short called *Hearts and Flowers* and a feature adapted from a Broadway play, the Civil War spy thriller *Secret Service*.[24] Even though the review appears in the Moving Pictures section, the *Variety* reviewer seems invested in highlighting the live elements of the show at the expense of the cinematic ones, noting that "American music and 'Secret Service' (reviewed in this issue), essentially an American drama, were the outstanding features of the program at the Rivoli this week."[25] As Mary Simonson suggests, there were many performance styles in the early twentieth century that engaged in intermedial performance.[26] This review reminds us that when performances mix media elements, critics often feel the need to separate and distinguish them.[27]

Hoffmann danced "The White Peacock" in the opening spot of her new vaudeville turn. It was eye-catching, with a costume that included a huge white fabric tail unfolding against a black backdrop. But it was not crowd-pleasing: "It strutted in silence and closed about the same way," noted the *Billboard* review of her Chicago act.[28] The later parts of her act, and even her "Dance of the Allies" that followed "The White Peacock," brought cheers and applause.[29] The Bolm dance fulfilled Hoffmann's aesthetic desires but left the audience cold. She still needed dances with populist appeal.

In Chicago for the kickoff to her 1919–1920 theatrical season, she bought a Harley-Davidson motorcycle, which included a diminutive sidecar with a cab enclosure. In figure 13.1, Gertrude poses in the sidecar, wearing a wide straw hat and smiling. Max Jr. sits on the motorcycle, bareheaded, wearing a casual suit and flowing tie. It is a charming but static image, in its depiction of a performer known for her mobility as a seat-belted passenger. Advertisements for Harley-Davidson appeared in newspapers that fall, often timed around Hoffmann's performances in the area. These advertisements do show her astride the motorcycle, a model described as "the feature-refined, womankind."[30] This motorcycle is not imagined as a vehicle for practical errands, nor is it one on which Hoffmann might indulge in the thrill of speed. Instead, it allows her to exercise in natural surroundings.[31] Her endorsement of a

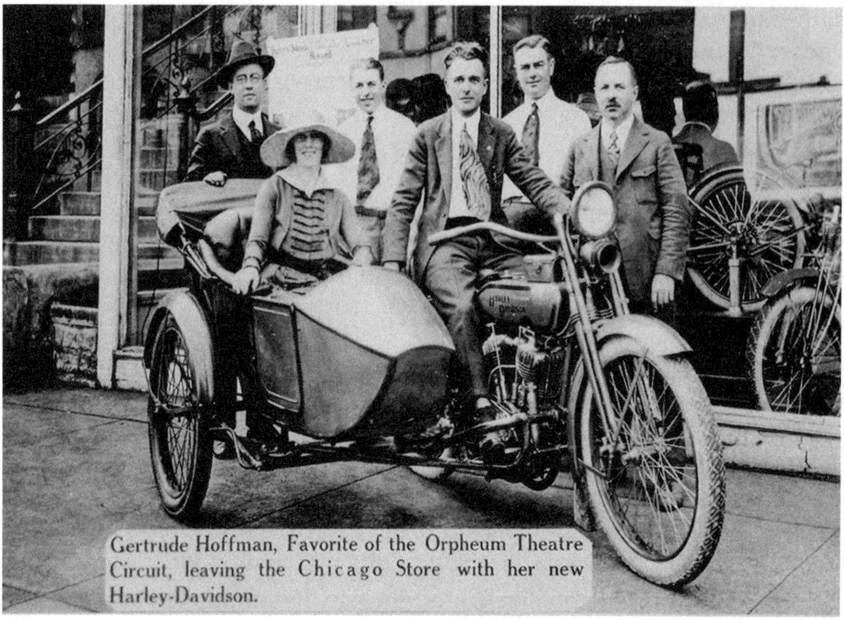
Gertrude Hoffman, Favorite of the Orpheum Theatre Circuit, leaving the Chicago Store with her new Harley-Davidson.

FIGURE 13.1. Promotional photograph of Gertrude Hoffmann outside a Harley-Davidson dealership. Collection of the author.

motorcycle still brought to mind the dangerous autonomy that was central to her celebrity image.

Gertrude Hoffmann had been performing for twenty years. An interview in a Minneapolis newspaper suggests that she was going through something of a midlife crisis. The Twin Cities loomed large in the Hoffmanns' history, often marking a place where their theatrical fortunes changed. Max joined the Bulger and Mathews troupe as its music director in Minneapolis, and Gertrude added her imitations to the *Saison des Ballets Russes* program there. This time through, she gave an extended interview with the *Minneapolis Journal* drama editor Carlton W. Miles in which she asked, "Is celebrity worth while?" This is a unique interview, both in the seriousness with which it treats Hoffmann and the length it devotes to her thinking aloud. The profile begins with a world-weary monologue:

> Glory, what does that amount to? Nothing. I've accomplished everything in the world that I wanted to accomplish. I've done all the things I planned to do. They are material things. Now that I have them I'm as unsatisfied as before. I want something bigger. What? I don't know. Perhaps I should like to live in a country where all the people were interested only in the arts—music, dancing, painting, sculpture,

> literature. I'm content to do just what I want in the future. On the other hand, I'll never be satisfied until I dance in the ballet at the Metropolitan.[32]

These sentiments ring true; she was someone who accomplished her career goals in short order. She had more success with lowbrow burlesques than with highbrow pantomimes, which must have been a disappointment. One part of Hoffmann's comments hints at her way forward. Her inchoate desire to abandon America for a pleasant life in a country that appreciates the arts clashes with her other career ambition, dancing in the corps de ballet at the Metropolitan Opera. Hoffmann may have been thinking about the new season at the opera house, which had recently been announced.[33] Richard Ordynski, her *Sumurun* collaborator, was the stage director at the Metropolitan, and Adolph Bolm was one of the ballet masters.[34] The men doing the work closest to her ideal of dance pantomime were employed at the Metropolitan Opera House; ergo, she should work there too.

In this interview, Hoffmann struggles with her sense of self as an aging woman in a field that favors the young.[35] With her fantasies of dancing in the opera ballet, Hoffmann engaged in nostalgia, remembering the first jobs she had held as a teenager in San Francisco. She claimed she felt the same in her mid-thirties as she had when she was seven years old, then noted that she could no longer play the same parts that she did in the past: "Perhaps you'll see me coming around here playing character roles soon," she says.[36] The Carlton Miles interview concludes with his discussion of Hoffmann's dissatisfied striving, which he calls "groping in the dark toward some unseen goal."[37] She sounds like a tragic heroine of the modern stage, torn between expectations that restrict her and ambitions that she can barely express:

> "I'm through with vaudeville after this season. I'm just drifting."
>
> And then she goes off on her daily motorcycle ride. "They tell me I've improved in appearance," she says. "Reason? Motorcycle rides, fresh air—and the fact that I no longer worry over things. I'm content." Is she? As the Ibsen characters universally say—"I wonder."[38]

Miles imagines Hoffmann as an Ibsen heroine, a vaudeville version of Hedda Gabler. It is tough to decide what to make of Miles and his indeterminate feeling, the sense that Hoffmann's contented face might mask a vexed brain. What if she were just having a bad day? There are no diaries or letters that detail her frame of mind in the fall of 1919, so this interview serves as an isolated, compelling data point.

Gertrude and Max Hoffmann continued on the Orpheum circuit, playing West Coast theaters and then circling back through the Plains states to Chicago. While the Hoffmanns were traveling, Max Jr. lived with Gertrude's mother Catherine and her sister Margaret on the Upper West Side of

Manhattan.[39] He was introduced to Norma Terris, who would later gain fame originating the role of Magnolia in *Show Boat*. To impress her, Max Jr. traveled to Havana, "to try to win a fortune in the gambling games of the Cuban capital."[40] The gambit failed before it began; he lost all but $4 playing poker on the boat ride there. A classmate paid for his return passage on the S.S. *Mexico*, which docked in New York on November 5, 1919.[41] Though he claimed to be twenty-two on the ship manifest, Max Jr. was seventeen.

Gertrude Hoffmann already had plenty of trouble to deal with on the road. A pretender sprang up in Ohio. Ads for a film called *A Perfect Model* claimed that "Gertrude Hoffman" would appear in person at the screenings. Some advertisements explained that she was "Cleveland celebrated artists' model," but others did not.[42] While she was performing in Los Angeles, Hoffmann received a letter from Dayton, Ohio, describing the act. The letter-writer could not believe that she "would play a cheap picture house" and found that "this so-called 'Gertrude Hoffman' was only a big woman lecturing on physical culture."[43] Hoffmann responded, writing to her lawyer and to the vaudeville circuit owner E. F. Albee.[44] She also took out advertisements in *Variety* warning exhibitors that her name was being used to advertise the film without her consent.[45] Hoffmann defended her intellectual property vigorously, in a reversal from the freewheeling days of her early career.

She sought new imitations for her act, showing a preference for the work of flamboyant Russian dramatic actresses. Hoffmann asked Alla Nazimova for permission to imitate her sword dance from the 1918 film *Eye for Eye*.[46] This imitation does not seem to have made it out of the planning stages. She did perform a send-up of Olga Petrova's melodramatic death scene from *The Shulamite*. Petrova, it should be noted, was ersatz Russian. Born Muriel Harding in London, she took on a Russian name and accent early in her career and maintained it throughout her life.[47] Both these scenes were borrowed from stories of cross-cultural love: in *Eye for Eye*, a sheik's daughter falls in love with a French naval officer; in *The Shulamite*, a South African farmer's wife attracts the attention of a visiting Englishman. Petrova took advantage of the publicity: she later visited Hoffmann's dressing room at the Palace, going through the scene with her in order to "give Miss Hoffmann some details which Mme. Petrova thought she should use."[48] Divas had to stick together.

Petrova played the Interstate Circuit of vaudeville houses in Texas, Arkansas, Louisiana, and Mississippi.[49] Owned by the St. Louis businessman Karl Hoblitzelle, the Interstate Circuit scheduled its vaudeville acts through the Keith–Albee organization.[50] This touring schedule was a smaller and less prestigious one than Hoffmann typically booked, with two-night stays in each city. It was a new market, though, in which big names could still draw big crowds. After she finished her southern Orpheum bookings, Hoffmann ventured into the Southwest. The act was well-received, but Hoffmann got into trouble outside of Wichita Falls. The sheriff in the small town of Burkburnett, Texas, saw the performer on her motorcycle and arrested her. He presumed that the vehicle was stolen.[51] After proving her identity and ownership, Hoffmann was released. When they took their Harley back to Brooklyn that spring, Max was fined for speeding as well.[52]

After this stint in the small time, Hoffmann returned to New York City. She refined her "White Peacock" dance and Petrova impersonations on the road. When she played the Palace once again, she was "the evening's hit."[53] A review of her performance gives more details on the Petrova act, which began with Hoffmann in her usual dressing-room alcove, wriggling into a corset and an old-fashioned ball gown.[54] While she put on these clothes, "the house had a giggle."[55] It is easy to imagine how the costume change might add commentary to her comedy. At the dawn of the age of the flapper, the idea of going backward to a time when women wore such complicated undergarments must have been laughable. This imitation would stand in stark contrast to those of scantily clad modern revue performers such as Ann Pennington.

Pennington was an icon of the Jazz Age. The petite dancer was known for her work with the *Ziegfeld Follies* and *George White's Scandals*; in 1926 she would introduce the "Black Bottom" dance to a white audience. With her Pennington impression, Hoffmann "showed class as a kicker"; Max's orchestra arrangements followed suit, including some blaring jazz solos.[56] She choreographed some jazz numbers for her dance troupe in the years to come, but her own dances were, for the most part, ballet and modern. She suggested that "classic dancing" might serve as a good substitute for alcohol.[57] "But don't jazz," she's quoted as saying, "the shimmy won't last. The ball-room dance of the future is going to be interpretative, something beautiful, nothing coarse and wiggly."[58] This seems out of character for a performer whose career was so intertwined with nightclubs and the social dancing that arose in them.

A rejection of social dances, especially those with an African American influence, can be found in the writings of ballet teachers from the period.[59] Hoffmann was soon to join their ranks. In May 1920 she participated in a ballet exhibition at Aeolian Hall, just north of Bryant Park. The program was pitched as "the first step in a nation-wide campaign to interest children in the art of ballet dancing."[60] The growing interest in ballet helped Hoffmann make the transition from performer to teacher and producer. Dance studies scholars have highlighted the long "interconnection of classical ballet and commercial theatrical dance" in American culture.[61] With her appearance at this recital, Hoffmann acknowledged the influence of ballet on her dances and a desire to share her love of dance with the next generation.

Her transition was a wise move. The year 1920 marked the beginning of the end for vaudeville's cultural dominance. "Toward the end of 1920, grosses at straight vaudeville houses began to sag badly," wrote Sime Silverman.[62] By 1926, only 3 percent of American theaters would stage live performances exclusively.[63] Inspired by Adolph Bolm and his fellow Russians, Gertrude Hoffmann drifted away from vaudeville and toward dance.

Chapter 14

✦

From Advanced Vaudeville to Cabaret

Just before Christmas in 1920, Max Hoffmann Jr. and Norma Terris applied for a marriage license.[1] They did not go through with it, in part since both were underage.[2] Max Hoffmann Sr. still dreamed of passing the conductor's baton to his son; he sent Max Jr. to a conservatory for six months.[3] The musical training did not take, so Gertrude Hoffmann prepared a double act for her son and his fiancée.[4] Billed as "Junior and Terris," the youngsters debuted in Asbury Park, New Jersey.[5] They then played the Twenty-Third Street theater, where Sime Silverman found them to be "a nice young couple with talent and an excellent turn," albeit one that needed a bit of refinement and trimming to be worthy of the big time.[6] Their billing allowed Max to be judged by his talent alone instead of trading on his family name for unearned publicity. The Hoffmann connection, however, was an open secret. One review uses near-eugenic language, congratulating Junior on his "breeding" and noting, "Blood will tell."[7] The details of the act show the influence of both Hoffmann parents: Terris does several imitations, and Junior plays the violin. Max and Norma toured the Interstate Circuit with their act that fall, finally marrying in Houston.[8]

Variety noted of Junior and Terris's act: "This turn is the first production work done by Miss Hoffmann other than for her own use."[9] This claim was not true, since Hoffmann did some work for hire in her dance directing days. It did highlight the broader industry's awareness that she was moving from a performing role to a producing one. Once she established her son in the family business, Gertrude Hoffmann turned her attention back to her own act. Her new vaudeville turn debuted that fall. Called *Gertrude Hoffmann and Her American Ballet*, it showed her commitment to dance and her desire to retreat from center stage. The act included more than a dozen dances, most of which were new.[10] These were all presented in a forty-five-minute set. Hoffmann performed in the opening pantomime and three dance duets with Leon Barte.[11] These included an *Arabian Nights*–inspired pantomime ballet, a Strauss waltz, and a mazurka.[12] The rest were done by her company, which included seven women and three men, many of whom would continue to dance with her for years to come. Some dances seemed like vaudeville specialties: a shimmy in ballet clothes, a toy soldier dance similar to the one still performed at Radio City Music Hall. Others were more highbrow. Perhaps inspired by Adolph Bolm's work with the Japanese dancer-choreographer Michio Ito, Hoffmann included a "Japanese Drum Dance" performed by Yashushi Wuriu.[13] The costuming adorned the dancers so beautifully that one review marveled, "They appear frequently to have stepped from the frame of some rare old masterpiece."[14] Even the lighting was carefully crafted.[15] Hoffmann took the aesthetic of her revues—fast-paced, varied, beautiful to look at—and applied it to dance.

Three of the dances in her program were created by Michel Fokine.[16] These Fokine dances gave Hoffmann legitimacy as a dancer, as Adolph Bolm's "The White Peacock" had done. Russian dances were trendy a decade earlier, but in the 1920s Americans were becoming more cognizant of ballet's styles, techniques, and big names.[17] Of course, Hoffmann had danced in several Fokine ballets before; this time, though, she gave him credit. Like Bolm, Fokine divided his time between performing concert dance and choreographing commissions for popular performers. He created a Russian dance for Gilda Gray, who became famous at the *Follies* for her American shimmy.[18]

Fokine had recently opened a dance studio in New York.[19] Hoffmann wanted to do the same, and she used her new tour both to advertise and recruit. She held classes in the cities where she toured, "explaining and demonstrating" to local ballet students.[20] The tour was pitched as a first step in "the formation of an all-American ballet."[21] Students who attended these morning classes could also try out for her company.[22] "Have You a Pavlowa or Mordkin in Your Home?" asked one advertisement in Cleveland.[23] A Philadelphia review from February 1922 noted that the company included local girls who "were recruited here last summer."[24] This was one way to guarantee a local audience's interest in repeat viewings.

Hoffmann took advantage of the national interest in ballet to find dancers who would be able to learn and perform her routines. She had a more personal motive for these local auditions as well. "I will never forget my childhood days and my burning desire to learn to dance," Hoffmann says in an interview with the *Vaudeville News*.[25] The illustration accompanying the story depicts Hoffmann in a balletic pose, with a long, elegant neck and thickly lashed, half-closed eyes. She continues:

> When I was a kiddie, my parents were too poor to gratify my ambition to learn the rudiments of the terpsichorean art. I resolved then that if I could ever afford it, I would build a school and dedicate it to poor children and tutor them myself, providing they displayed the least bit of talent. . . . Success came to me after a hard struggle. My progress was retarded because of lack of opportunity. That is another reason why I want to establish a school.[26]

Hoffmann regretted her lack of formal dance training. The youngest child of a single mother, she needed to find a paying job as soon as possible. With the open calls on tour, Hoffmann gave ambitious young women like herself the option to see the newspaper advertisement, audition, and be cast.

Gertrude Hoffmann and Her American Ballet toured the Keith vaudeville circuit that fall, facing stiffer competition thanks to the Shubert brothers. The theatrical industry suffered from the 1920 depression, but the Shubert Organization used this economic slump to enter vaudeville and compete against the monolithic syndicate run by E. F. Albee.[27] Shubert Advanced Vaudeville was launched September 1921.[28] The Keith–Albee and Orpheum circuits held a monopoly on big-time vaudeville houses, but the Shuberts began to oppose them directly, with their own stars playing the same towns at the same times. They planned to play vaudeville bills at twenty-two theaters that were straight theatrical or burlesque houses. The Shuberts paid high salaries to lure big names away.[29] Some of the theaters on their circuit were too small to break even on ticket sales.[30] This dangerous combination made the first season of Shubert Vaudeville "a colossal financial failure."[31] Hoffmann held her own when her act went up against Shubert Vaudeville headliners including Marie Dressler (in Philadelphia) and Nora Bayes (in Pittsburgh).[32]

Early 1922 offered exciting, even vaudevillian, theatrical events in more highbrow venues. The composer John Alden Carpenter collaborated with Adolph Bolm on a ballet called *Krazy Kat: A Jazz Pantomime*. The dance was first performed at Town Hall in New York City January 20 and 21, 1922.[33] In the popular comic strip, Ignatz the mouse tormented Krazy and threw bricks at his head.[34] The ballet opens with Krazy sleeping; the score is a parody of *Prélude à l'après-midi d'un faune*, "designated in the score as 'The Afternoon Nap of a Faun.'"[35] Krazy awakens from a nap to see a poster for a Grand Ball, finds ballet clothes and dresses in them, and dances ecstatically—first in a ballet style, then a Spanish dance. A "mysterious stranger" offers Krazy a catnip bouquet; he engages in "a wild frenzy of jazz dancing."[36] The stranger is revealed as Ignatz; he hits Krazy with a brick, and the cat passes out once more.[37] Bolm danced the role of Krazy wearing a full mask. The ballet was an important modernist collaboration, "the first of the composer's work to trade in patently lowbrow forms and the first piece of art music to use the word *jazz* in its title."[38] Hoffmann did not attend the premiere because she was performing in Boston. In some respects, though, her career laid the groundwork for this kind of artistic cross-pollination. The phrase "jazz pantomime" suggests the ways that her revues spanned popular and highbrow, old-fashioned and up-to-date. Her program, like the *Krazy Kat* ballet, brought the logic of variety to bear in the world of art dance. In fact, her program presented the very same styles of dance: Russian, Spanish, and jazz. Carpenter and Bolm, like Hoffmann, were drawing from the culture at large. The mixing of high and low can be seen in popular performance of the 1920s as much as in avant-garde work.

Hoffmann had a more direct connection to the other international modernist performance debuting that winter. *La Chauve-Souris*, a "Russian vaudeville" hosted by Nikita Balieff was brought to New York City by Hoffmann's former manager Morris Gest.[39] Her image appeared on the curtain as part of a massive illustration by Ralph Barton where he caricatured the "first-nighters" expected to see the show.[40] Drawn from legitimate theater, vaudeville, and dance, as well as literature, music, politics, and high society, the curtain provided a visual who's who of the day's celebrities. Hoffmann appears in the sixth row. Her large eyes and rosy cheeks dominate in her caricature, along with her auburn hair, center-parted and arranged in two buns. Hoffmann may have attended one of the *Chauve-Souris* performances: she was booked to perform at the Riverside Theatre that week but left the bill on a Wednesday complaining of illness.[41] That Saturday, when *Chauve-Souris* opened, the singer Belle Baker was still filling in for Hoffmann.[42] Of course, Hoffmann might have been sick the whole time but, if she did play hooky, it would have been for a show like *Chauve-Souris*.

She returned to the stage soon after *Chauve-Souris* opened, playing the Bushwick Theatre. In an interview with the *Brooklyn Daily Eagle*, she recants earlier claims that jazz dancing would not last: "To organize an American ballet and not recognize our own peculiar art of dancing would be stupid and pedantic. Americans are curiously ashamed and self-conscious about this barbaric music and dancing."[43] Here Hoffmann acknowledges what Brenda Dixon Gottschild calls the "Africanist presence" in American performance, though she does so in the primitivist language of the day.[44] In order to recognize the value of African American culture she needs to see it through the eyes of European artists who are the arbiters of value: jazz, she says, "is far more appreciated abroad. Foreign composers look to the negro melodies as one of the most interesting factors in the art of music. The new world symphony [by Antonín Dvořák] is based upon them, and it is considered a masterpiece."[45] It sounds like the influx of jazz-inspired high art changed Hoffmann's mind.

Critics celebrated Hoffmann's act for its "dance melange," which brought jazz dancing into dialogue with pointe and pantomime. At the same time, though, they complained about her appearance on vaudeville bills with too much dancing. A successful vaudeville bill was supposed to balance different types of acts.[46] When she played Boston in February, the critic Len Libbey called it "one of the saddest bits of booking, as far as variety is concerned, of the season. Of the eight acts, six depend on either singing or dancing or a combination of both."[47] When she played the Palace in April, the reviewer noted the lack of a comedian in the first half of the show.[48] Vaudeville was losing the variety of performance types that defined it as a form.[49]

The Shuberts struggled to maintain their vaudeville circuit. They were "caught between motion picture interests and the Albee octopus."[50] They regrouped for the second season, signing new stars to take over failing units. Hoffmann signed a contract with Arthur Klein where she agreed to star in a new revue for the Shuberts called *Hello Everybody*.[51] The Four Marx Brothers signed with Shubert Vaudeville that season as well, even as the Shuberts sued their uncle Al Shean (and his partner Ed Gallagher) for breach of contract.[52] A splashy two-page spread in October 1922 tried to pitch Shubert Vaudeville as the next big thing.[53] The Shuberts' vaudeville units were neither innovative nor inevitable. For Gertrude Hoffmann, though, they provided one last chance to tour in vaudeville as well as a model for the kind of work she would do after the experiment ended.

Hello Everybody debuted at the Central Theatre in Jersey City, New Jersey.[54] Hoffmann performed double duty, appearing before the intermission in a dance turn, and afterward in a musical comedy revue.[55] The split format let her do the serious dancing she loved as well as the imitations, songs, and comic sketches that the audience loved. She was supported by the comedians Harry and Willie Lander, along with most of the dancers who toured with her in *Gertrude Hoffmann and Her American Ballet*. The dance program included two numbers that added novelty to her act. One was a "Moving Picture Scene" in which members of the company played popular movie stars. This scene remediated cinema, the major threat to live performance in the era. It took on the characteristics of film, such as its types (the vamp) and its styles of movement (slapstick).[56] It ended with a "Cinema Ballet," unifying all these elements.[57] The other was an athletic number, in which female members of the company participated in three fencing drills.[58] Although fencing may sound unusual on a dance program, it would become a signature routine of her dance troupe in the years to come.

The show opened the vaudeville season at the Garrick Theater in Chicago.[59] The unit played shows in Ohio, Missouri, Kentucky, and Maryland, with split weeks in Indiana and Pennsylvania. They opened in New York City on Christmas Day. Michel Fokine added a few numbers to the New York program, including a version of *Les Sylphides* (now billed to him) and a Christmas ballet.[60] Max Hoffmann Jr. and Norma Terris played for a month in a Nora Bayes show called *Queen O' Hearts*.[61] They found another job in Lew Leslie's cabaret act, which opened in January 1923.[62] In a matter of months, Max's mother would follow suit.

Hello Everybody toured the Northeast. The Hoffmanns were closer to home, but their schedule was worse. Arthur Klein booked his units to play alternate weeks at the Shubert Vaudeville houses. On their weeks off, the units could perform only if they found bookings at independent houses.[63] Shubert Vaudeville had lost $3 million by this point.[64] Hoffman's act soldiered on, playing a split week in western Massachusetts, followed by an extended booking at the Majestic Theatre in Boston.[65]

While the show played Boston, the dancer Harriet Fowler was stricken with appendicitis. Coverage of this illness provides the first published evidence of Gertrude Hoffmann's religious beliefs; because she held "Christian Science views" and served as Fowler's guardian, Hoffmann did not want her to have an operation.[66] Thankfully she relented, and Fowler recovered under the care of the Bay State Hotel's owners.[67] Hoffmann's Christian Science beliefs were shared with many of vaudeville's leading ladies, including Eva Tanguay and Nora Bayes.[68]

By March, the writing was on the wall. Cast members received half salaries; one told the stage manager, "[I] must be paid every Saturday just like the stage hands, with no cuts nor stalling."[69] *Hello Everybody* closed in Boston on March 17. On their train ride home, Gertrude Hoffmann paid the remaining salaries for her dancers and musicians.[70] Shubert Vaudeville ended its "disastrous season," but reports in the press claimed that Lee Shubert "has not entirely abandoned the idea of an opposition vaudeville circuit" and might continue it that fall.[71] Those pretenses were abandoned for good by August 1923.[72]

Gertrude Hoffmann and most of the company found a stopgap. Like Max Jr., she took her talents from the vaudeville stage to the cabaret. Ernie Young, the owner of the Marigold Garden nightclub in Chicago, offered a new show to Hoffmann and "the bulk of the Shubert unit." A news story about the deal refers to her dancers as "16 Tiller Girls," confusing them with another all-girl dance troupe. The story promises that the new act will have "a lot of surprises," including "nude pictures on the order of Ali Ben Haggin tableaux."[73] That would be Ben Ali Haggin, who painted, costumed, and designed "living pictures" for the *Ziegfeld Follies*. Notably, the promised nudity is no longer Hoffmann's, but that of her young female dancers.

Vaudeville was becoming a mode of performance and not just a venue. As big-time vaudeville theaters struggled to compete, performers found work in Hollywood, but also in revues and nightclubs. *Hello Everybody* played the Marigold Garden for six weeks to great success. Hoffmann's change of venue was trendsetting: "The outlying places of amusement where dining and dancing is the rule are offering big vaudeville attractions," according to the *New York Clipper*, and Irene Castle was said to be the next on tap for a stint in the cabarets.[74] The end of Shubert Advanced Vaudeville was in a sense the end of Hoffmann's career as a vaudeville star as well. When *Hello Everybody* moved to the Marigold Garden, the show changed. The acts where she was front and center were pruned to make way for her "romping girls."[75] They were featured in old favorites such as the "sleigh bells" and "bathing" numbers. A new number called "Up in the Air" would earn the dance troupe, dubbed the "Gertrude Hoffmann Girls" a place in the *Ziegfeld Follies* that fall. Gertrude Hoffmann was retreating from the spotlight.

Part V

Offstage, 1923–1966

Chapter 15

✦

The Gertrude Hoffmann Girls, at Home and Abroad

A turning point came in 1923. That year, Gertrude Hoffmann wrote of herself, "[She] began to neglect her personal stage career unnecessarily . . . she continued to be expressed through her girls."[1] For most of her life, Hoffmann had focused on honing her solo performance. Now her energy was rerouted into training large groups of young women and devising work for them. Hoffmann performed a handful of times in the years to come, at benefits and in nightclub acts. Her "personal stage career," though, had ended.

"Her girls" were part of her dance troupe, the Gertrude Hoffmann Girls. Hoffmann followed in the footsteps of many solo female performers who then founded dance troupes such as Isadora Duncan, Loie Fuller, and Ruth St. Denis. Hoffmann taught them, choreographed routines for them, toured with them, and loaned them out to other shows. She worked with them in the United States and Europe from the end of Advanced Vaudeville to the beginning of World War II.

She tried to secure an act for these girls on the roof of the Shuberts' Century Theatre in the summer of 1923. In a lengthy telegram to Lee Shubert, Hoffmann described her plans for an evening's entertainment that would rival the Folies Bergère and the Moulin Rouge.[2] Shubert received her plans with enthusiasm: he replied the following day, saying he knew she was "capable of giving colorful entertainment to the public" and that the Shuberts "would be interested in doing business."[3] The proposed collaboration did not pan out that summer: Lee was sick with tonsillitis in late May and J. J. was focused on their new *Passing Show* production.[4] Since her summer plans fell through, she rested in Freeport, Long Island.

A quaint seaside village that was at the same time accessible from Manhattan, Freeport served much the same purpose in the early twentieth century that the Hamptons do today. The town was a popular off-season spot for vaudeville entertainers.[5] According to Fred Allen, "The stars first established summer homes at Freeport, and then the smalltimers precipitated a real-estate boom."[6] Freeport was home to an organization called the LIGHTS Club, which stood for "Long Island Good Hearted Thespian Society."[7] In 1916, the LIGHTS Club opened a clubhouse for show-business types; they also fielded a baseball team and a polo club.[8] Since vaudeville performers were nearly always on the road in December, they hosted Christmas on the Fourth of July.[9] Max Hoffmann was a charter member of the LIGHTS Club, and Gertrude appeared in their benefit performances.[10]

This Long Island village provided the wandering Hoffmanns with a sense of community. They rented out their Sea Gate home and bought land in Freeport in 1921.[11] By the summer of 1923, they had moved in to their "big roomy home with plenty of ground around it," which included an old barn and an apple orchard.[12] The family called it "the farm."[13] Max Hoffmann opened a music school a few blocks from the Freeport Long Island Railroad stop.[14] He called for the village to found a boys' drum and bugle corps; music lessons would take place in their barn, and prep-school graduate Max Jr. would teach the military drills.[15]

Gertrude Hoffmann followed suit by opening a Freeport dance conservatory, though not as soon as anticipated. A local newspaper announced the groundbreaking for her studio in October 1923.[16] "At the present time," the story notes, "she is staging some ensemble numbers for the Ziegfeld Follies and eighteen of her pupils are in the cast."[17] Hoffmann had choreographed and performed in revues for more than a decade, and by 1923 the revue format was wildly popular.[18] She knew how to assemble one of its vital elements: a graceful group of young women.[19] Over the next years, the Gertrude Hoffmann Girls epitomized the modern American girl, both in their stage shows and in their offstage publicity. They were young, athletic, wholesome, and white.[20] Their stage shows shaped the understanding of Americanness and femininity throughout the 1920s.

The Gertrude Hoffmann Girls made their debut in the *Ziegfeld Follies of 1923*. They performed aerial acrobatics in a number called "Webbing," seen in figure 15.1. Twelve ropes were lowered from rigging near the front of the stage. Hoffmann Girls ascended the ropes until they formed three rows. Suspended by one foot, upside down, and sideways, they moved through a bevy of patterns, sometimes holding on to one rope and sometimes to two. The number ended with the girls swinging out over the audience.[21]

Their act was a hit: the *Follies* dance director Ned Wayburn was "jealous" of the Hoffmann Girls' reception.[22] Hoffmann's diary references some conspiracy between Wayburn and a few stagehands that may have resulted in the webbing number being cut for time at one point.[23] Wayburn and Hoffmann had butted heads for nearly two decades, so this claim seems credible. Their dispute was short-lived, though, since the Hoffmann Girls were invited to perform their act abroad. Hoffmann gloated that her girls were "the only ones sought for London."[24] Throughout her career she had borrowed from Europe, but now European shows wanted her work.

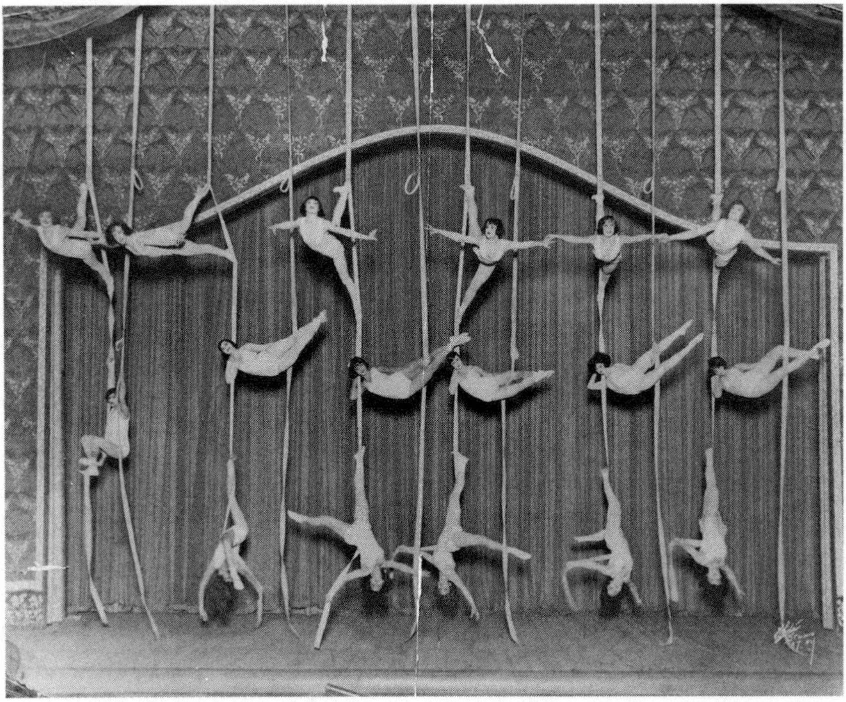

FIGURE 15.1. The Gertrude Hoffmann Girls in their "Webbing" number from the *Ziegfeld Follies of 1923*. Max and Gertrude Hoffmann Photograph Collection, Special Collections and University Archives, Wake Forest University, Winston-Salem, N.C.

In 1924 the Hoffmann Girls performed in a revue called *Leap Year* at the London Hippodrome. The music hall comedian George Robey played the lead. *Variety* reported that their act was altered due to its initial indecency: "The Lord Chamberlain" was said to have "notified the management of the Hippodrome to place more clothes on the dance troupe," and to have insisted they "modify their wiggling splits and contortions."[25] They were the "outstanding hit" of the show, even if this was so because reviewers admired their legs more than their gymnastics.[26]

Hoffmann attended Christian Science services while they were abroad. She was in London at the same time as Miss Juliet (Juliet Delf), a fellow American vaudeville performer and follower of Mary Baker Eddy. In a letter to one of the former Hoffmann Girls in 1951, Hoffmann reminisces about venting to Juliet as they drove home: "We were the hit of London, but here was I complaining—When she let me out, Juliet let me have it good, she roared like a lion and said, 'Gertrude Hoffmann, you had better start each day to count your blessings and every minute be grateful to God for all good.'"[27] She admired Delf's fierce optimism and tried her best to practice it.

Gertrude Hoffmann returned to New York City on August 12, but she did not stay home for long. The Hoffmann Girls secured an even more noteworthy European booking. Fire had destroyed the Moulin Rouge music hall in February 1915.[28] When it reopened in December 1924, they were featured in the "semi-American revue" called "New York Montmartre."[29] The Paris edition of the *New York Herald* described the swiftness of the routines, joking that the Hoffmann Girls "whizz through their astounding act at a relative rate of speed calculated to make George M. Cohan call for Mr. Einstein's help."[30] Carrying on the style of Hoffmann's solo shows, the Hoffmann Girls impressed the crowds with their variety and stamina. The *Herald* review continues: "At the end of Act I seven of the eighteen vie with each other in a dance competition offering all the best features of buck and wing, jazz and toe dancing. It stopped the show on the first night—and with due cause."[31] This review highlights the balance between the individual and the group that played out over the course of their routines. In some numbers, they worked together to create a stage picture. In others, they showed off their skills as dancers, competing for applause.

The Gertrude Hoffmann Girls developed a performance style unique to all-girl dance troupes of the period. Athleticism was important, but so was personality. This sets them apart from the chorus of Ziegfeld girls who were "matched, like pearls."[32] The Tiller Girls were similarly dependent on uniformity. In his famous essay "The Mass Ornament," the German cultural critic Siegfried Kracauer sees the Tiller Girls as "girl clusters" or as sets of body parts, but never as individuals.[33] When the Gertrude Hoffmann Girls returned to the United States, a Shubert press release highlighted this difference: "The Gertrude Hoffmann troupe is the first to rebel against the machine-like, precisional type of dancing that Tiller made so famous. The audiences of Paris, London and New York have gotten tired watching the rhythmic lifting and falling of legs, always in time and to the beat like piston rods."[34] With their rhythmic regularity, the Tiller Girls were out of step with Jazz Age dancing, while the Hoffmann Girls worked against the mechanical rhythm through syncopation. The surrealist poet Paul Éluard extended this idea into his art. He began his poem "Les Gertrude Hoffmann Girls" with a stanza listing all their first names. Names alone comprise the first three lines; the fourth describes Florence as "toute nue" (in the nude), then lists the remaining three girls' names. These lines are written in perfect alexandrines, the classical French poetic line with six two-beat phrases, a pause, and six more two-beat phrases. The Gertrude Hoffmann Girls could be unique and at the same time fit into a larger pattern.

Dance critics responded to the Hoffmann Girls with measured enthusiasm. They recognized the troupe's representativeness—both of American identity and of modern life—but they could not quite acknowledge their work as art.

The dance critic André Levinson wrote an essay (translated and published in *Theatre Arts* in August 1928) that credited the troupe with bringing the chorus to the forefront of the Paris revue.[35] He notes that the Hoffmann Girls "stylize exercise," but then insists that this stylization of sport is not the same as dance.[36] The Hoffmann Girls extend the imitative work of their mentor into the realm of group performance. Levinson calls their fencing numbers "imitation"; the same was true of solo dances that mimicked animals such as leopards and peacocks. Hoffmann continued to be expressed through her girls because they combined commercial dance and imitations, her two specialties.

When the Hoffmann Girls played a vaudeville engagement at the Scala Theatre in Berlin in 1925, critics echoed the French association between feminine sportiness and American identity.[37] Karl von Wiegand, a newspaper correspondent who wrote about Weimar Germany for American audiences, notes that the "eighteen dancing, prancing Gertrude Hoffman girls" have been warmly received, both by audiences and by German intellectuals. They have been met with both "approving applause" and "long and weighty essays in newspapers." Wiegand observes that the most American things about the Hoffmann Girls are their slender figures. This description of their body type, along with the one critique that they are "not quite erotic enough in their manner" suggests that they follow the pattern of desexualization that critics have noted as a part of German Girlkultur.[38] Earlier all-girl dance troupes featured curvy, substantial women (like the British Blondes or the French revue dancers of the Moulin Rouge), but these dancers had streamlined, adolescent bodies.

The Hoffmann Girls moved through European capitals, embodying a modern way of living.[39] According to Wiegand, Berlin women tried to emulate them by wearing the sporty American fashions. He describes an interesting displacement: German women are "stepping out in flapper costume designed for pert little college girls in the tall grass regions of those United States."[40] While male critics may have disavowed the sexuality of the Hoffmann Girls, female audience members took great pleasure in the new image of femininity that they saw represented onstage.[41] They wanted to try it on for themselves.

The Gertrude Hoffmann Girls epitomized America when they performed in Europe. When they returned home, they booked a spot in a Winter Garden show that leveraged their European pedigree. The Shuberts staged two previous *Artists and Models* revues.[42] They followed this success with *Artists and Models* 1925, which was dubbed "the Paris edition." What was particularly Parisian about this revue? The "Incomparable" Hoffmann Girls, who were billed on the first page of the program as "Direct from a Year at the Moulin Rouge, Paris, and a Year at the Hippodrome, London."[43] The theater critic Percy Hammond cheered on the Hoffmann Girls and the Shubert brothers in a nationalistic stretch of his review. The Hoffmann Girls had been "making Paris really and truly Parisian" when they played there, he wrote.[44] Now "they are in a better show in the Winter Garden than they were when I saw them not long ago, in the American county fair proceedings at the Moulin

Rouge."[45] American girls could produce "Parisianness" better than their Gallic counterparts, it would seem, but when French producers tried to represent America the results were amateurish.

Broadway audiences were eager to see the bohemian lifestyle represented onstage: the first *Artists and Models* revue developed from performances put on in Greenwich Village. But they wanted to see this nominally European spectacle produced by Americans with an American cast.[46] American girls who came into contact with France were more appealing because they could be seen as both titillating and wholesome. *Artists and Models* 1925 was full of scenes in which women were objectified; in perhaps the most egregious example, the chorus girls who had long been known as "chickens" were turned on a human rotisserie over an open flame.[47]

Offstage, the Hoffmann Girls served as moral exemplars. They were, according to one newspaper article, "a new model in chorus girls."[48] They did not drink, smoke, stay out late, or date men they met at the stage door. Gertrude Hoffmann encouraged them to channel their energy and ambition into their careers, putting off marriage until their character developed. She was their choreographer, producer, and den mother.

Once they returned to New York City, she took on another role in an official capacity—dance teacher. In their nonperforming hours, members of the dance troupe trained with Hoffmann and with William J. Hermann, a "physical director, gymnast, acrobat, club swinger and swordsman."[49] While associated with Hermann, Hoffmann visited circuses for inspiration. At Playland amusement park in Westchester County, New York, Hoffmann tried to interview the acrobat and aerialist Tiny Kline. Kline respected Hermann's work, but she resented Hoffmann's intrusive questions: "She sought the know-how so she might copy my act. The very cheek of her!" she wrote.[50] Ivan Tarasoff, a former member of Diaghilev's Ballets Russes company, joined Hoffmann's faculty soon after.[51] An ad proclaimed Hoffmann, Hermann, and Tarasoff "recognized leaders in their respective arts," who "have formed the dance's strongest teaching triumvirate."[52] By the mid-1920s, New York City dance teachers recognized the demand for training in a variety of performance styles.[53] In addition to "Stage Dancing" and ballet, their studio offered classes in "Producing," "Acrobatics," and "Fencing."[54] They offered at least one acting class as well.[55]

On her American Ballet tour of 1921, Hoffmann sought new pupils through classes she taught in the morning. Pupils who were quick at picking up the steps may have been asked to sign a contract. To find more dancers in 1926, she was more direct. A classified ad in the *New York Daily News* requested that "good looking, shapely girls age 16 to 20" visit her studio for possible casting in "future Gertrude Hoffmann troupes at home and abroad."[56] Interested parties were asked to "apply with bathing suits" and to make their application "to Gertrude Hoffmann personally."[57] It is likely that this caveat was made to assure prospective Hoffmann Girls of the job's legitimacy.

While some Hoffmann Girls performed in *Artists and Models*, others filled in the choruses of Shubert shows around town. Gertrude Hoffmann provided eighteen additional dancers to J. J. Shubert for $1,500 per week.[58] In the fall of 1925, her dancers performed in the companies of *Big Boy* (an Al Jolson vehicle) and *Gay Paree*.[59] By the end of the year, she had hired and trained an additional troupe of performers for another Shubert revue, *A Night in Paris*.[60] The show played in the Casino de Paris on the roof of the Century Theatre. Nine years before, that roof garden theater had been called the Cocoanut Grove; Gertrude Hoffmann performed there in *Dance and Grow Thin*. Norma Terris was featured in *A Night in Paris*, giving "Impressions of Broadway Stars" and singing the song "Fascinating Lady."[61] Instead of the original eighteen Gertrude Hoffmann Girls, this show featured thirty-six. A program played on their European association, calling them "Les Reines [Queens] de Paris."[62] A second troupe of Hoffmann Girls traveled to Paris in June 1926, sailing for Paris on the S.S. *Hamburg*.[63] They came back in July, ready to perform in *A Night in Paris* when it moved to Broadway. Hoffmann's dancers seemed to need a European tour before they could provide spicy revue numbers to a Broadway audience.

Gertrude Hoffmann had other things to focus on. Her mother, who had been living with Gertrude and Max in Freeport, died of pneumonia at the age of seventy-four.[64] The funeral was held at the Church of the Ascension on the Upper West Side of Manhattan, presumably Catherine Hay's home parish since it was near a previous address. Margaret, the oldest sister with whom Catherine Hay kept in close contact, was traveling in Europe when her mother passed away. Gertrude Hoffmann's brother George and sister Rose, along with Rose's husband Robert, were present.[65] As the youngest in her family, Gertrude was the last to spend time in her mother's house in San Francisco. She remembered sitting on a stool at the age of six or so, listening to her mother talk to her friends about money, the "change of life," men.[66] Did they discuss the ways women dealt with death?

Catherine Hay never worked in the theater, but she made Gertrude Hoffmann's life imaginable. Hay sewed costumes for variety performers, introducing her daughter to the work that went into making a show spectacular. With her oversight of the young Kitty's house cleaning, she instilled a thoroughness and attention to detail. According to a letter that Gertrude sent to a former Hoffmann girl, Catherine raised her children to be tolerant: "I never (thank God) heard anything of nationalities or religions spoken of in our house. And so when I left home to go out into the world, I was free."[67] Whether Catherine Hay's open-mindedness was intrinsic or in response to the discrimination she felt as a divorcée, she passed it on to her daughter.

While Hoffmann recovered from her mother's death, she went on teaching and staging dances. Working with the Shuberts became a family affair. Max Hoffmann Jr. was cast in *Gay Paree* (1926), a Winter Garden production starring Sophie Tucker and Chic Sale. Max Sr. took on the role of musical director for the next "international revue" put on by the Shuberts. *A Night in Spain* starred several performers of note, including the future Stooge Shemp Howard and the Betty Boop inspiration Helen Kane.[68] As in *Artists and Models*, Norma Terris had a featured number. Terris would not remain family for long: she and Max Jr. soon divorced.

In *Night in Spain*, the Gertrude Hoffmann Girls shared the stage with the Allan K. Foster Girls. Although her troupe may have diminished in importance, Hoffmann's profile was elevated. For *Artists and Models*, she had only been given credit for the dances in which the Hoffmann Girls appeared.[69] For *A Night in Spain*, though, she shared credit as choreographer for the whole show.[70] The Hoffmann Girls pursued the kind of dance that interested their choreographer—athletic, sometimes sexy and sometimes funny, always imitative. They took up her work as a transatlantic embodiment of modern American womanhood. Hoffmann dancers found work both at home (in touring Shubert productions) and abroad (in a London revue called *Shake Your Feet*). They transmitted Gertrude Hoffmann's work in both directions, communicating Americanness to Europe and Europeanness to America.

By the late 1920s, all-girl dance troupes were a dime a dozen. *Murray Anderson's Almanac* of 1929 included a dance number with a mouthful of a title: "Tiller, Foster, Hoffman, Hale and Albertina Rasch."[71] This number featured one representative "girl" from each of these dance troupes. But by the time Anderson's show opened, Hoffmann had retreated from touring. She returned to life in Freeport, where she lay low for the next few years. Her local newspaper advertised that the promised dance studio would open on April 6, 1929.[72]

Chapter 16

Modern Dance and Floor Shows

By 1929, Gertrude and Max Hoffmann were both living and teaching in Freeport. Her dance studio, like Max's conservatory, was within walking distance of the Freeport Long Island Railroad stop. She taught children, women who wished to limber up and lose weight, as well as "Business Girls desiring to go on the stage."[1] One anecdote even suggests that Hoffmann's work with kids in Freeport inspired the plot of the Rodgers and Hart musical *Babes in Arms*.[2] The Long Island actors' colony full of out-of-work vaudevillians and their children was the avowed inspiration for the musical's setting.[3] She worked within the same paradigm as that show, trying to strike a balance between highlighting the freshness of her performers and developing (and even commodifying) their talent.[4]

Gertrude lost another family member in 1930, her brother George.[5] George Hay worked with Gertrude on and off throughout her vaudeville career. He helped her with costume changes as early as 1911 and served as her stage manager in 1914. Hay lived on Long Island near his brother-in-law and sister and was present when their mother died. George also passed away at the Hoffmann home on South Bayview Avenue. Reverend John O'Toole led a requiem mass in his memory at the local Catholic Church, Our Holy Redeemer. She stayed in touch with her two sisters who lived nearby: Rose, who was married, and Margaret, a single bookkeeper.

Throughout the 1930s, Hoffmann joined the call to promote American dance as an art. In 1930, the dancer Margaret Severn founded a combination studio-dormitory-employment bureau called the Dancers' Club. Their stationery called it a "business and social headquarters for professional dancers, teachers, and students."[6] Gertrude Hoffmann was among the founding members, as were the leading lights of ballet and modern dance. Severn also seems to have looked to Hoffmann's curriculum as an inspiration for her own. An issue of the *Dancers' Club News* announced a new fencing class.[7] Severn danced in Keith–Albee vaudeville houses in New York City at the same time the Hoffmann Girls performed their fencing act in *Artists and Models*, so it is likely that she would have associated this training with Hoffmann.[8]

Because she no longer toured, Gertrude Hoffmann had more free time to attend the performances of other dancers. She was particularly interested in the development of modern concert dance. In her diary, Hoffmann records the transition of the choreographer and performer Doris Humphrey. She wrote off Humphrey's early performances as "Nearly Duncan-Amateur, chasing butterflies and veils." Humphrey (or "Humphries" as Hoffmann repeatedly wrote) moved quickly in her estimation: "6 months later—modern dance."[9] Hoffmann may be compressing her timeline here, but the assessment stands. Humphrey performed a scarf dance with the Denishawn Group in the earlier years of her career; once she broke with Ruth St. Denis and Ted Shawn, her choreography developed in abstract, innovative directions.[10]

Hoffmann sought out writings on modern dance in this period as well, haunting the one shop that stocked books from European choreographers. She wrote that Charles Weidman, Humphrey's longtime collaborator, was a regular at this bookshop as well. She held the German choreographers Rudolph Laban and Mary Wigman in particular esteem, writing that Germany was the "beginning of Modern Dance I think in World, copied here + added to by [Martha] Graham + Doris + Charles."[11]

Mary Wigman's first tour of the United States evoked intense reaction among dancers and enthusiasts in New York City.[12] Wigman inspired Hoffmann to craft and perform a solo dance piece, something she had not done for a decade. The dance was a direct parody of Wigman, drawing on Hoffmann's mimicry skills, which were even rustier. John Martin described "a battery of percussion instruments" accompanying Wigman's debut, which included "drums, gongs, cymbals, tom-toms, gamelon."[13] Hoffmann scored her response with a wood block, tympani, and gongs, but also a ratchet and a siren. Wigman was known for dances rooted in gestures that expressed intense emotional states.[14] The comedy of Hoffmann's piece comes from forcing the audience to read her gestures as literally as possible. A bird whistle was followed by the annotation, "She listens"; she scratched her leg to the noise of sandpaper.[15] At the end of the dance, she followed a pattern of repetition and variation. She held up one finger to the sound of a gong, walked for ten counts, and repeated this pairing of gesture and music. Then she mimed rowing for eight beats and did sit-ups for another eight. This exercise was followed by a whine; when she held her finger again, the sound that ended the piece was not a gong but a fart.[16] Hoffmann's dance succeeded because it maintained Wigman's style while reversing all of her principles. She thus contributed to the "domestication of Wigman" that took place in American dance circles during the 1930s.[17] Any of the externalized emotion central to Expressionism was stripped away, and the tension and release came in the form of physical exercise. The highbrow was brought low with rude humor.

For the first time since the *Saison des Ballets Russes* tour, Hoffmann combined her love of cutting-edge dance performance with her skill as a physical comedian. Her performance was part of a benefit for the Dancers' Club that took place in December 1932. The "Monster Dance Performance" was given on a Sunday evening. It featured forty-six dance acts, with performers ranging from Ruth St. Denis and her temple dancers to the tap dance master Bill Robinson.[18]

Curiously, Hoffmann's appearance on the program is not listed as a Wigman parody. She follows performance #41, a dance by Rosamund Birchby titled "Eastern Idols (authentic)."[19] Birchby was accompanied by several Indian musicians playing sitar, tabla, and the like. Hoffmann's performance titled "Satyrical" is listed as #41a, suggesting that it should be read as a direct response to Birchby's. (This numbering also shows how Hoffmann's parody was still being framed as secondary, not creative work in its own right.) Nevertheless, John Martin singled out Hoffmann's "masterly burlesque of Mary Wigman" in his review of the benefit for the next day's *New York Times*. She was overwhelmed by this review and sent a telegram to express her thanks: "COMING FROM AMERICAS FOREMOST CRITIC OF THE DANCE IT MEANS EVERYTHING I AM DEEPLY GRATEFUL."[20] Hoffmann resented the harsh dismissals that had come from the New York theater critic George Jean Nathan during her solo career. The critics who most appreciated her work then wrote in Chicago and points farther west. Martin's appreciation was in a sense her moment of critical redemption.

Hoffmann looked for girls for a "new theatrical production" as early as October 1932.[21] With his review of her benefit performance, John Martin validated her desire to recommence producing and performing. But vaudeville bookings had dried up. Even the Palace Theatre changed its program, alternating mixed bills of vaudeville and a feature film with bills of movies alone.[22] In 1933 she got back to work, developing dances that could serve as movie prologues. That spring, a new group of Gertrude Hoffmann Girls danced in the prefilm programs at midtown Manhattan movie theaters.

The United States was in the depths of the Great Depression. How did the Hoffmann Girls play differently in this new economic era? The cultural critic Siegfried Kracauer said that the precision dancers in Weimar Germany performed a phantom optimism, dancing as if they still believed in "never-ending prosperity."[23] Like the chorus girls wearing coins and singing "We're in the Money" in Busby Berkeley's *Gold Diggers of 1933*, the Hoffmann Girls embodied wish fulfillment. They helped remind New Yorkers of the immediate past when the economy had flourished and pleasure reigned.

An ad in *Variety* celebrated the Hoffmann Girls' success and promised that Hoffmann herself was preparing a return to the stage to "do her well-known imitations and dances."[24] This did not come to pass. The Hoffmann Girls played to mixed reviews that shared one central theme: their work was far different from that of the synchronized dancers who typically preceded feature films. Eugene Burr at *Billboard* called their work "difficult and beautifully executed," saying that it was "a welcome relief from Broadway's overabundance of precision units."[25] A *Variety* review of their work at the RKO Roxy

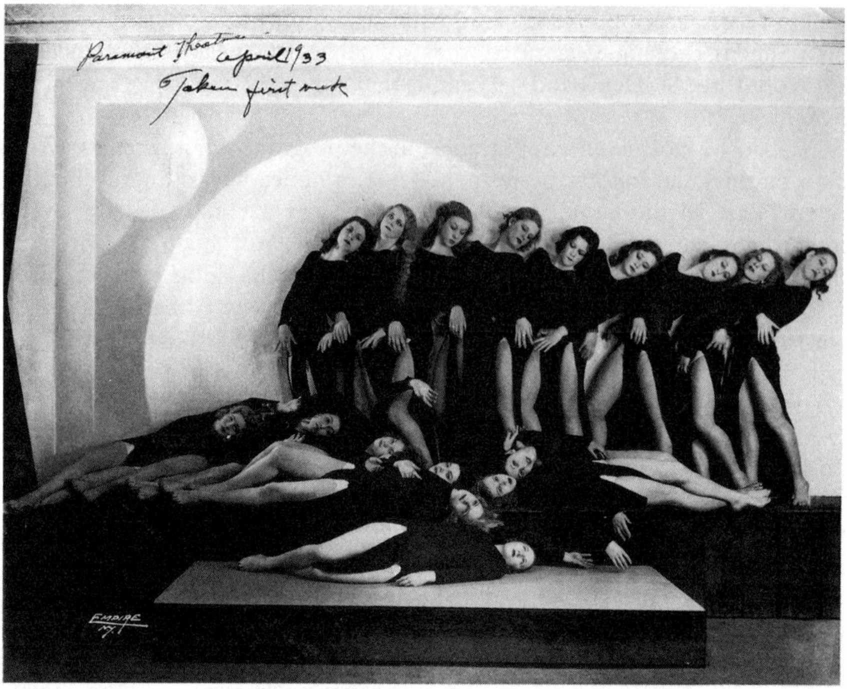

FIGURE 16.1. The Gertrude Hoffmann Girls in a number from the 1930s, likely "Over the Waves." Max and Gertrude Hoffmann Photograph Collection, Special Collections and University Archives, Wake Forest University, Winston-Salem, N.C.

compares them to the house's precision dance group the Roxyettes—now known as the Rockettes.[26] The Hoffmann Girls complicated the critical understanding of the all-girl dance troupe phenomenon then, as they do now.

With the spring performances of the Hoffmann Girls, we can see the new influences on Hoffmann's work. Their May 12 show at the RKO Roxy included a number called "Over the Waves." The *Variety* reviewer "Char" found it to be "a very odd routine, but staged and lighted effectively, with [the] idea of girls being under water forcefully limned."[27] Between this description and Hoffmann's avowed interest in Doris Humphrey, this dance seems to respond to Humphrey's 1928 dance *Water Study*.[28] She may also have been drawing on the asymmetrical choreography of Albertina Rasch, whose work in *The Band Wagon* recently made a big splash.[29] In figure 16.1, nearly half the company lies on the floor in uneven arrangement, with their tipped heads and elongated legs set off against the black of their dresses. The other dancers stand, to the right of center, with their torsos and heads tilted to the right. The Hoffmann Girls were never precision dancers, but this picture is nonetheless striking for its languid irregularity. Imitation had always been Hoffmann's artistic modus operandi, and this image suggests her new subject for mimicry was modern dance.

While Gertrude Hoffmann worked with her dancers, Max Hoffmann Jr. continued to rebel against his parent's longtime union. He married the vaudevillian Thelma White in 1930 and divorced her in 1932. White was best known for her appearance in the anti-marijuana camp classic film *Reefer Madness* (1936). Helen Kane became the third Mrs. Max Hoffmann Jr. in 1933. That summer, they both starred in a musical called *Shady Lady*, with Max Sr. as music director. "The heat and the show's mediocrity" kept audiences away.[30] It closed after thirty performances.[31] That marriage was equally brief, ending in 1935. His marriage to Luana Walters, a Hollywood actress known for her roles in Westerns, lasted longer: they were married in 1936 and remained so until Max Hoffmann Jr.'s untimely death in 1945.

After a few months in movie theaters, the Gertrude Hoffmann Girls found a more permanent venue: the Paramount Grill, a restaurant and nightclub in the basement of midtown Manhattan's Paramount Hotel. Their floor show opened October 19, 1933.[32] Hoffmann had produced and performed in Chicago's nightclubs before, but here she faced a changed entertainment landscape. Burlesque houses had opened on Forty-Second Street.[33] Gertrude Hoffmann's name was no longer synonymous with the daring and risqué: patrons were warned in the Paramount Grill *Variety* review that Hoffmann Girls "don't go in for nudity."[34] The older Hoffmann Girls routines were nevertheless well-received when performed by this new crop of dancers. The "Webbing" routine was called "perhaps the first real novelty to show up in the night club field in a long while," and their fencing act was deemed an "old favorite."[35] Their warm reception at the Paramount Grill again highlights the differences between precision dance work and the work of this troupe. While precision dance is presentational and frontally directed, the Hoffmann Girls' work seemed to be more successful in an immersive environment.

A promotional picture, seen in figure 16.2, shows them in the same costumes they wore on movie theater stages, long-sleeved dark dresses with modest necklines and high slits. This type of dress seems to be what Kate Elswit calls an "artifact of dance spectatorship," one that shows how commercial dance makers watched modern dance and translated its practices into the realm of the nightclub revue.[36] The dresses are severe and plain, though still revealing—Martha Graham meets femme fatale. In fact, the Hoffmann Girls are dressed similarly to Fanny Brice in her 1936 Follies dance parody "Modernistic Moe."[37] Their costumes sketched a kind of generic dance modernism, one that is carried on into the 1950s with the *White Christmas* number "Choreography." In this promotional photo the Hoffmann Girls are unsmiling, each contorting an arm so she can splay her fingers over her forehead. But here they are arranged symmetrically, showing their bare legs, with

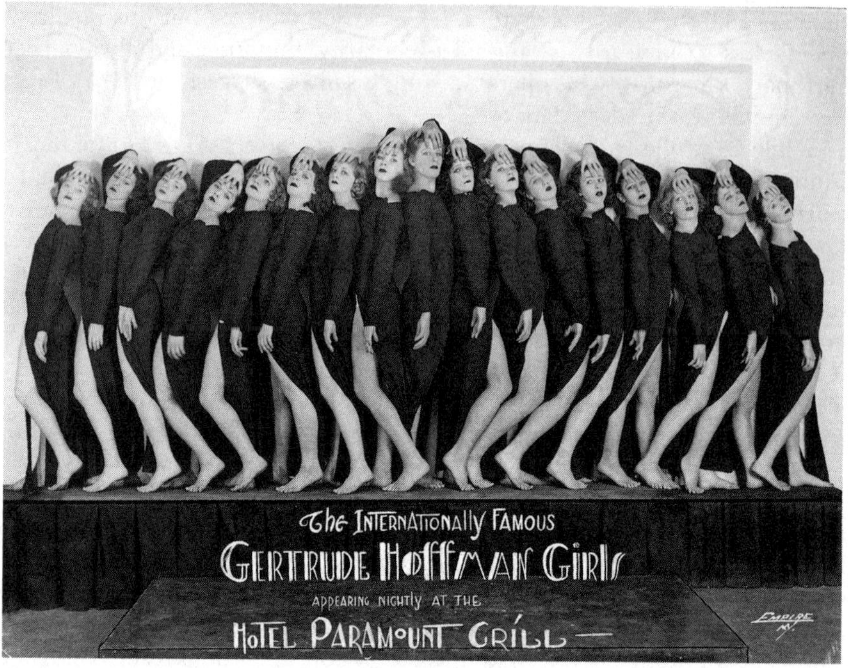
The Internationally Famous
Gertrude Hoffman Girls
Appearing Nightly at the
Hotel Paramount Grill —

FIGURE 16.2. The Gertrude Hoffmann Girls in a promotional photograph for their show at the Hotel Paramount Grill. Gertrude Hoffmann Collection—Brooklyn Public Library—Brooklyn Collection.

the tallest girl at the center. Taken as a whole, the photo presents a pastiche of modern and precision dance.

Late in their run at the Paramount Grill, Gertrude Hoffmann joined the act. She did not perform the imitations promised months earlier. Instead, she did a few ballroom dance numbers with a partner.[38] She wore a red gown and performed a rumba that "brings down the house (and brings in a half dozen baskets of flowers)."[39] Critics discussed her age and her long career. One columnist claimed that when she received her bouquets on opening night, she fainted.[40] Hoffmann's dancing was still up to par, but her appearance also drew on the burgeoning nostalgia for vaudeville's golden age.

Prohibition was repealed on December 5, 1933. Hoffmann did not stick around at the American nightclubs; instead, she parlayed success at the Paramount Grill into another international booking. On February 1, 1934, she signed a contract for the group to perform at the Municipal Casino in Cannes.[41] Gertrude and Max Hoffmann and a troupe of Gertrude Hoffmann Girls sailed for France. Many of Hoffmann's dance studio pupils from Freeport joined this tour; while they were traveling, they abided by the same "boarding school rules" that Hoffmann insisted upon for her dancers.[42] But

Hoffmann Girls could look fierce as well. When they arrived at Cannes, the dancers carried their own fencing equipment off the train. The theater owners met them at the station and "nearly passed out" at the sight of that many young women armed with sabers.[43]

Their reception in France was positive. Hoffmann's papers include several reviews in French written during this tour. One says that the Hoffmann Girls act helps the reviewer reconsider the power of music-hall performance.[44] Another impressed her so much that she had a portion of it translated. The section related to her work is bracketed and underlined in pencil, with the translation attached: "The creator who has composed this picture of an inflaming colour and movement and a strict and almost brutal class, is a genius."[45] The Hoffmann Girls stayed in Cannes for several months and then booked a summer gig at the Casino de Paris, co-headlining with the French comedienne Cécile Sorel.[46]

The Hoffmann Girls returned to the United States in August 1934. They performed for four weeks at the Michigan Theatre in Detroit. This was another house where vaudeville acts performed before a feature film. In their month in Detroit, the Hoffmann Girls shared the stage with the Bob Hope company and the Three Garland Sisters.[47] Frances, the youngest and most talented, would soon change her first name to Judy and sign a contract with MGM. The Hoffmann Girls failed to make the leap to film that their vaudeville costars managed. Hoffmann wanted the movies to be the next step: "We're waiting for the call to play in the picture 'Follies Bergere,'" she said.[48] Hoffmann traveled west to pursue this plan; a Parisian friend wished her a happy new year on a postcard mailed to a Hollywood address.[49]

The year 1935 was a tough one, full of opportunities that fizzled. The booker Alex Gerber signed up the eighteen Gertrude Hoffmann Girls for a South American tour that did not pan out.[50] They toured upstate, playing stage shows before feature films in Binghamton and Rome, New York.[51] The Castle Theatre in Long Beach, Long Island, attempted a straight vaudeville program over Labor Day weekend with the Hoffmann Girls among their featured acts. The weather failed to cooperate, and the actors netted "peanuts."[52] Hoffmann tried to cobble together work for her dance troupe, but venues were becoming scarcer and competition was fiercer.

Hoffmann rejected one obvious place to seek work. The Federal Theatre Project (FTP) was established in August 1935 as part of the Works Progress Administration.[53] The relief program included support for dancers; Doris Humphrey and Charles Weidman were among the modern dancers in Hoffmann's circle who contributed to the FTP's dance program.[54] Perhaps because she spent so much of her life on the popular stage, Gertrude Hoffmann wrote in her diaries that "subsidized theatre" was "no good."[55] She expressed her scorn in interviews as well, saying, "It makes the girls lazy. They can get these government jobs where they have to rehearse only a few hours a day. They stick to these jobs because they are sure and they don't learn anything about dancing. They won't take regular jobs even at higher salaries because they are afraid the jobs won't last."[56] Her distaste for the WPA reveals one of Hoffman's beliefs about how theater got made. Performing was always a social business, one in which she knew the impresarios funding her work and could banter and bargain with them face to face. The WPA took away the personal touch.

Though wary of federal charity, Hoffmann continued to volunteer with organizations that sought to broaden the reach of dance. She cosigned a letter calling for a Dance Congress and Festival to support the variety of dance arts being practiced in the United States.[57] The weeklong series of performances and conversations brought together practitioners of folk dance, modern dance, and commercial dance on the theater and variety stages. Hoffmann was scheduled to perform as a part of the Sunday night program, but she canceled at the last minute.[58]

She went back to work for the Shubert brothers in the summer of 1936. For the previous few years, J. J. Shubert had staged summer productions of their operettas at outdoor concert venues.[59] He brought *Blossom Time* and *The Student Prince* to Jones Beach on Long Island. Hoffmann choreographed the ballets that ran with both shows.[60] Jones Beach Stadium held 10,000 people, making this the largest venue by far where Hoffmann staged dances. Her contributions played well, adding "a welcome note of color and movement" to the insubstantial operettas.[61]

That fall, Hoffmann returned to a familiar city. She choreographed the floor show for the College Inn, the restaurant in the Hotel Sherman. *Variety* reported how many former vaudeville acts were booked in Chicago nightclubs that season. The College Inn Show for October 1936 "reads like a regular variety bill of 1926," the article noted.[62] Vaudevillians could still find places to perform before a live audience, but their acts were seen as old-fashioned, out of date.

Ironically, this was an era during which Hoffmann's choreography was most innovative. Her dances and viewing practices suggest that she had developed an interest in modern dance of the black diaspora. As part of the College Inn floor show in 1937, the Hoffmann Girls performed dances inspired by Harlem and the Bahamas.[63] In spite of her distaste for subsidized theater, Hoffmann loved *Bassa Moona*, a dance opera that was produced by the Federal Theatre Project and directed by the Nigerian immigrant Momodu Johnson.[64] The dances in *Bassa Moona* were framed by the narrative of a royal wedding and they each had a designated cultural meaning—"dances of sacrifice, worship, martial prowess, and possession."[65] A story in the African American newspaper the *New York Age* described her response: "Gertrude Hoffman, one of the greatest exponents of interpretative dancing, witnessed a performance of 'Bassa Moona,' the African dance drama now playing and the WPA Negro Theatre, and stated, 'The dancers in this show gave the greatest interpretation of rhythmic dancing, with no instruments except the tom-toms, that I have ever seen."[66] Her interest in African diasporic dance continued into the 1940s, when she attended a matinee performance by Katherine Dunham's company.[67]

Gertrude Hoffmann returned to New York City for another nightclub job. The International Casino opened in Times Square in fall 1937.[68] The restaurant and theater seated 2,500 people and occupied a full city block of Broadway—from West Forty-Fourth to West Forty-Fifth Street.[69] The Hoffmann Girls performed with the International Casino floor show for the next two years. In this era, Hoffmann worked with Clifford C. Fischer, a booking agent and producer of revues. The International Casino closed in January 1939, but Fischer and Hoffmann kept working together. She contracted to provide twelve Hoffmann Girls for what he called "Folies Bergere of 1939" and what *Variety* called a "vaudfilm tour."[70] This show combined two types of performance that were central to the Hoffman Girls oeuvre: the Parisian-style nightclub show and the vaudeville movie prologue. The work done by the Hoffmann Girls throughout the 1920s and 1930s shows just how flexible the revue format was, and just how many different types of venues booked revue-style shows. Critics have discussed the "vaudeville aesthetic" in radio, film, and television.[71] Hoffmann's work in this period suggests that historians of performance ought to pay more attention to how this aesthetic evolved for dancers, especially all-girl dance troupes. The Hoffmann Girls demonstrated that revue acts could transfer to a cabaret or a preshow performance on a movie theater stage.

While the Hoffmanns still lived in Freeport, one thing changed in their village. The LIGHTS Clubhouse, a central gathering place for the vaudevillians who had long been a part of the town, burned down on February 9, 1939. Only one fireman was injured, and the unnamed *Nassau Daily Review* reporter engaged in a flight of fancy, describing the blaze in terms of its showmanship: "The old building, deserted for many years, staged a spectacular last performance such as would have delighted the hearts of the theatre folk whose laughter once rang through its halls. There was a capacity audience, an arresting show, the fountain and even fireworks, which popped and boomed as the flames ignited them. The last act mystified police and firemen, who had not known that there was anything of that nature stored in the place."[72] Although it was long deserted, the clubhouse managed to perform a last show worthy of its past. One of the biggest celebrations held there was Christmas on the Fourth of July. This fire reversed that, setting off fireworks in midwinter.

The Hoffmanns took one more trip abroad to join a London revue, in spite of looming war. The Hoffmann Girls were booked for *The Crazy Show*, with Max Hoffmann as the music director. They sailed to London on August 8, 1939, and played previews at the Hippodrome in Brighton at the end of the month.[73] Hitler invaded Poland on September 1, and England's prime minister Neville Chamberlain declared war on Germany on September 3. Although the Hoffmann Girls were supposed to play in the London show through the end of the year, they sailed home from Southampton a week and a half later.[74] It would be the last trip abroad for both Max and Gertrude Hoffmann.

Chapter 17

✦

Remembering

When Gertrude Hoffmann returned to New York in the fall of 1939, she went back to teaching dance at her Manhattan studio. She also reverted to one of her oldest creative habits—celebrity imitation. Her diaries from this period brim with comic monologues in the voices of then-popular stage and screen actresses. Three films released in late 1939 seem to have rekindled Hoffmann's desire to imitate. Bette Davis starred in *The Private Lives of Elizabeth and Essex*, Greta Garbo in *Ninotchka*, and Marlene Dietrich in *Destry Rides Again*. These films marked a resurgence of powerful and interesting divas, figures so iconic that they were worth parodying. She wrote parodies that joked about the frequency with which actresses played Elizabeth I, as well as Garbo and Dietrich's world-weariness.[1]

These parodies also helped Hoffmann imagine alternate paths that her career might have taken. A draft script offers the following lead-in to her imitations: "I'd love to act in a drama / They never give me a chance / And the only way that I can act in one / Is to imitate somebody else."[2] To make matters worse, there was an actress named Gertrude W. Hoffmann who *did* play parts in Hollywood dramas during this era. A German émigré, she became best known as the next-door neighbor on the television show *My Little Margie*. The archival traces that Hoffmann left of her viewing practices and imagined performances in this era show a woman who felt disappointed by the arc of her career.

Her diaries from late 1939 and 1940 suggest she was still thinking about the dancers she watched as source material for reproduction. Their steps may have inspired dance combinations taught in her studio classes; the costumes, drawn with color and fabric choice noted, may have helped her costume the Hoffmann Girls with whom she still worked. Hoffmann's notes often included the few alterations that she would make in the dances she watched—a different bit of business with a costume, or a striking pose that should have been held for an additional beat.[3] Perhaps this was simply a personal diary that put to use her remarkable memory for production design and choreography.

Even before the United States entered World War II, the war in Europe influenced Hoffmann's imagined performances. She clipped a newspaper article about Europe's fashionable café society, which "because of the exigencies of war" had recently "been forced to move en masse to New York."[4] These are not pitiful exiles, though: they entertain themselves in swanky restaurants and nightclubs on the Upper East Side of Manhattan. The war-era café society inspired her script for a "one woman fashion show."[5] While some of the types parodied in this sketch could be New York society women from any period, others are glamor girls whose lives reveal the impact of war and displacement. An "Oriental Jitter Bug from the Streets of Cairo" wears finger cymbals that are "a military secret," while a "fashion girl that dotes on lace and lingerie" waltzes alone, "dreaming of her bombadier [*sic*] in the air corps of the U.S.A."[6] The last figure in this sketch "was a Can Can dancer at the Moulin Rouge in Paris."[7] The narration goes into further detail: "I met her there some years ago—She is now a refugee and we met again in New York recently."[8] A later journal includes notes for a cabaret show with a nostalgic French theme: lyrics to "The Last Time I Saw Paris" and "Place Pigalle" sit beside the names of the characteristically Parisian performers Maurice Chevalier and Sarah Bernhardt.[9] Paris was a formative city in Hoffmann's career, so it is easy to imagine her emotional connection. Journals from this period still focus on her work, so any response to the war can only be intuited through her plans for performance.

In the spring of 1940, Gertrude Hoffmann's Manhattan dance studio was on the same block of West Fifty-Sixth Street as her apartment; it was also around the corner from Carnegie Hall. Eleanor King, a dancer in the Humphrey–Weidman group, found Hoffmann's studio to be a "dependable place for work."[10] This was especially true compared to the Ruth St. Denis studio where King had studied; there, her barre work took place in a cluttered space, where the floor was covered in cracker crumbs and parakeet feathers.[11] The English choreographer Anthony Tudor taught classes at Hoffmann's studio as well.[12] Hoffmann still taught her own classes there, chiefly ballet and stage dance if her notes for in-class routines are good evidence. Here as in other parts of her career, her taste and the ways she facilitated the sharing of other dancers' work had a greater influence than did her own practice.

Dorothy Bird, a performer who moved between Broadway, ballet, and modern dance, shared several stories about her work with Gertrude Hoffmann. One anecdote shows the rivalry between Hoffmann and Agnes de Mille. The two women had known each other for a decade through their work for the Dancers' Club, and even before that de Mille had taken classes with Hoffmann's former Russian ballet partner Theodore Kosloff.[13] "In response to a request by Agnes de Mille," Bird writes, "I started teaching a Graham class in Gertrude Hoffman's studio. Everyone was curious about Martha's work, since she never allowed outsiders into her studio."[14] Bird describes a moment when she was trying to explain details of the floor work, and de Mille asked her to hurry on to the next steps; as a choreographer looking for inspiration, she presumably wanted an overview of all the characteristic movements in

Graham's dances. "Meanwhile," she writes, "Gertrude Hoffman was frantically signaling to me, 'Don't let Agnes tell you what to do!'"[15] Hoffmann may have wanted to assert her right to run the class in her studio as she wished, but it is likely that she was also watching the demonstration in the mindset of a dance teacher who wanted pupils to learn how to do the steps. De Mille of course choreographed *Oklahoma!* only a few years after this exchange.[16] The women valued different parts of the dance. Hoffmann felt that de Mille had highbrow ambitions but was not an especially good technical dancer.[17] Hoffmann suspected that de Mille thought her dancing and her studio were both too commercial. This feeling bears out in the brief mention of Hoffmann in *Dance to the Piper*, the first volume of Agnes de Mille's autobiography. There, Hoffmann is described as "an enterprising American, who saw the value of beating the Russians to New York with their own ballets."[18] Hoffmann's talent, to de Mille, is entrepreneurial and not artistic.

Hoffmann's studio helped her pursue both her aesthetic and commercial ambitions. In the era when burlesque was on the rise, she often found nightclub jobs for her pupils. Dorothy Bird accepted an offer from Hoffmann for a booking in a West Coast nightclub but backed out when she found out that she would have to dance topless.[19] Hoffmann responded, "Why not? Are you ashamed? You have nothing to be ashamed about. You have beautiful breasts!"[20] Her comfort with the nude female form persisted. She made notes for striptease routines that riffed on Gypsy Rose Lee and *The Mikado*.[21] She sketched a stripper's costume that include a net bra covered in fringe and wrote next to it, "fringe flys [*sic*] up, shows breasts, showy for turns [and] bends, *effective*."[22] In 1952 *Billboard* notes that the dancer Gaby de Lys has moved from "niteries and musicals" to "burly strip," with Hoffmann's help.[23] A later article describes de Lys using "a bare-feet ballerina technique" during her striptease.[24] Hoffmann's aesthetic plays out in de Lys's act.

Dance was gaining cultural value as an all-American art form.[25] In February 1942, the Museum of the City of New York mounted an exhibition called *Dancing through Two Centuries, 1740–1940*.[26] The display of dance's long history in New York City included artifacts from the Museum of Modern Art's dance archives. Narratives about dance's development in New York City saw the arrival of Russian dance as a turning point, so Hoffmann's Russian ballet production made an appearance among the playbills and photographs. Critics disagreed about its prominence within the exhibit: Walter Terry found that there was "quite enough material" on Gertrude Hoffmann, while John Martin said the program for the *Saison des Ballets Russes* was hidden in a corner.[27]

Hoffmann recognized the ways American dance history was being narrated and wished to contribute to the story being told. She outlined and wrote narration for a ballet on the life of Michel Fokine.[28] Her imagined ballet begins with a scene "ala Petrouchka": parents take their children to audition for the imperial ballet school, performing peasant dances to communicate their excitement and rustic background. This scene was meant to illustrate "how ballet dancing began from folk dancing."[29] She incorporated several important stages of the Russian ballet's development, from Léon Bakst meeting Diaghilev and other painters and composers, to the arrival of Isadora Duncan in St. Petersburg, to Diaghilev moving his troupe to Paris.[30] In this period, Hoffmann is invested in telling the history of performance through performance.[31] Though her notes are sparse, they suggest her understanding of the ways that dance changes over time, both in terms of style and technique and in terms of the kinds of stories that a medium is best equipped to tell. She had always been drawn to Fokine's ballets, and she reached a point in her career where she felt the power of retrospective storytelling as a means of claiming an artist's legacy. Hoffmann ended her notes on the Fokine ballet with the assertion that "He Lives On."[32]

Her notes for this work in progress suggest that she was in regular contact with Fokine's wife and partner Vera Fokina. When she wonders which dancers and choreographers were trained as part of the Imperial Ballet, she writes, "Fokina should know."[33] Her notes about the later chapters in Fokine's life emphasize his stage successes with his wife, such as their Metropolitan Opera performance produced by Sol Hurok. She also imagines Fokina as Fokine's connection to his past: "In private life he carried on the customs of Imperialist Russia, Fokina his Czarina."[34] The rhyme is cheeky, and it leaves the power dynamics of the relationship ambiguous: Is Fokine the czar who rules as an equal or a subject bound to obey her? She may have been drawn to their longtime partnership and collaboration since it mirrored her work with Max.

Michel Fokine and Hoffmann's former manager and coproducer Morris Gest died within months of one another in 1942. Morris Gest was described in his obituary as a "showman in the grand manner" who produced expensive, over-the-top theatrical spectacles that often lost a great deal of money.[35] His management of Hoffmann during her "Salome" days was mentioned as an early success that legitimated his taste and authority. Hoffmann's acts of copying appeared in Fokine's obituary as well: "Although Fokine did not cross the Atlantic himself," it reads, it was "Gertrude Hoffmann, who presented the Fokine ballets 'Les Sylphides,' 'Schéhérazade,' and 'Cléopâtre' here in the Summer" of 1911.[36] This narrative highlights how dance moved across the Atlantic in the 1900s and 1910s, often floating free of the composers and performers who created it. Hoffmann remained fiercely proud of bringing the Russian ballet productions to the United States. The coverage of Fokine's life and death likely reinforced her belief that this would be her lasting contribution to the history of dance.

Max Hoffmann was also reckoning with his creative past. He reconnected with Raymond Hubbell, a fellow composer with whom he had worked more than forty years earlier in Chicago.[37] A new film called *My Gal Sal* was coming out, written by Theodore Dreiser about his brother Paul Dresser who was the most popular songwriter of the 1890s. Hubbell and Hoffmann had both worked with Dresser in his heyday. The following year, Max contacted his congressional representative to inquire about a list of his copyrights.[38] His congressman was Sol Bloom, himself a former songwriter and sheet music salesman with a connection to the Chicago music industry in the Gay Nineties. Copyright had always been a fraught issue for Max and Gertrude: they claimed it when they were being copied, but they also pushed back against its limits when their imitations succeeded.

American theatrical culture was deep in the throes of nostalgia during the mid-1940s.[39] The critic David Hasbany sees a "nostalgic sensibility" at work in the shows of this period, one that helped audiences escape the stress of contemporary life in the same way they did during the later nostalgia boom of the late 1960s and 1970s.[40] Max Hoffmann played a small role in this wartime look backward: he returned to the Broadway theater pit, playing violin in the orchestra for *Oklahoma!* and filling in as conductor.[41] *Variety* and local newspapers published columns listing what had played in theaters that week in past decades; Gertrude Hoffmann often made an appearance in these columns, and she clipped and scrapbooked references to her earlier triumphs.[42]

In this atmosphere, Gertrude Hoffmann planned her comeback act, a stage show that would demonstrate her skills as a dancer and comedian as well as her long history in the entertainment business. The program varied in different drafts, but it always included dances and celebrity imitations. Hoffmann imagined returning to dances that were part of her vaudeville repertoire, works by Isadora Duncan and Maud Allan.[43] She also added new acts that she had never performed in public, such as an imitation of Carmelita Maracci, who synthesized ballet and Spanish dance.[44] She planned to send up stage and screen stars including Ethel Merman, Mae West, and Gertrude Lawrence.[45] Her papers include listings of the outfits she would need for each turn, along with estimated costs for hiring the necessary backup dancers and musicians.[46] In her book *Moving Performances*, Jeanne Scheper considers how the divas of the twentieth-century stage tried to shape their own public reception and reputation.[47] Hoffmann engaged in similar practices of self-archiving by rewriting and reorganizing her comeback act. Her retrospective performance is in one sense her attempt to craft an archive.

A *Variety* article on her planned show was front-page news in August 1944. She shared column inches with stories about Tokyo Rose and Dwight Eisenhower, along with coverage of Mae West's newest stage vehicle *Catherine Was Great*.[48] Details in the Hoffmann story suggest how far her plans were from coming to fruition: "She has readied a routine with a girl ensemble background which at present runs four and one-half hours. Aware that the turn is much over-time, Miss Hoffman says she cannot cut anything out because 'it's all too good.'"[49] She no longer had to hone her act with the shrewd editorial eye of a vaudeville performer. Notes from another notebook suggest she tried to edit the program by shortening the length of the dances she performed.[50] This performance took on too much symbolic weight: it needed to show off her greatest hits and prove that she kept up with the new trends. She could not make a cut.

Hoffmann never performed her comeback show, though she kept writing and revising it through the end of the decade. It is what the theater scholar Pannill Camp calls a "performance nonevent."[51] The imagined retrospective that exists in bits and pieces from the mid-1930s to the late 1940s fits into Hoffmann's long history of revue performances. As early as her 1910 act, Hoffmann was thinking about the pressures of celebrity and the ways that imitations must change over time in her before-and-after number, "It Isn't That Way Anymore." She wanted to revive this structure in her 1940s act, imagining "former stars" as they appeared both "long ago and now."[52] One of these stars was Ethel Barrymore, whom Hoffmann imitated in 1910. She wanted to do a comic bit in which the commanding actress sang a popular song of the swing era, "I'm Stepping Out with a Memory Tonight."[53] Nearly three decades before Stephen Sondheim's *Follies*, Gertrude Hoffmann imagined staging work that juxtaposed women stars in the present with their younger, more glamorous selves.

After his divorce from Helen Kane in 1935, Max Hoffmann Jr. worked in Hollywood, mostly playing uncredited roles in westerns and gangster films. He returned to stage performance during World War II. Like his parents, Max Hoffmann Jr. was well-received in Chicago: in April 1942, an old-fashioned farce called *Good Night Ladies* opened at the Blackstone Theatre, with Hoffmann in a supporting role.[54] He stayed with that show for nearly three years: it played for more than one hundred weeks in Chicago and then transferred to New York, where it closed on March 24, 1945.[55] Max Hoffmann Jr. was found dead in a hotel room a week later.[56]

Good Night Ladies had transferred to Boston, where Hoffmann and his wife Luana Walters were due to appear. Newspaper accounts report that Walters "found him in a state of collapse," and stated that Max Jr. "had been suffering from a stomach ailment."[57] The Hoffmanns received heartfelt condolence letters about their loss. An old friend from their days in Virginia reminisced about Max Jr.'s birth in Norfolk.[58] Reina Gest, who lost her husband Morris a few years earlier, wrote a letter in which she empathized with their heartbreak.[59] A note from Gertrude's friend Ann Cary was addressed to Max Sr. alone. It discussed his mourning in relation to Christian Science principles and ended with the injunction, "Do not malpractice on yourself."[60] According to the beliefs of Christian Science (which it is not clear Max followed), he could have been engaging in emotional negligence by blaming himself for his son's death, or perhaps wishing that he had been the one to die instead. By 1945, Gertrude Hoffmann was committed to the tenets of Christian Science. Her papers notably lack any of her thoughts about her son's death. Any personal archive will have gaps, of course, but perhaps this one should be read through her beliefs. Mourning the loss of your son's physical life would contradict the idea that all of God's creation is perfect. Putting those feelings into words would be a form of "error" that Christian Scientists sought to avoid.

Max Hoffmann Jr. followed his parents' lead: replacing his mother's drafted dance partners, learning violin like his father, even performing in a song-and-dance act with his first wife. He arguably superseded his parents in fame since he appeared in movies, something that Gertrude Hoffmann wished to do but never achieved for herself. But he never found stability in his private life to counteract the ups and downs of celebrity. Max Hoffmann Jr.'s four marriages stand in stark contrast to his parents' sixty-year union. His parents kept working after their son's death: Max Sr. in the *Oklahoma!* pit, Gertrude at her dance studio. The show went on.

World War II ended, and the city that had been the Hoffmanns' home for the past forty years started to transform. Industries relocated to the suburbs, and so did white, middle-class New Yorkers.[61] Midtown Manhattan underwent as much construction in the postwar era as it had at the turn of the twentieth century. Instead of the subway, now Times Square saw the rise of sleek, modern office buildings.[62] New York City was coming into its own as a metropolis that represented a new kind of modernity, one associated with new kinds of mass culture. The city no longer felt like home.

The Hoffmanns began to consider relocating to Los Angeles. Gertrude's sister Rose and brother-in-law Bob had moved to Sherman Oaks, a neighborhood in the San Fernando Valley, in 1942.[63] Charlotte Schley, the Hoffmanns' former next-door neighbor in Freeport and onetime secretary for the Hoffmann dance studio, had relocated to nearby Van Nuys. (Schley's daughters Helen and Frances had taken classes at the dancing school and performed with the Hoffmann Girls troupe in the 1930s.[64]) In 1948, Gertrude Hoffmann sent a Christmas card to her old friend Mary Jones in which she mentioned the possible move. Jones sent a quick reply to say she thought it was good idea.[65] She seemed confident that Hoffmann would find work in the movies and that Max could conduct orchestras recording motion picture soundtracks.[66]

Mary's son Starr West Jones expressed an interest in writing Gertrude Hoffmann's biography. Jones had served in the army during World War II, taken journalism courses on the GI Bill, and started writing for *Guideposts*, the inspirational magazine founded by Norman Vincent Peale.[67] His mother sent a letter of support in May 1951, asking Hoffmann to share her stories with him.[68] Mary's letter was followed a week later by a note from Starr Jones in which he requested a supper date and included samples of his writing.[69] Work on the memoir continued. A note from 1953 reads, "Carton marked 'BOOK' containing all foreign press notices and photos that may be used for the book 'Tales of Hoffmann.'"[70] Whether this book was to be written by Jones or by Hoffmann herself is unclear.

She had not been feeling well. The letter from Mary Jones mentions a "physical handicap" that "has come to [her]," but in good Christian Science fashion it denies that handicap any power over her friend.[71] Later that year,

Hoffmann was struck by another blow. Her sister Rose died on November 25 in her Sherman Oaks home.[72] She was Gertrude's closest sibling in age, and the one with whom she shared the experience of early auditions and performances. (Later, George and Margaret became more central to her life and work.) Though Rose and Bob had lived in Los Angeles since the 1940s, they had kept in touch with affectionate holiday cards.[73] Rose left half ownership of the house to her sister, and Bob welcomed the Hoffmanns to move in with him.[74]

A move to Los Angeles seemed imminent. The Hoffmanns began to downsize, selling the land surrounding their Freeport house and putting their collected costumes and music in storage.[75] A letter from 1953 suggests further progress: Gertrude Hoffmann asked lots of questions about Los Angeles in a letter to her friend Charlotte Schley—where they could swim, what it would take to buy a car, how close Van Nuys was to Hollywood. In her response Schley assures her that Van Nuys is "like Freeport—only larger" and that she and her daughter will do their best to help the Hoffmanns adjust.[76] Nothing came of it until nearly a decade later.

That year Hoffmann's old rival Eva Tanguay was the subject of an undistinguished biopic, *The I Don't Care Girl*, starring Mitzi Gaynor as the mercurial performer.[77] Another former vaudevillian, George Jessel, produced and starred in it.[78] Hoffmann writes in an earlier journal about the ways that *The Great Ziegfeld* got Florenz Ziegfeld's character wrong. "Most movies . . . always give the leading character the opposite of what they are," she muses.[79] But in the 1950s, nostalgic musicals and biopics were constructing the public history of vaudeville—a history in which she very much wanted to be included. The media historian George C. Custen sees in the six films that Jessel produced the creation of a mythology "that vaudeville was the only legitimate form of entertainment, and that the era of vaudeville was a privileged, halcyon time."[80] With Hoffmann already in a nostalgic, retrospective mode, this romantic vision of the past must have been compelling.

Their next move took the Hoffmanns the length of a city block, from their apartment to the Great Northern Hotel. Gertrude Hoffmann was seventy years old, and Max was eighty-two. Living in a hotel room, they could depend on the staff for meal preparation and cleaning duties. Gertrude Hoffmann kept a careful list of the hotel staff and their jobs, likely so she could remember their names and tip them at Christmas. Next to the name of a bell captain named Russel she notes, "carried me up"![81] Max still had some pull on Broadway; he got tickets for friends to see *Pipe Dream*, a Rodgers and Hammerstein musical based on the John Steinbeck novel *Cannery Row*.[82] They had sold their Freeport house by this time; the son of a former Hoffmann girl remembers hearing that his mother picked them up from the hotel and drove them to Jones Beach for an outing.[83]

As a result of her professional life, Gertrude Hoffmann was a night owl. At the Great Northern Hotel, she liked to stay up on Tuesdays until 11:00 P.M.

to watch a local talk show called *Night Beat*.[84] Mike Wallace, who did not yet have a national audience, would interview newsworthy figures of the day, many of whom came from Broadway. One episode featured Ben Gazzara, who had recently played Brick in *Cat on a Hot Tin Roof*. Gazzara trained with Lee Strasberg at the Actors Studio; his discussion of method acting led Hoffmann to think about old and new techniques: "He [i.e., Gazzara] told that if a new actor asks why this or why that concerning acting that the old timer will answer O you people—why do you ask such ?'s."[85] She responded to Gazzara's dismissals: "Well the old timer had learned his trade through long experience, all these so-called emotional reactions came to the fore as he went on carrying a spear or Richelieu's train or suping in a mob scene."[86] The "he" applied to the theoretical old-timer is disingenuous, since all these examples of "his" long experience are taken from Hoffmann's days as a supernumerary in San Francisco. Hoffmann had mixed feelings about the Actors Studio "method" as she understood it. She doubted the idea that one's understanding of a character must be rooted in personal experience. Her performance as Salome was a success, she wrote, regardless of the fact that her "mother was not a Herodias."[87] She did express appreciation for one Actors Studio principle: "The one thing they go after & do is to strip the person of all self-consciousness [and] fear of criticism—Yes—I believe that is called for as a natural move."[88] She must have looked at the Actors Studio through a dual lens, as a stage performer and teacher who reckoned with strategies for getting the best performance out of her students.

She paid close attention to the representation of vaudeville on television and in movies of the day. On another *Night Beat* episode, Wallace interviewed Rosie Dolly, half of the Jazz Age singing and dancing duo The Dolly Sisters. (Rosie's sister Jenny had died by suicide in 1941.) Hoffmann responded incredulously to Rosie's cavalier discussion of the wealth and world travel that were part of her life. "Rose tossed off 65,000.00 as tho she had always been accustomed to millions. . . . I wondered why she did not give the 65,000.00 towards the education of girls striving for a place in the theater or to any real cause which might help probable Dolly Sisters."[89] This lament echoes Hoffmann's long-ago wish to start a dancing school for girls who could not otherwise afford to take lessons. Hoffmann herself could have done so much, the diary entry suggests, with the money the Dolly Sisters frittered away in gambling losses and jewelry. To be fair, it should be noted that Rosie Dolly spent much of her later life and her fortune supporting Hungarian children.[90] This interview must have shocked Hoffmann because it failed to acknowledge her role in the sisters' success: she was, after all, the first person to give them a job.[91] George Jessel produced a movie about the sisters in 1947, and that too had glossed over the role Hoffmann played in making them stars.

A biopic of Elsie Janis was in the works in summer 1959.[92] She was another vaudeville star whose path had crossed with the Hoffmanns. When a teenaged Janis made her Wistaria Grove Roof debut in 1905, Gertrude Hoffmann was the venue's dance director and Max its music director. Hoffmann copied out the beginning of news report on *The Elsie Janis Story*, following it with a question: "Write your idea? To Doris Day. Her husband is [the movie producer] Martin Melcher."[93] She had two connections to the Hollywood power couple: they were friendly with Charlotte Greenwood, who warmly remembered the Hoffmanns from her days in New York City, and Melcher was an avid Christian Scientist.[94] That fall, *Pillow Talk* opened and Day, paired with Rock Hudson, became a megastar.

Around the same time, Hoffmann used a letter to sketch out the idea of a biopic based on her life. "Dear Lucille Ball," it begins, "Would you be interested in doing a film of another's life experience in the theatre world."[95] With this letter, as with much of the work from the last twenty years of her life, Hoffmann is both trying to write herself into this theatrical past and to ensure that she will survive beyond it.

It was not a bad idea. At that time, Desilu Studios was seeking solo projects for Ball, and they were looking at types of stories similar to the one Hoffmann tells. A memo suggests that Lucille Ball might wish to play Fanny Brice, the prohibition-era nightclub hostess Texas Guinan, or Gladys Hurlbut, a stock theater performer.[96] Hoffmann identifies a shared theatrical language that connects the two women, one of pantomime and comic imitation. She writes, "Your panto with Red Skelton also Bullfight gave me the idea to try interesting you to do me."[97] Hoffmann identifies these two moments of vaudeville-style performance in the *Lucy-Desi Comedy Hour*: she imitates Skelton in his pantomime of eating a meal as the "Freddy the Freeloader" character during the "Lucy Goes to Alaska" episode from 1959. She performs as a matador in the "Lucy Goes to Mexico" episode from 1958. These two performances are themselves reminiscences and repetitions of previous performances—the "bullfight dance" on *I Love Lucy* and the pairing of Skelton and Ball in the 1943 MGM musical *Du Barry Was a Lady*. Both of these doubled moments in Ball's career are moments of imitation and physical comedy. The humor arises from her skill in mimicking the movements—of a matador, of a sad clown—and the ways those movements mismatch what we are expecting from the body of either a glamorous movie star or a hapless housewife.

The second page of this letter to Lucille Ball is written in pencil on a paper napkin, as if to further emphasize its ephemerality. It is here that Hoffmann attempts to articulate what is unique about her career. She writes: "Imitations—musical—dramatic—satire—dance—burlesques I did a bit of everything. Contrast and versatility was a big part of my success."[98] This description explains why Gertrude Hoffmann's life did not fit into the framework of 1950s celebrity and storytelling. Lucille Ball may have done "a bit of everything" herself—starting as a showgirl, playing vamps in Hollywood B movies, and making a huge hit as a TV star. Ball remains a star, remains *Lucy* because fans perceive a consistent personality beneath the changes.

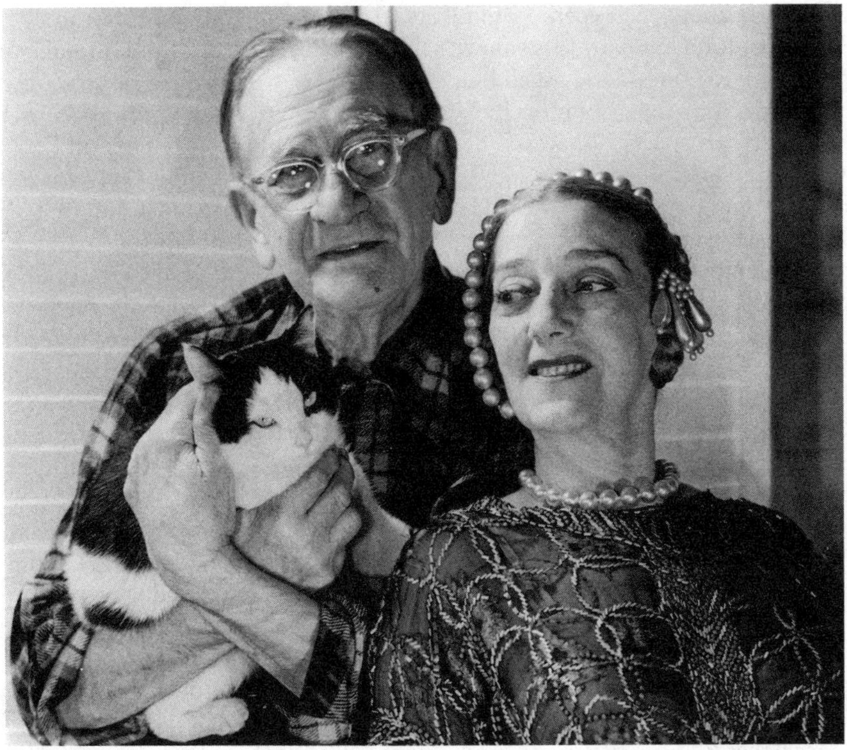

FIGURE 17.1. Max and Gertrude Hoffmann with a cat. Max and Gertrude Hoffmann Photograph Collection, Special Collections and University Archives, Wake Forest University, Winston-Salem, N.C.

The Hoffmanns finally moved west in 1961. They rented an apartment in Hollywood. It was near a park, and a short walk from movie palaces on Hollywood Boulevard like the Egyptian and El Capitan. A Christian Science church stood less than a mile away. They got a pet, a black and white cat that seemed to have a particular affection for Max. The living space in their tiny apartment was dominated by a television. In figure 17.1, Max looks his nearly ninety years. Gertrude is younger, in her seventies, and she keeps up her appearance with makeup, jewelry, and a beaded dress. She strikes a theatrical pose, with her body turned to the right and her head to the left.

Max longed to return to New York City and go back to work. In August 1962, he wrote J.J. Shubert (in a labored, shaky hand), offering his services as a musician or arranger and enclosing a self-addressed, stamped envelope so they could mail him a railroad ticket.[99] Gertrude broke her hip a month later; though she had several insurance policies to pay for medical costs, she was still concerned about the expense and joked, "Think I will vote for Medicare."[100] She wrote John Shubert, J.J.'s son who had taken over the day-to-day management of the business, and asked him to confirm her employment history if the insurance company got in touch. Gertrude's letter was more optimistic about her career prospects out west: she said she was "writing sketches and acts to sell to television and films."[101] Max eventually moved to the Convalescent Hospital and Home for the Retired twelve miles away in Encino, California.[102] There, he died of a heart attack on May 21, 1963.[103] His obituary in *Variety* described him as the "musical director for the Shuberts' shows in New York for years"; it also mentioned his work with the *Ziegfeld Follies* and his songwriting career.[104] "Surviving," it concluded, "is his wife, former dancer Gertrude Hoffman."[105] He and Gertrude had been married for more than sixty years.

How did Gertrude Hoffmann fill her days without Max? She must have kept up her correspondence; when the *Dance Magazine* writer John Dougherty obtained a grant to write a book on Adolph Bolm, he got in touch with her at the Hollywood address.[106] Perhaps she followed the rise of Barbra Streisand: her ascent to superstardom playing vaudevillian Fanny Brice in *Funny Girl* was covered extensively in the *Los Angeles Times* throughout 1964. Hoffmann may have written more about her life in San Francisco during her last years, but she dated her journals inconsistently. Her sister Margaret moved in.

Whether she went to a Reading Room or listened to a radio show on the topic, Hoffmann almost certainly kept up with the lesson-sermons of the Christian Science church. The weekly selections from the King James Bible and Mary Baker Eddy's *Science and Health with Key to the Scriptures* are published in the *Christian Science Quarterly*. Followers read and meditate on those passages in relation to the topic, one of twenty-six rotating themes chosen by Eddy as central themes of Christian Science.[107] "Probation After Death" was the theme for the lesson-sermon on Sunday October 23, 1966. For Christian Scientists, the probation that people went through was a daily testing of their beliefs; the idea of a final judgment was an error, since it artificially separated life from death. The passages to be read that week asked Christian Scientists to trust in God and to move beyond an understanding rooted in the material world.[108] Gertrude Hoffmann died of a heart attack on Friday, October 21, 1966. One hopes those passages gave her some comfort in her final days.

A few trade papers reported her death, and some of their information was dismissive of her achievements or flat-out wrong. The *Variety* obituary called her "a leading dancer of the 1920s," missing the mark by a decade or two.[109] *Dance News* dated Hoffmann's borrowed Ballets Russes opening four months late.[110] *Variety* mentions her controversial performance as Salome: "It was then considered daring even to dance barefoot."[111] In the age of the go-go dancer, this description places her squarely in another era. Gertrude Hoffmann wanted to bring her life to the movie screen at the time when vaudeville was mythologized, but she died when the signifiers of her life were being recovered as camp.

Her obituaries consider Hoffmann's impact on American ballet to varying degrees. In *Dance News*, she was called a "dancer, impresario, and, above all, [a] shrewd business woman."[112] This echoes Agnes de Mille's assessment of Hoffmann as "an enterprising American."[113] While the dance magazines found her business sense noteworthy, *Variety* felt the same about her dance training: "In her time she had some of the aura of a Martha Graham. Later she conducted a dance studio."[114] Her credentials as the producer of the first fully staged Ballets Russes performances in America are glossed over by *Variety*: it mentions that she "at one time had an act that specialized in Russian dances."[115] As might be expected, her borrowed Ballets Russes featured more prominently in her *Dance News* obituary. The piece discusses the lack of credit to Michel Fokine and her faulty crediting of Theodore Kosloff's role in *Schéhérazade* "as the Favorite Arab (sic!) of Zobeide."[116] That exclamatory "sic" feels flippant, seeming proof that she lacked knowledge about the Ballets Russes. Gertrude Hoffmann's taste at times outstripped her talent, but when *La Saison des Ballets Russes* opened in 1911, she was the American who knew the most about Diaghilev's ballets as *productions*: the choreography, the costumes, the set designs, the programs, and the history.

Gertrude Hoffmann never settled on one identity. On Max Hoffmann's death certificate, her listed occupation was "actress"; on her own death certificate, it was "dancer."[117]As the youngest child of a single mother, she could not afford to have a singular calling. She was multitalented and practical: if she could not perform, she directed dances; if she could not choreograph, she taught. Many performers and teachers, including Adolph Bolm and Michel Fokine, did the same thing. In this era, dance and vaudeville were interdependent. Hoffmann crossed back and forth between them, and in the end neither side knew quite where she belonged.

Conclusion

Gertrude Hoffmann personified American vaudeville at its height. She shifted the popular conception of what vaudeville was and did. She showed how dance and spectacle were unavoidably intertwined with other forms of modern variety performance. Her work carried on the tricks and the training of her apprenticeship even as it responded to emergent trends. She put the coterie audiences of transatlantic modernism in dialogue with the broader American public. Her critical reputation decentered New York City and highlighted the ways that reputations could be made on the road and on the West Coast as much as in the East. A vaudeville performer's skill set determined that performer's career in the longer term. After the variety theater ceased to be a viable form of public entertainment, stars with compelling, original personalities were able to make the move into film and (eventually) television.[1] Performers like Hoffmann who were best at planning large, spectacular numbers moved into working for revues and staging nightclub floor shows. This branch in the genealogy of vaudeville is less personality-driven and more collective, less comic but more dazzling.

This was an era when, as the historian Susan Glenn notes, "Theater mattered to women."[2] Gertrude Hoffmann's life paints a clear picture of the freedom and the restrictions that came with such a life. She was able to become an auteur, but only by plying a trade dismissed as mere spectacle. She worked her way up to stardom, but she also never got the respect she felt she deserved. She used costumes of otherness to claim freedom for herself onstage, but when offstage she insisted upon the privileges of Progressive Era white womanhood. Her life story reveals a female performer's career and archive in all its complexities.[3]

Gertrude Hoffmann's work embodies the nuanced and nonlinear relationship of performance to time and tradition.[4] A cover song can succeed where the original failed; cultural references to a book or movie can precede and shape interpretations of the artifact itself. Her production impersonations mark a key moment in the mediated modern era, after mass print culture pervaded American society but before broadcast media had done the same. Newspapers and magazines could popularize a scandalous dance happening elsewhere, but only live performance could bring it before the local audience.

Today, the imitation craze continues online.[5] Amateur videos re-create scenes from Hollywood films shot-for-shot with handmade props.[6] The comedian Celeste Barber copies celebrity selfies on Instagram, highlighting the discrepancies between their bodies (and wardrobes and houses and partners) and her own.[7] Hoffmann's biography helps contemporary audiences to see the long history and continued vitality of live performance as a site for imitation and reimagining. The critical response to her work in her own time also prefigures contemporary dialogue about cultural appropriation. Imitation is a form of transmission, an act of love and theft.

Biographers are mimics too, taking gestures and traces of another person and trying to bring them convincingly to life. So, I will end with my visit to her grave, imitating Alice Walker in search of Zora Neale Hurston perhaps, or Hermione Lee bringing a silk flower for Edith Wharton. I arrived at the cemetery and asked the attendant where to go. He dubiously asked if I was family; no, a writer, I said. Her remains were inaccessible, kept below the mausoleum level in an area where visitors were prohibited. I circled the small memorial park twice: even though I did not have the exact coordinates, I knew I had passed somewhere near her.

NOTES

In articles and advertisements, Gertrude Hoffmann's surname is spelled with a single *n* nearly as often as it is spelled with a double *n*. When her name appears in a source as "Gertrude Hoffman" I retain the variant spelling in quoted material. Unsigned newspaper articles are cited in full in the notes but are not included in the bibliography.

Introduction

1. "Person to Person (Tommy Armour; Moss Hart & Kitty Carlisle)," CBS, May 8, 1959, Paley Center for Media, https://www.paleycenter.org/collection/item/?q=murrow&p=5&item=T:07497.

2. Quotations and details in the rest of the paragraph are taken from Gertrude and Max Hoffmann, box 2, folder 21: Personal notebooks, Red notebook, Gertrude and Max Hoffmann Papers (MS 608), Z. Smith Reynolds Library Special Collections and Archives, Wake Forest University, Winston-Salem, N.C. (hereafter GMHP).

3. Ibid.

4. For a discussion of America's brand of theatrical populism, see Trav S.D, *No Applause—Just Throw Money: The Book That Made Vaudeville Famous* (New York: Faber and Faber, 2005), 274.

5. Barbara Naomi Cohen, "The Borrowed Art of Gertrude Hoffmann," *Dance Data* 2 (1977): 2–11; Susan A. Glenn, *Female Spectacle: The Theatrical Roots of Modern Feminism* (Cambridge, Mass.: Harvard University Press, 2000); Mary Simonson, *Body Knowledge: Performance, Intermediality, and American Entertainment at the Turn of the Twentieth Century* (Oxford: Oxford University Press, 2013), 33–36; Marlis Schweitzer, "The Salome Epidemic," in *The Oxford Handbook of Dance and Theater*, ed. Nadine George-Graves (Oxford: Oxford University Press, 2015), 890–921.

Chapter 1

1. Lawrence Estavan and Edmond McAdoo Gagey, eds., *Theatre Buildings: Part 1*, San Francisco Theatre Research 15 (San Francisco: Work Projects Administration, Northern California, 1940).

2. Gertrude and Max Hoffmann, box 2, folder 21: Personal notebooks, Red notebook, GMHP.

3. For a discussion of the sacralization of culture at the turn of the twentieth century, see Lawrence Levine, *Highbrow/Lowbrow: The Emergence of Cultural Hierarchy in America* (Cambridge, Mass.: Harvard University Press, 1990).

4. Julia A. Walker, *Expressionism and Modernism in the American Theatre: Bodies, Voices, Words* (Cambridge: Cambridge University Press, 2005), 90.

5. Estavan and Gagey, *Theatre Buildings: Part 1*.

6. *Twelfth Census of the United States, 1900*, under "Catherine G. Hayes," microfilm roll no. T623, RG 29, National Archives and Records Administration, Washington, D.C. Accessed through "1900 United States Federal Census," ancestry.com. Barbara Cohen-Stratyner, the first author to publish an article on Hoffmann, gives her birth year as 1886. Armond Fields gives the date as 1885. Barbara Cohen-Stratyner, "Hoffman, Gertrude (1886–1966)," *Routledge Encyclopedia of Modernism* (2016), https://www.rem.routledge.com/articles/hoffman-gertrude-1886-1966; Armond Fields, *Women Vaudeville Stars: Eighty Biographical Profiles* (Jefferson, N.C.: McFarland, 2012), 189.

7. U.S. Bureau of the Census. "Availability of 1890 Census," https://www.census.gov/history/www/genealogy/decennial_census_records/availability_of_1890_census.html.

8. See Mary Russo, "Aging and the Scandal of Anachronism," in *Figuring Age: Women, Bodies, Generations*, ed. Kathleen M. Woodward, Theories of Contemporary Culture (Bloomington: Indiana University Press, 1999), 20–33.

9. These include Fields, *Women Vaudeville Stars*; Anthony Slide, *The Encyclopedia of Vaudeville* (Jackson: University Press of Mississippi, 2012).

10. "Catharine Beecher," National Women's History Museum, https://www.womenshistory.org/education-resources/biographies/catharine-esther-beecher.

11. For a discussion of Delsarte's influence on American modern dance, see Elizabeth Kendall, *Where She Danced: The Birth of American Art-Dance* (Berkeley: University of California Press, 1979); Carrie J. Preston, *Modernism's Mythic Pose: Gender, Genre, Solo Performance* (Oxford: Oxford University Press, 2011); Walker, *Expressionism and Modernism*.

12. Gertrude and Max Hoffmann, box 2, folder 23: Performance Notes, GMHP.

13. Ibid.

14. Ibid.

15. Federal Writers Project of the Works Progress Administration, *San Francisco in the 1930s: The WPA Guide to the City by the Bay* (Berkeley: University of California Press, 2011), 177.

16. All the details in this paragraph are taken from Gertrude and Max Hoffmann, box 2, folder 21: Personal notebooks, Red notebook, GMHP.

17. David S. Shields, "Studio, Elite," Broadway Photographs, http://broadway.cas.sc.edu/content/studio-elite.

18. Gertrude and Max Hoffmann, box 2, folder 21: Personal notebooks, Red notebook, GMHP.

19. Amelia Ransome Neville, "Fin de Siecle," in *More San Francisco Memoirs 1852–1899: The Ripening Years*, ed. Malcolm E. Barker (San Francisco: Londonborn Publications, 1996), 289–93, 292.

20. Ian McIniss, email message to the author, July 19, 2016.

21. Edith Sparks, *Capital Intentions: Female Proprietors in San Francisco, 1850–1920* (Chapel Hill: University of North Carolina Press, 2006), 25.

22. Ibid.

23. "People's Palace Music Hall," advertisement, *San Francisco Call*, July 15, 1894.

24. Gertrude and Max Hoffmann, box 2, folder 21: Personal notebooks, Red notebook, GMHP.

25. Ibid.

26. Ibid.

27. "Mismated Couples," *San Francisco Call*, December 16, 1893.

28. *Twelfth Census of the United States, 1900*, under "Catherine G. Hayes." Accessed through ancestry.com.

29. Gertrude and Max Hoffmann, box 2, folder 21: Personal notebooks, Red notebook, GMHP.

30. "Female Help Wanted," *San Francisco Call*, May 8, 1895.

31. "From Convent to Salome," *Inter Ocean*, December 20, 1908.

32. Kendall, *Where She Danced*, 4, 6.

33. Ibid., 6.

34. "Old Favorites Are Welcomed," *San Francisco Call*, June 22, 1897.

35. Gertrude and Max Hoffmann, box 2, folder 21: Personal notebooks, Red notebook, GMHP.

36. Grace Kinglsey, "Rialto," *Los Angeles Daily Times*, March 14, 1916.

37. Gillian B. Anderson, "Synchronized Music: The Influence of Pantomime on Moving Pictures," *Music and the Moving Image* 8, no. 3 (2015): 3–39, 12.

38. Ashton Stevens, "Our Own Little Theatrical Monopoly," *San Francisco Call*, December 19, 1897, 36.

39. "A Love Story Embellished with Flitting Fairies Is the Delightful Feature of the Orpheum Pantomime," *San Francisco Call*, December 21, 1897, 14.

40. Gertrude Hoffmann, "Gertrude Hoffmann: Experiences and Credits," box 1, folder 1, Gertrude Hoffmann Collection, Brooklyn Public Library, Brooklyn Collection (hereafter GHC).

41. Jerome A. Hart, *In Our Second Century: From an Editor's Note-Book* (San Francisco: Pioneer Press, 1931), 425

42. James R. Smith, *San Francisco's Lost Landmarks* (Fresno, Calif.: Quill Driver Books, 2005), 108.

43. Alfred Metzger, "History of the Tivoli Opera House, 1879–1899," *Pacific Coast Musical Review*, September 25, 1915, 7.

44. "The Children's Hospital Matinee at the Orpheum," *San Francisco Call*, January 19, 1899; "Thespians' Munificent Gift of Gold," *San Francisco Call*, August 18, 1899.

45. Cover of Souvenir Programme Benefit given by the Columbia, Orpheum, California, Alcazar, Tivoli, Grand Opera House and the Chutes Theater for the Reception of the Returning United States Volunteers at the Orpehum Theater on Thursday, Aug. 17, 1899, Museum of Performance and Design, Performing Arts Library, Online Archive of California, http://oac.cdlib.org/ark:/13030/c8k935gc/?brand=oac4.

46. Gray Brechin, *Imperial San Francisco: Urban Power, Earthly Ruin, with a New Preface* (Berkeley: University of California Press, 2006), 133.

47. Bonnie M. Miller, *From Liberation to Conquest: The Visual and Popular Cultures of the Spanish-American War of 1898* (Amherst: University of Massachusetts Press, 2011), 111–12.

48. "Thespians' Munificent Gift of Gold."

49. "Myriads of Scintillating Lights Turn Night into Day as If by a Wizard's Wand," *San Francisco Call*, August 27, 1899, 2. Kirsten Silva Gruesz, "America," in *Keywords for American Cultural Studies*, ed. Bruce Burgett and Glenn Hendler, 21–25 (New York: New York University Press, 2014).

50. "Chorus Goes into Society: Ballet Row over the Mardi Gras," *San Francisco Call*, February 7, 1899, 14.

51. "He Waved His Gilded Wand and Dull Care Vanished," *San Francisco Call*, February 15, 1899, 12.

52. "Chorus Goes into Society: Ballet Row over the Mardi Gras," *San Francisco Call*, February 7, 1899, 14.

53. Her fellow Tivoli ballet girl Irene Duval, by contrast, feels the need to defend her honor. In the next day's paper, she suggests that Gertrude made up the story that she met Ed Greenway there. The line between ballet girl and prostitute was a vanishingly small one, so I find it interesting that only Duval feels the need to proclaim her innocence. "Never Was in the Tivoli Wine Room," *San Francisco Call*, February 8, 1899, 14.

54. Anthony Walter, "The Thousand and Second Tale," *San Francisco Call*, October 22, 1911, Editorial/Dramatic/Society, 27.

55. Robinson Locke, "Scrapbooks / Gertrude Hoffman," series 1, reel 24, vols. 273–74, 273:102, Robinson Locke Collection, Billy Rose Theatre Division, New York Public Library for the Performing Arts (hereafter RLC, BRTD, NYPLPA).

56. Gertrude and Max Hoffmann, box 2, folder 21: Personal notebooks, Red notebook, GMHP.

57. "Morosco's Is Transformed," *San Francisco Chronicle*, March 6, 1899, 7.

58. Gertrude and Max Hoffmann, box 2, folder 21: Personal notebooks, Red notebook, GMHP.

59. "Personal Mention," *San Francisco Dramatic Review*, December 9, 1899, 5.

60. Gertrude and Max Hoffmann, box 2, folder 21: Personal notebooks, Red notebook, GMHP.

61. Preston, *Modernism's Mythic Pose*, 80.

62. Gertrude and Max Hoffmann, box 2, folder 21: Personal notebooks, Red notebook, GMHP.

63. Ibid.

64. "New York Success Not Sufficient for This City," *San Francisco Call*, March 13, 1900, 12.

65. "At the Local Theaters: The Alcazar," *San Francisco Dramatic Review*, December 9, 1899, 6.

66. "Haddon Chambers' Play Wears Well," *San Francisco Call*, June 5, 1900, 4.

67. Locke, "Scrapbooks / Gertrude Hoffman," 273:67, RLC, BRTD, NYPLPA.

68. Gertrude and Max Hoffmann, box 2, folder 21: Personal notebooks, Red notebook, GMHP.

69. It is also possible that Hoffmann is conflating the two times she starred with Roberts. She appeared in 1898 as Florence Roberts's page in *Richelieu*. By 1900, she was established as a chorus member with a specialty in Spanish dances.

70. "Florence Roberts Takes Opposite View to Mary Anderson," *San Francisco Dramatic Review*, February 6, 1909, 16.

71. Lee Coyle, *George Ade* (New York: Twayne, 1964), 53.

72. "Stage Gossip: Last Week of Dunne and Ryley's Comedians," *Argonaut*, August 6, 1900, 11.

73. "Just of Passing Interest," *San Francisco Dramatic Review*, June 30, 1900; "Just of Passing Interest," *San Francisco Dramatic Review*, August 18, 1900.

Chapter 2

1. Gertrude and Max Hoffmann, box 2, folder 29: Max Hoffman, Personal and Performance notebooks, GMHP.

2. Ibid.

3. Ibid.

4. Ibid.

5. Ibid.

6. Ibid.

7. James Weldon Johnson, *The Autobiography of an Ex-Colored Man* (New York: Hill and Wang, 1991), 82.

8. Isidore Witmark and Isaac Goldberg, *The Story of the House of Witmark: From Ragtime to Swingtime* (New York: L. Furman, 1939), 170.

9. Burton William Peretti, *Lift Every Voice: The History of African American Music* (Lanham, Md.: Rowman and Littlefield, 2009), 60–62.

10. Edward A. Berlin, *Ragtime: A Musical and Cultural History* (Berkeley: University of California Press, 1984), 66.

11. "Free Concert," advertisement, *Saint Paul Globe*, January 28, 1898, 8.

12. Gertrude and Max Hoffmann, box 2, folder 29: Max Hoffman, Personal and Performance notebooks, GMHP.

13. Chas. K. (Charles Kassell) Harris, *After the Ball: Forty Years of Melody; An Autobiography* (New York: Frank-Maurice, 1926), 203, http://archive.org/details/afterballfortyye00harr.

14. Witmark and Goldberg, *Story of the House of Witmark*, 170–71.

15. Ibid., 170.

16. Konrad Schiecke, *Downtown Chicago's Historic Movie Theatres* (Jefferson, N.C.: McFarland, 2011), 49.

17. Witmark and Goldberg, *Story of the House of Witmark*, 169

18. "A Rag Baby," advertisement, *Leader-Telegram*, May 10, 1900.

19. Gertrude and Max Hoffmann, box 2, folder 21: Personal notebooks, Red notebook, GMHP

20. Anthony Walter, "The Thousand and Second Tale," *San Francisco Call*, October 22, 1911, Editorial/Dramatic/Society, 27.

21. Gertrude and Max Hoffmann, box 2, folder 33: Max Hoffmann, Apartment Inventory and Packing Lists, 1953, Red notebook, GMHP.

22. Ibid.

23. Lee Coyle, *George Ade* (New York: Twayne, 1964).

24. ""Dramatic and Musical: Variety Farce at the Victoria the Only Novelty. Mr. Goodwin in 'When We Were Twenty-One' and Mr. Willard in 'The Middleman'—Gossip of the Stage," *New York Times*, January 22, 1901, 6.

25. Robinson Locke, "Scrapbooks/Gertrude Hoffman," series 1, reel 24, vols. 273–74, 273:67–68, RLC, BRTD, NYPLPA.

26. Ibid.

27. "Gertrude Hoffman Is 'Coming Back,'" *Richmond Times Dispatch*, August 5, 1913, 12.

28. Ibid.

29. Gertrude and Max Hoffmann, box 2, folder 21: Personal notebooks, Red notebook, GMHP.

30. Ibid.

31. Gladys Hurlbut, *Next Week East Lynne! A Famous Stock Company Leading Lady Recounts Her Hilarious Experiences on the Gum-and-Gimlet Circuit* (New York: E. P. Dutton, 1950), 145–50.

32. "Two Negroes Shot," *Times Dispatch*, April 7, 1901, 22. The headline refers to the most important news coming out of Norfolk, Virginia, in the story; Gertrude and Max's marriage appears in the second paragraph, and the Yale baseball game's cancellation rounds out the story.

33. Ibid.

34. Gertrude and Max Hoffmann, box 2, folder 21: Personal notebooks, Red notebook, GMHP.

35. Hurlbut, *Next Week East Lynne!* 25.

36. Gertrude and Max Hoffmann, box 2, folder 21: Personal notebooks, Red notebook, GMHP.

37. For extensive coverage of Wells's career, see Eric Jay Dewberry, "Jake Wells Enterprises and the Development of Urban Entertainments in the South, 1890–1925" (Ph.D. diss., Georgia State University, 2010). For close attention to the exhibition practices in one city on the Wells circuit, see Terry Lindvall, "Cinema Virtue, Cinema Vice: Race, Religion, and Film Exhibition in Norfolk, Virginia, 1908–1922," in *Hollywood in the Neighborhood: Historical Case Studies of Local Moviegoing*, ed. Kathryn Fuller-Seeley (Berkeley: University of California Press, 2008), 91–103.

38. Lindvall, "Cinema Virtue, Cinema Vice."

39. Ibid.

40. Information on the Bijou Musical Comedy Company and their first shows in Virginia is easily accessible on the Virginia Chronicle website, https://virginiachronicle.com, particularly in issues of the *Richmond Dispatch*.

41. "Summer Amusement," *Richmond Dispatch*, April 28, 1901, 6.

42. Gertrude Hoffmann, "Gertrude Hoffmann: Experiences and Credits," box 1, folder 1, GHC.

43. "Theatres," *Atlanta Constitution*, May 19, 1902, 7.

44. G. Hoffmann, "Gertrude Hoffmann: Experiences and Credits," GHC.

45. "In Manhattan," *Brooklyn Life*, September 6, 1902, 40

46. "At the Theatres Next Week," *Evening World*, August 19, 1902, 7.

47. Ibid.

48. "Vaudeville Houses," *Brooklyn Daily Eagle*, August 31, 1902, 36, 37.

49. David E. Chinitz, *T. S. Eliot and the Cultural Divide* (Chicago: University of Chicago Press, 2005), 115.

50. Ibid., 116; Eugene Levy, *James Weldon Johnson: Black Leader, Black Voice* (Chicago: University of Chicago Press, 1976), 86.

51. Chinitz, *T. S. Eliot*, 116.

52. "Sadie My Creole Lady," sheet music, Duke University Libraries, Digital Collections, http://library.duke.edu/digitalcollections/hasm_b0438/.

53. For the history of "coon shouting" and its association with white women's performance in this era, see Pamela Brown Lavitt, "First of the Red Hot Mamas: 'Coon Shouting' and the Jewish Ziegfeld Girl," *American Jewish History* 87, no. 4 (1999): 253–90; Lori Lynne Brooks, "'To Be Black Is to Be Funny': 'Coon-Shouting' and the Melancholic Production of the White Comedienne," *Women and Performance: A Journal of Feminist Theory* 25, no. 1 (January 2, 2015): 1–22.

54. Susan A. Glenn, *Female Spectacle: The Theatrical Roots of Modern Feminism* (Cambridge, Mass.: Harvard University Press, 2000), 54.

55. "Footlight Flashes," *Philadelphia Inquirer*, May 24, 1903, 33.

Chapter 3

1. Robinson Locke, "Scrapbooks / Gertrude Hoffman," series 1, reel 24, vols. 273–74, 273:103, RLC, BRTD, NYPLPA.

2. Barbara Stratyner, *Ned Wayburn and the Dance Routine: From Vaudeville to the Ziegfeld Follies* (Madison: University of Wisconsin Press, 1996), 21.

3. "New York's Incredible Lost Rooftop Theatres," March 17, 2017, http://www.messynessychic.com/2017/03/17/new-yorks-incredible-lost-rooftop-theatres/.

4. Vincent Sheean, *The Amazing Oscar Hammerstein: The Life and Exploits of an Impresario* (London: Weidenfeld and Nicolson, 1956), 108.

5. "Plays and Players," *Theatre Magazine*, July 1904, 160.

6. Gertrude and Max Hoffmann, box 2, folder 21: Personal Notebooks, Red notebook, GMHP.

7. Ibid.

8. *State Population Census Schedules, 1905*, under "Gertrude Hoffman," New York State Archives, Albany, New York. Accessed through "New York State Census, 1905," ancestry.com.

9. "Notes of the Stage," *New York Daily Tribune*, August 12, 1903, 4.

10. "Baby Steals Buggy and Tries Auto: Maxmillion Hoffmann, Three Years Old, Has Penchant for Free Rides," *San Francisco Chronicle*, March 17, 1905, box 1, folder 2, GHC.

11. Ibid.

12. Barbara Cohen-Stratyner, "Hoffman, Gertrude (1886–1966)," *Routledge Encyclopedia of Modernism*, 2016. https://www.rem.routledge.com/articles/hoffman-gertrude-1886-1966.

13. Locke, "Scrapbooks / Gertrude Hoffman," 273:2, RLC, BRTD, NYPLPA.

14. Ibid.

15. G. Hoffmann, "Gertrude Hoffmann: Experiences and Credits," n.d., box 1, folder 1, GHC.

16. "At the Casino," *Times Dispatch*, June 26, 1904, image 18.

17. The comic trio comprised George Bickel, Harry Watson Jr., and George Wrothe. "Me, Him, and I Program," October 31, 1904, Belknap Playbills and Programs Collection. Special and Area Studies Collection, George A. Smathers Library, University of Florida, Gainesville (hereafter BPP).

18. Chas. K. (Charles Kassel) Harris, *After the Ball: Forty Years of Melody; an Autobiography* (New York: Frank-Maurice, 1926), 203, http://archive.org/details/afterballfortyye00harr.

19. Locke, "Scrapbooks / Gertrude Hoffman," 273:2, RLC, BRTD, NYPLPA.

20. Gertrude and Max Hoffmann, box 2, folder 21: Personal notebooks, Red notebook, GMHP.

21. Max Page, *The Creative Destruction of Manhattan, 1900–1940* (Chicago: University of Chicago Press, 2001).

22. Stratyner, *Ned Wayburn and the Dance Routine*, 15.

23. Locke, "Scrapbooks / Gertrude Hoffman," 273:2, RLC, BRTD, NYPLPA.

24. Ibid.

25. Gertrude and Max Hoffmann, box 2, folder 21: Personal notebooks, Brown notebook with first line "To Al Roon—Hotel Ansonia, GMHP.

26. Ibid.

27. Chicot, "'Corks' on Girl Acts," *Variety*, December 23, 1905, 7.

28. G. Hoffman, "Gertrude Hoffmann: Experiences and Credit," box 1, folder 1, GHC.

29. Rachel Shteir, *Striptease: The Untold History of the Girlie Show* (New York: Oxford University Press, 2005), 33.

30. Frank Cullen, *Vaudeville, Old and New: An Encyclopedia of Variety Performers in America*, with Florence Hackman and Donald McNeilly, 2 vols. (New York: Routledge, 2006), 1:252–53.

31. "Agent's Own 'Girl Act,'" *Variety*, September 1, 1906, 5.

32. "The Pullman Girls," *Variety*, February 24, 1906, 7.

33. Ibid.

34. "New Acts of the Week: In the Swim," *Variety*, March 24, 1906, 6.

Chapter 4

1. Grant Hayter-Menzies, *Charlotte Greenwood: The Life and Career of the Comic Star of Vaudeville, Radio and Film* (Jefferson, N.C.: McFarland, 2007), 41.

2. Gertrude and Max Hoffmann, box 2, folder 21: Personal notebooks, Red notebook, GMHP.

3. Ibid.

4. The back of this photo is labeled "Gertrude Hoffman, K&P 125th St. Dec. 9th," so it's likely that it shows her costume for the December 1907 run of shows. White Studios, *Gertrude Hoffmann Imitating Eddie Foy as Sister Anne in Mr. Bluebeard*, GHC.

5. Robinson Locke, "Scrapbooks / Gertrude Hoffman," series 1, reel 24, vols. 273–74, 273:3, RLC, BRTD, NYPLPA.

6. Gertrude and Max Hoffmann, box 2, folder 21: Personal notebooks, Brown notebook with first line "To Al Roon—Hotel Ansonia," GMHP.

7. "Shows of the Week: Metropolis Roof," *Variety*, August 4, 1906, 11.

8. "Shows of the Week: Metropolis Roof," *Variety*, August 11, 1906, 9.

9. "Shows of the Week: Metropolis Roof," August 4, 1906, 11.

10. Eve Golden, *Anna Held and the Birth of Ziegfeld's Broadway* (Lexington: University Press of Kentucky, 2000), 106.

11. Gertrude and Max Hoffmann, box 2, folder 21: Personal notebooks, Brown notebook with first line "To Al Roon—Hotel Ansonia," GMHP.

12. Ibid.

13. Locke, "Scrapbooks / Gertrude Hoffman," 273:4, RLC, BRTD, NYPLPA.

14. "The Parisian Model Program," December 24, 1906, BPP.

15. Gertrude and Max Hoffmann, box 2, folder 21: Personal notebooks, Brown notebook with first line "To Al Roon—Hotel Ansonia," GMHP.

16. Ibid.

17. Golden, *Anna Held.*

18. Ibid., 33

19. Susan A. Glenn, *Female Spectacle: The Theatrical Roots of Modern Feminism* (Cambridge, Mass: Harvard University Press, 2000), 79.

20. Ibid.

21. Jonathan Goldman, *Modernism Is the Literature of Celebrity* (Austin: University of Texas Press, 2011), 31.

22. Gertrude and Max Hoffmann, box 2, folder 21: Personal notebooks, Brown notebook with first line "To Al Roon—Hotel Ansonia," GMHP.

23. Ethel Lloyd Patterson, "'It Is So Silly, All This Fuss,' Says Anna Held, as She Tells about Her Full-Grown Daughter," *Evening World*, September 24, 1908, 3.

24. Ethan Mordden, *Ziegfeld: The Man Who Invented Show Business* (New York: St. Martin's Press, 2008), 63.

25. Golden, *Anna Held*, 108.

26. Rhonda K. Garelick, *Electric Salome: Loie Fuller's Performance of Modernism* (Princeton, N.J.: Princeton University Press, 2007), 118–55.

27. For more on the plot of *A Parisian Model*, see John Franceschina, *Harry B. Smith: Dean of American Librettists* (New York: Routledge, 2003).

28. "The Parisian Model Program," April 15, 1907, BPP.

29. Locke, "Scrapbooks / Gertrude Hoffman," 273:3, RLC, BRTD, NYPLPA.

30. "The Parisian Model Program," April 15, 1907.

31. Barbara Stratyner, *Ned Wayburn and the Dance Routine: From Vaudeville to the Ziegfeld Follies* (Madison: University of Wisconsin Press, 1996), 38.

32. Hoffmann, box 2, folder 21: Personal notebooks, Brown notebook with first line "To Al Roon—Hotel Ansonia," GMHP.

33. Ibid.

34. Gertrude and Max Hoffmann, box 2, folder 21: Personal notebooks, Red notebook, GMHP.

35. See Charles Dana Gibson, "The Gibson Girl's America: Drawings by Charles Dana Gibson; Creating an Ideal," March 30, 2013, online exhibition, Library of Congress, Washington, D.C., http://www.loc.gov/exhibits/gibson-girls-america/creating-an-ideal.html; Frank Marotti, "Gibson Girl," in *Fashion and Merchandising Fads*, ed. Frank Hoffmann and Beulah B. Ramirez (New York: Routledge, 2014), 100–104.

36. For a discussion of this intertextual moment, see Jennifer Schmidt, "Unruly Reproductions: The Embodied Art of Mimicry in Vaudeville," *Journal of American Drama and Theatre* 31, no. 3, https://jadtjournal.org/2019/05/13/unruly-reproductions-the-embodied-art-of-mimicry-in-vaudeville/.

37. For a history of statue posing in relation to solo female performance, see Carrie J. Preston, *Modernism's Mythic Pose: Gender, Genre, Solo Performance* (Oxford: Oxford University Press, 2011). For a discussion of tableaux vivants and suffrage performance, see Mary Chapman, *Making Noise, Making News: Suffrage Print Culture and U.S. Modernism* (Oxford: Oxford University Press, 2014).

38. Gertrude and Max Hoffmann, box 2, folder 21: Personal notebooks, Brown notebook with first line "To Al Roon—Hotel Ansonia," GMHP.

39. "No Parisian Model Score," *New York Times*, May 14, 1907, 11.

40. "Hoffman Seeks Injunction," *New York Dramatic Mirror*, June 1, 1907, 15.

41. "No Parisian Model Score," 11.

42. Gertrude and Max Hoffmann, box 2, folder 21: Personal notebooks, Red notebook, GMHP.

43. Ibid.

44. "No Parisian Model Score," 11.

45. Gertrude and Max Hoffmann, box 2, folder 21: Personal notebooks, Red notebook, GMHP.

46. "No Parisian Model Score," 11.

47. Gertrude and Max Hoffmann, box 2, folder 21: Personal notebooks, Red notebook, GMHP.

48. "Charge against Max Hoffman Fails," *New York Times*, May 16, 1907, 7.

49. Gertrude and Max Hoffmann, box 2, folder 21: Personal notebooks, Red notebook, GMHP.

50. Ibid.

51. Ibid.

52. "Charge against Max Hoffman Fails," 7.

53. "Plays and Players," *Elmira Gazette and Free Press*, May 27, 1907, 6.

54. "'The Honeymooners'—Act II," Edward B. Marks Music Co. Collection, George M. Cohan Collection, MCNY, 6.

55. Ibid., 20.

56. The title of this song anticipates the last show Cohan wrote, *The Musical Comedy Man*. He was working on the show when he died in 1942, and the title song appeared in the biographical musical about his life, *George M*.

57. Though the third act is missing from the Museum of the City of New York script, I have extrapolated this claim from reviews and the storyline in the first and second acts.

58. Franklin Fyles, "The Critical First-Nighters," *Salt Lake Herald*, June 9, 1907, Magazine, 15.

59. Locke, "Scrapbooks / Gertrude Hoffman," 273:7, RLC, BRTD, NYPLPA.

60. Ibid., 273:6.

61. Ibid., 273:9.

62. Ibid., 273:12.

63. In later incarnations, Hoffmann would use the Gertrude Hoffmann Girls and other comedians who were part of her revue as a buffer for her costume changes. But in this period of her career, when she was working with a small cast, these tweaks show her directorial ambitions in action.

64. Caroline Scurfield Caffin, *Vaudeville: The Book* (New York: M. Kennerley, 1914), 142.

65. Locke, "Scrapbooks / Gertrude Hoffman," 273:10, RLC, BRTD, NYPLPA.

66. Ibid., 273:11.

67. Caffin, *Vaudeville*, 150.

68. "The New Plays: George M. Cohan Up in the Air with 'The Honeymooners,'" *Evening World*, June 4, 1907, 13.

69. Locke, "Scrapbooks / Gertrude Hoffman," 273:12, RLC, BRTD, NYPLPA.

70. This is especially true of Elsie Janis, who began as a mimic and then succeeded as an actress and screenwriter.

71. Alan Dale, "A Diaphanous Dancer," *Cosmopolitan* 56 (December 1913): 117–18, 118.

72. Ibid.

73. "Mr. and Mrs. Max Hoffman," *Variety*, December 21, 1907, 3.

74. Ibid.

75. For a full biography of Tanguay, see Andrew L. Erdman, *Queen of Vaudeville: The Story of Eva Tanguay* (Ithaca, N.Y.: Cornell University Press, 2012).

76. Jody Rosen, "Vanishing Act," *Slate*, December 1, 2009, http://www.slate.com/articles/arts/music_box/2009/12/vanishing_act.html.

Chapter 5

1. Susan A. Glenn, *Female Spectacle: The Theatrical Roots of Modern Feminism* (Cambridge, Mass: Harvard University Press, 2000), 88–95. For the association of mimesis with primitive subjects, see Michael Taussig, *Mimesis and Alterity: A Particular History of the Senses* (New York: Routledge, 1993), 207–13.

2. Sime Silverman, "The Girl Question," *Variety*, January 11, 1908, 17.

3. For a full discussion of imitative performance by women in this period, see chapter 3 of Glenn, *Female Spectacle*.

4. Franklin Fyles, "Broadway Roof Gardens Open in Summer Rivalry," *Chicago Sunday Tribune*, June 9, 1907, Drama.

5. Ibid.

6. Thank you to Marlis Schweitzer for this formulation. Her early reading of this chapter helped shape this and the project as a whole.

7. "Variety Theatres: Alhambra Theatre," *New-York Tribune*, March 1, 1908.

8. "Act II, Scene Seven (Salome from San Francisco), Undated," series 1, box 1, folder 16, Morris Gest Papers, Harry Ransom Center, University of Texas at Austin (hereafter MGP), www.lib.utexas.edu/taro/uthrc/00740/00740-P.html.

9. Robinson Locke, "Scrapbooks / Gertrude Hoffman," series 1, reel 24, vols. 273–74, 273:17, RLC, BRTD, NYPLPA.

10. Glenn, *Female Spectacle*, 80.

11. Locke, "Scrapbooks / Gertrude Hoffman," 273:13, RLC, BRTD, NYPLPA.

12. "Act II, Scene Seven (Salome from San Francisco)," MGP.

13. Anthea Kraut's work, which I discuss later in this chapter, analyzes the ways that the distinction between "vernacular" performance and performance worthy of copyright has been shaped by ideas about racial and class hierarchy. Vaudeville was lower class, and tap dancing was associated with African American performers.

14. Robert W. Snyder, *The Voice of the City: Vaudeville and Popular Culture in New York* (New York: Oxford University Press, 1989), 60.

15. "Artist's Forum," *Variety*, January 25, 1908, 9.

16. Eligibility to register one's material in the Protected Materials Department was, according to Steve Allen, one of the inducements to join National Vaudeville Artists, Inc. See Fred Allen, "A Tribute to Vaudeville's Golden Era," *Life Magazine*, November 12, 1956, 83. In addition, *Variety* opened its own Protected Materials Department

around the same time. See "Variety Protected Materials Department Collection," Collection MSS 017, Emerson College Archives and Special Collections, http://atom.emerson.edu/index.php/variety-protected-materials-department-collection-2.

17. "Act II, Scene Seven (Salome from San Francisco)."

18. "United's Unsettled State," *Variety*, February 29, 1908, 8.

19. "Act II, Scene Seven (Salome from San Francisco)."

20. Locke, "Scrapbooks / Gertrude Hoffman," 273:16, RLC, BRTD, NYPLPA.

21. Judith Hamera, *Unfinished Business: Michael Jackson, Detroit, and the Figural Economy of American Deindustrialization* (Oxford: Oxford University Press, 2017), 38.

22. Harry Lauder was also a mimic, albeit one of Scottish types rather than celebrities. See Marlis Schweitzer and Daniel Guadagnolo, "Feeling Scottish: Affect, Mimicry, and Vaudeville's 'Inimitable' Harry Lauder," *Journal of Dramatic Theory and Criticism* 26, no. 2 (July 13, 2012): 145–60.

23. Locke, "Scrapbooks / Gertrude Hoffman," 273:16, RLC, BRTD, NYPLPA.

24. Ibid.

25. "White Rats' Ball," *Variety*, March 21, 1908, 8; "K.-P. Employees Give Ball," *Variety*, March 28, 1908, 7.

26. "'The Merry Widow' Proves Captivating; Wins Instant Approval in American Debut at the New Amsterdam Theatre. Repeats Foreign Success Miss Ethel Jackson Plays the Widow with Spirit—Famous Waltz Charms Large Audience," *New York Times*, October 22, 1907, 9.

27. Marlis Schweitzer, *Transatlantic Broadway: The Infrastructural Politics of Global Performance* (Basingstoke, Eng.: Palgrave Macmillan, 2015), 30.

28. "Warning!! ('The Merry Widow' Advertisement)," *New York Clipper*, December 28, 1907, Illinois Digital Newspaper Collections, 15.

29. "Won't Burlesque 'The Merry Widow': Edgar Smith Quits Joe Weber, Not Liking the Latter's Plan for a Show. Doesn't Want to Infringe and Can't See, Whatever the State of Copyright May Be, How to Carry Out Instructions in Any Other Way," *New York Times*, December 18, 1907, 9.

30. Ibid.

31. Robert Spoo, *Without Copyrights: Piracy, Publishing, and the Public Domain*, (Oxford: Oxford University Press, 2016), 32–33.

32. Schweitzer, *Transatlantic Broadway*, 31

33. "'Merry Widow' in Burlesque," *Variety*, January 4, 1908, 6.

34. See Marlis Schweitzer, "'Darn That Merry Widow Hat': The On- and Offstage Life of a Theatrical Commodity, circa 1907–1908," *Theatre Survey* 50, no. 2 (November 2009): 189–221n32, as well as *Brown v. Select Theatres Corporation*, 56 F. Supp. 438 (D. Mass. 1944), https://www.leagle.com/decision/194449456fsupp4381384.

35. "Did 'Mlle Modiste' and 'The Merry Widow' Compare Notes?" *New York Evening Telegram*, October 25, 1907, sec. M, 8.

36. Victor Herbert, "Victor Herbert Defends 'Mlle. Modiste,'" *Evening Telegram*, October 28, 1907, 8.

37. Matthew White Jr., "'The Merry Widow' Travestied," *Munsey's Magazine* 38, no. 6 (March 1908): 820–21.

38. "New York Theaters," *Washington Herald*, April 19, 1908, 4.

39. White, "'The Merry Widow' Travestied."

40. "Is the Merry Widow Waltz a Child of Mendelssohn's Brain?" *Washington Times*, March 22, 1908, Magazine, 4, 8–9.

41. For dancing with a dummy, see Sime Silverman, "Mabel Hite Soon," *Variety*, January 11, 1908, 4. For dancing with volunteers, see Rush, "Virginia Earl," *Variety*, February 29, 1908, 14.

42. "Shapiro 1908 Song Crop," *Variety*, February 1, 1908, 38.

43. Ibid.

44. Peyton Boyle, *The Federal Reporter* (St. Paul: West, 1908), 585.

45. Ibid.

46. Ibid.

47. "The Drama in the Law of Copyright," *Harvard Law Review* 44, no. 4 (1931): 628–33, 628.

48. Boyle, *Federal Reporter*, 585.

49. Anthea Kraut, *Choreographing Copyright: Race, Gender, and Intellectual Property Rights in American Dance* (Oxford: Oxford University Press, 2015), xi.

50. Paul Goldstein, *Goldstein on Copyright* (New York: Aspen, 2005), sec. 2.10.

51. Kraut, *Choreographing Copyright*, 83.

52. Ibid., 27–28, 215–16.

53. *Henry W. Savage v. Gertrude Hoffman*, United States Circuit Court for the Southern District of New York, Case no. 2–192.

54. "'Merry Widow' Not Original?" *New York Sun*, April 8, 1908, 7.

55. "The Law and the 'Merry Widow,'" *Star-Gazette*, April 16, 1908 (rpt. from *New York Press*), 6.

56. Ibid.

57. J. L., "Is the Merry Widow as Young as She Says?" *Theatre*, May 1908, 119; "The Dubious Past of 'The Merry Widow,'" *Current Literature* 44, no. 6 (June 1908): 651–52.

58. "Dubious Past of 'The Merry Widow.'"

59. See Derek Miller's discussion of this case in Derek Miller, *Copyright and the Value of Performance, 1770–1911*, Theatre and Performance Theory (Cambridge: Cambridge University Press, 2018), 142–43.

60. *Savage v. Hoffmann*, 159 F. 584 (C. C. S. D. N. Y 1908), https://www.ravellaw.com/opinions/48bdbd192738073a5f25a22d06a3b143.

Chapter 6

1. "Mysterious American Dancing Girl in Poses That Captivated Europe," *Evening World*, April 20, 1908, 3.

2. See Amy Koritz, "Dancing the Orient for England: Maud Allan's 'The Vision of Salome,'" *Theatre Journal* 46, no. 1 (1994): 63–78.

3. Harriet Coffin, "All Sorts and Kinds of Salomes," *Theatre*, April 1909, 130.

4. Sharon Marcus, "Salomé!! Sarah Bernhardt, Oscar Wilde, and the Drama of Celebrity," *PMLA* 126, no. 4 (2011): 999–1021.

5. For an extensive history of Wilde's Salome, see Petra Dierkes-Thrun, *Salome's Modernity: Oscar Wilde and the Aesthetics of Transgression* (Ann Arbor: University of Michigan Press, 2011).

6. Grant Hayter-Menzies, *Charlotte Greenwood: The Life and Career of the Comic Star of Vaudeville, Radio and Film* (Jefferson, N.C.: McFarland, 2007), 4.

7. Previous critics have suggested that Froelich moved on to perform her dance in vaudeville immediately after this show closed. Margaret Araneo's dissertation convincingly argues that this was likely not the case and that Froelich performed her Salome dance in 1908. Margaret Araneo, "Nervous Salomes: New York Salomania and the Neurological Condition of Modernité" (Ph.D. diss., City University of New York, 2017), ProQuest Dissertations and Theses Full Text (1899182112), 124–25.

8. John Yohalem, "The Salome Scandals of 1907," *Opera News*, https://www.operanews.com/operanews/issue/article.aspx?id=174&issueID=9&archive=true.

9. Araneo, "Nervous Salomes," 126–27.

10. Gertrude and Max Hoffmann, box 13, folder 1, Programs and Publications: Various Programs: Follies of 1907, GMHP.

11. Elizabeth Kendall, *Where She Danced: The Birth of American Art-Dance* (Berkeley: University of California Press, 1979), 75.

12. Franklin Fyles, "New York's First Melodrama," *Salt Lake Herald*, August 4, 1907, Magazine, 5.

13. See Marlis Schweitzer, *Transatlantic Broadway: The Infrastructural Politics of Global Performance* (Basingstoke, Eng.: Palgrave Macmillan, 2015), especially chapter 1, "Networking the Waves: Ocean Liners, Impresarios, and Broadway's Atlantic Expansion," 37–68.

14. "Act II, Scene Seven (Salome from San Francisco), Undated," series 1, box 1, folder 16, MGP.

15. Ibid.

16. Robinson Locke, "Scrapbooks / Gertrude Hoffman," series 1, reel 24, vols. 273–74, 273:19, RLC, BRTD, NYPLPA.

17. "Notes," *Variety*, May 9, 1908, 10.

18. "Act II, Article Transcripts and Notes on Polaire and Gertrude Hoffman, 1913, Undated," series 1, box 2, folder 5, MGP.

19. Locke, "Scrapbooks / Gertrude Hoffman," 273:26, RLC, BRTD, NYPLPA.

20. Ibid. This is far different from an account of Gertrude Hoffmann watching Hawaiian dancer Doraldina's nightclub performance, where she and Max not only had "a ringside seat" but she also reportedly "moved onto the floor in order to get a better view of the dancer." Grace Kingsley, "An All-Star Interview," *Los Angeles Sunday Times*, October 17, 1920, sec. 3.

21. Schweitzer, *Transatlantic Broadway*, 151–52.

22. Mary Simonson, *Body Knowledge: Performance, Intermediality, and American Entertainment at the Turn of the Twentieth Century* (Oxford: Oxford University Press, 2013), 36.

23. My analysis is informed by Penny Farfan's discussion of doubling in the work of Loie Fuller; where Farfan identifies Fuller with the queer uncanny, I see Hoffmann's doubling as more informed by technologies of reproduction that were increasingly vital in modern mass culture. Penny Farfan, *Performing Queer Modernism* (Oxford: Oxford University Press, 2017), 27–40.

24. "Act II, Scene Seven (Salome from San Francisco)."

25. Gertrude and Max Hoffmann, box 2, folder 26: Performance and Music Notes, GMHP.

26. Locke, "Scrapbooks / Gertrude Hoffman," 273:22, RLC, BRTD, NYPLPA.
27. Ibid., 273:23.
28. See W. R. Titterton, "The Maud Allan Myth," *New Age: A Weekly Review of Politics, Literature, and Art* 3, no. 9 (June 27, 1908): 171–72. Via Modernist Journals Project.
29. There is some disagreement about this part of the dance. A few critics say the prop is taken from an onstage cistern or well, while others describe her finding the head in the shadows. It is possible that the onstage well was removed from the act after an early performance, as Schweitzer suggests. Marlis Schweitzer, "The Salome Epidemic," in *The Oxford Handbook of Dance and Theater*, ed. Nadine George-Graves (Oxford: Oxford University Press, 2015), 890–921, 915. Since the vast majority of reviews say Hoffmann concludes her performance by kissing the head and collapsing on the ground, I assume that approximates the end. Only one review says that she ends by throwing the head down the well—the *New York Times* review mentioned by Schweitzer.
30. Locke, "Scrapbooks / Gertrude Hoffman," 273:24, RLC, BRTD, NYPLPA.
31. Ibid.
32. Simonson, *Body Knowledge*, 34.
33. Franklin Fyles, "New York Is Dancing Mad," *Washington Post*, July 26, 1908, 3.
34. Marvin Carlson, *The Haunted Stage: The Theatre as Memory Machine* (Ann Arbor: University of Michigan Press, 2003), 59.
35. Locke, "Scrapbooks / Gertrude Hoffman," 273:24, RLC, BRTD, NYPLPA.
36. Ibid.
37. "Summer Shows at the Roof Gardens: Hammerstein's Roof. Gertrude Hoffman and Variety," *Theatre*, August 1908, 201, vii.
38. Kendall, *Where She Danced*, 76.
39. Locke, "Scrapbooks / Gertrude Hoffman," 273:26, RLC, BRTD, NYPLPA.
40. Ibid.
41. Ibid.
42. Schweitzer, "Salome Epidemic."
43. Locke, "Scrapbooks / Gertrude Hoffman," 273:24, RLC, BRTD, NYPLPA.
44. University of Toronto, "Sartorial," *The Varsity*, November 24, 1908.
45. Fyles, "New York Is Dancing Mad."
46. Locke, "Scrapbooks / Gertrude Hoffman,"273:25.
47. Glenn, *Female Spectacle*, 104.
48. Locke, "Scrapbooks / Gertrude Hoffman," 273:46, RLC, BRTD, NYPLPA.
49. "Act II, Scene Seven (Salome from San Francisco)."
50. Gertrude and Max Hoffmann, box 2, folder 21: Personal notebooks, GMHP.
51. Locke, "Scrapbooks / Gertrude Hoffman," 273:27, RLC, BRTD, NYPLPA.
52. "Act II, Scene Seven (Salome from San Francisco)"; and Locke, "Scrapbooks / Gertrude Hoffman," 273:28, RLC, BRTD, NYPLPA.
53. Andrew L. Erdman, *Blue Vaudeville: Sex, Morals and the Mass Marketing of Amusement, 1895–1915* (Jefferson, N.C.: McFarland, 2004), 108.
54. In "Salome Epidemic," 911, Schweitzer lists many of the important Salome articles of the past twenty years.
55. Locke, "Scrapbook / Mlle. Dazie," series 1, reel 13, 147: 39, RLC, BRTD, NYPLPA.

56. David S. Shields, "Frank C. Bangs," Broadway Photographs, broadway.cas.sc.edu/content/frank-c-bangs.

57. David Mayer, "'Quote the Words to Prompt the Attitudes': The Victorian Performer, the Photographer, and the Photograph," *Theatre Survey* 43, no. 2 (2002): 223–51, 228.

58. "Summer Shows at the Roof Gardens," 200–201, vii.

59. "The Theatre Magazine Post Cards," advertisement, *Theatre*, September 1908, xii.

60. Penny Farfan, "The Picture Postcard Is a Sign of the Times," *Theatre History Studies* 32 (January 2012): 93–119, 99.

61. For a discussion of similar reactions to *Merry Widow* postcards, see "'My Word, How He Is Kissing Her!': The Material Culture of Theatrical Promotion," in Schweitzer, *Transatlantic Broadway*, 146–89.

62. Locke, "Scrapbooks / Gertrude Hoffman," 273:32–33, RLC, BRTD, NYPLPA.

63. "Act II, Article Transcripts and Notes on Polaire."

64. "Loie Fuller," special issue, *Dance Index* 1, no. 3 (March 1942), 47, http://archive.org/details/danceindexunse_1.

65. "Early General Correspondence (1908–1910)," box 74, folder 3, Early General Correspondence, the Shubert Archive, New York (hereafter TSA).

66. Schweitzer, *Transatlantic Broadway*, 161.

67. Charles W. Collins, "The Mimic World," *Chicago Inter Ocean*, December 23, 1908, 6.

68. "Early General Correspondence (1908–1910)."

69. John Martin Papers, series 4: Programs and Playbills, box 18, folder 2, 1910–1919, John Martin Papers, Jerome Robbins Dance Division, the New York Public Library of the Performing Arts, Dorothy and Lewis B. Cullman Center (hereafter, JMP, JRDD, NYPLPA).

70. "Early General Correspondence (1908–1910)."

71. Schweitzer, *Transatlantic Broadway*, 160.

72. Schweitzer, "Salome Epidemic," 909.

73. "Early General Correspondence (1908–1910)" and "Act II, Article Transcripts and Notes on Polaire."

74. See Jeremy C. Young, *The Age of Charisma: Leaders, Followers, and Emotions in American Society, 1870–1940* (Cambridge: Cambridge University Press, 2016), especially 111, for discussion of Billy Sunday's usage of vaudeville and baseball techniques.

75. The Hoffmanns returned via Southampton on the *Kronprinzessin Cecilie* on June 30, 1909. Ship Manifest, S.S. *Kronprincessin Cecilie*, Liberty Ellis Foundation, June 30, 1909, https://www.libertyellisfoundation.org/passenger-details/czoxMjoiMTAxNjM1MDEwMTI5Ijs=/czo4OiJtYW5pZmVzdCI7.

76. William Winter, *The Life of David Belasco* (New York: Moffat, Yard, 1918), 298.

77. Gertrude and Max Hoffmann, box 2, folder 21: Personal notebooks, GMHP.

78. Ibid.

79. Locke, "Scrapbooks / Gertrude Hoffman," 273:52, RLC, BRTD, NYPLPA.

80. Ibid., 273:53. For a discussion of Hoffmann's response, see Morgan Stevens-Garmon, "Gertrude Hoffman and the Dance That Offended Public Decency,"

Museum of the City of New York (hereafter MCNY), https://www.mcny.org/story/gertrude-hoffman.

81. "Act II, Article Transcripts and Notes on Polaire."

82. Locke, "Scrapbooks / Gertrude Hoffman," 273:56, RLC, BRTD, NYPLPA.

83. Ibid., 273:55.

84. Jane Desmond, "Dancing Out the Difference: Cultural Imperialism and Ruth St. Denis's 'Radha' of 1906," *Signs* 17, no. 1 (1991): 28–49, 30.

85. See Kendall, *Where She Danced*; Desmond, "Dancing Out the Difference." One fascinating counterexample to this trend is Priya Srinivasan, *Sweating Saris: Indian Dance as Transnational Labor* (Philadelphia: Temple University Press, 2011). Srinivasan considers the labor of Indian dancers who inspired and worked with St. Denis.

86. Desmond, "Dancing Out the Difference," 38.

87. Ibid., 39.

88. Ibid., 32.

89. Locke, "Scrapbooks / Gertrude Hoffman," 273:57, RLC, BRTD, NYPLPA.

90. Kendall, *Where She Danced*, 75.

91. Elin Diamond, *Unmaking Mimesis: Essays on Feminism and Theater* (New York: Routledge, 1997), 105.

92. Gertrude Stein, *Last Operas and Plays* (Baltimore: Johns Hopkins University Press, 1995), xxix–xxx.

93. Locke, "Scrapbooks / Gertrude Hoffman," 273:58, RLC, BRTD, NYPLPA.

94. "Maud Allan Does 'Salome': A Milder Siren Than Her Vaudeville Rivals," *The Sun*, January 30, 1910, 6.

95. "Act II, Article Transcripts and Notes on Polaire."

Chapter 7

1. Robinson Locke, "Scrapbooks / Gertrude Hoffman," series 1, reel 24, vols. 273–74, 273:61, RLC, BRTD, NYPLPA.

2. For a sentimental look back at the era, see Robert Baral, *Revue: A Nostalgic Reprise of the Great Broadway Period* (New York: Fleet, 1962). A more recent history of the form is Lee Allyn Davis, *Scandals and Follies: The Rise and Fall of the Great Broadway Revue* (New York: Limelight Editions, 2000). Maya Cantu thinks through the relation of highbrow and lowbrow culture in a later revue, the Garrick Gaieties, with her article "'Gilding the Guild': Art Theatre, the Broadway Revue and Cultural Parody in The Garrick Gaieties (1925–1930)," *Studies in Musical Theatre* 7, no. 1 (March 1, 2013): 45–60.

3. "Act II, Article Transcripts and Notes on Polaire and Gertrude Hoffman, 1913, Undated," series 1, box 2, folder 5, MGP.

4. Ibid.

5. Locke, "Scrapbooks / Gertrude Hoffman," 273:61, RLC, BRTD, NYPLPA.

6. Ibid.

7. Ibid., 273:69.

8. Ibid.

9. "Hoffman, Gertrude, Clippings, 1906–1937," series 1, box 11, folder 22, MGP.

10. Ibid.

11. Alan Dale, "A Diaphanous Dancer," *Cosmopolitan* 56 (December 1913): 118.

12. "Hoffman, Gertrude, Clippings, 1906–1937."

13. Locke, "Scrapbooks / Gertrude Hoffman," 273:56, RLC, BRTD, NYPLPA.

14. Frank Cullen, *Vaudeville, Old and New: An Encyclopedia of Variety Performers in America*, 2 vols. (New York: Routledge, 2006), 1:692. Alice Lloyd's sister was Marie Lloyd, the wildly popular British music-hall performer.

15. Trina Robbins, *Nell Brinkley and the New Woman in the Early 20th Century* (Jefferson, N.C: McFarland, 2001).

16. "Act II, Article Transcripts and Notes on Polaire."

17. Born Annette Marie Sarah Kellermann, she is typically referred to as "Annette Kellerman" both in contemporaneous coverage and present-day criticism.

18. In an early version of the act, she followed this with a duet, playing Nora Bayes while her performing partner Lee Chapin played Bayes's partner Jack Norworth. See Locke, "Scrapbooks / Gertrude Hoffman," 273:61, RLC, BRTD, NYPLPA.

19. Kathleen B. Casey, *The Prettiest Girl on Stage Is a Man: Race and Gender Benders in American Vaudeville* (Knoxville: University of Tennessee Press, 2015), xxv.

20. Locke, "Scrapbooks / Gertrude Hoffman," 273:69, RLC, BRTD, NYPLPA.

21. M. Alison Kibler, *Rank Ladies: Gender and Cultural Hierarchy in American Vaudeville* (Chapel Hill: University of North Carolina Press, 1999), 123.

22. Locke, "Scrapbooks / Gertrude Hoffman," 273:61, RLC, BRTD, NYPLPA.

23. Valleri J. Hohman, *Russian Culture and Theatrical Performance in America, 1891–1933* (New York: Palgrave Macmillan, 2011), 65.

24. Carl Van Vechten, "Anna Pavlowa a Wonderful Dancer," *New York Times*, March 1, 1910, 9.

25. Ibid.

26. Carl Van Vechten, "Russian Dancers in Amazing Feats," *New York Times*, March 2, 1910, 9.

27. "Dancer a Sensation," *Variety*, March 5, 1910, 4.

28. "Russian Dancers to Return in Fall," *New York Times*, April 6, 1910, 11.

29. "'Chantecler' for New York," *Variety*, March 12, 1910, 3.

30. Locke, "Scrapbooks / Gertrude Hoffman," 273:64, RLC, BRTD, NYPLPA.

31. Ibid., 273:65.

32. Locke, "Scrapbooks / Gertrude Hoffman,"," 273:70, 71, 74, 77, RLC, BRTD, NYPLPA.

33. Ibid., 273:70.

34. Ibid., 273:71.

35. Ibid.

36. Ibid., 273:79.

37. Ibid.

38. Ibid., 273:82.

39. Ibid.

40. Ibid.

Chapter 8

1. "Eddie Leonard Objects," *Variety*, March 19, 1910, 40.

2. Ibid.

3. Gertrude and Max Hoffmann, box 13, folder 5: Saison Ballet Russes-Original and American; Tableau de La Troupe-Programs, GMHP.

4. "Back from a Road Tour of Twenty-Seven Weeks," *Variety*, March 2, 1912, 7.

5. Hanna Järvinen, "Failed Impressions: Diaghilev's Ballets Russes in America, 1916," *Dance Research Journal* 42, no. 2 (2010): 76–108, 79.

6. Oliver M. Sayler and Marjorie Barkentin, "On Your Toes—America! The Story of the First Ballet Russe," *Dance Data*, no. 2 (1977): 20–27, 22.

7. Anthea Kraut, *Choreographing Copyright: Race, Gender, and Intellectual Property Rights in American Dance* (Oxford: Oxford University Press, 2015).

8. Robert Spoo, *Without Copyrights: Piracy, Publishing, and the Public Domain* (Oxford: Oxford University Press, 2013), 4.

9. All details of Hoffmann's backstage visit to the Châtelet Theatre are taken from "Act II, Article Transcripts and Notes on Polaire and Gertrude Hoffman, 1913, Undated," series 1, box 2, folder 5, MGP.

10. Ibid.

11. Robinson Locke, "Scrapbooks / Gertrude Hoffman," series 1, reel 24, vols. 273–74, 273:66, RLC, BRTD, NYPLPA.

12. Details in this paragraph are all approximations based on a transcription of material from "Act II, Article Transcripts and Notes on Polaire."

13. "Hoffman, Gertrude, Clippings, 1906–1937," series 1, box 11, folder 22, MGP.

14. Locke, "Scrapbooks / Gertrude Hoffman," 273:68, RLC, BRTD, NYPLPA.

15. "Act II, Article Transcripts and Notes on Polaire."

16. Ibid.

17. For a capsule biography of Ida Rubinstein, see Lynn Garafola, "Ida Rubinstein," Jewish Women's Archive, https://jwa.org/encyclopedia/article/rubinstein-ida. For a book-length biography, see Vicki Woolf, *Dancing in the Vortex: The Story of Ida Rubinstein* (New York: Routledge, 2013).

18. Charles S. Mayer, "Ida Rubinstein: A Twentieth-Century Cleopatra," *Dance Research Journal* 20, no. 2 (1988): 33–35, 33.

19. "'Winter Garden Advertisement' Display Ad 47—No Title," *New York Times*, June 11, 1911, Drama-Resorts-Music, X3.

20. Lincoln Kirstein, *Dance: A Short History of Classic Theatrical Dancing* (Trenton, N.J.: Princeton Book, 1969), 355.

21. Sayler and Barkentin, "On Your Toes—America!" 22.

22. "Act II, Article Transcripts and Notes on Polaire."

23. Ibid.

24. Ibid.

25. Carolyn Lowrey, *The First One Hundred Noted Men and Women of the Screen* (New York: Moffat, Yard, 1920), 96.

26. "Act II, Article Transcripts and Notes on Polaire."

27. Ibid.

28. See Carrie J. Preston, *Learning to Kneel: Noh, Modernism, and Journeys in Teaching* (New York: Columbia University Press, 2016).

29. Gertrude Hoffmann, "How the Russian Ballet Was Brought to America," *New York City American*, June 25, 1911, box 11, folder 6, GMHP.

30. Locke, "Scrapbooks / Gertrude Hoffman," 273:69, RLC, BRTD, NYPLPA.

31. Ibid., 273:68, 69.

32. Ibid., 273:69.

33. "Russian Dancers Arrive in Furs," *New York Times*, September 28, 1910, 11.
34. "Russian Dancers Again Triumph Here," *New York Times*, October 16, 1910, 13.
35. Ibid.
36. "In the Theaters," *Indianapolis Star*, October 23, 1910, 20.
37. Valleri J. Hohman, *Russian Culture and Theatrical Performance in America, 1891–1933* (New York: Palgrave Macmillan, 2011), 81.
38. "Act II, Article Transcripts and Notes on Polaire."
39. "Mlle. Bianci," *Variety*, September 3, 1910, 12.
40. Sime Silverman, "Danses Classique Russe," *Variety*, September 10, 1910, 16.
41. Hohman, *Russian Culture*, 82.
42. Barbara Naomi Cohen, "The Borrowed Art of Gertrude Hoffmann," *Dance Data* 2 (1977): 2–11, 11.
43. Sayler and Barkentin, "On Your Toes—America!" 22.
44. Ibid.
45. "Gertie Hoffmann's Surprise," *Variety*, June 10, 1911, 4.
46. "'Winter Garden Advertisement' Display Ad 47—No Title."
47. Ibid.
48. Ibid.
49. Cohen, "Borrowed Art of Gertrude Hoffmann," 7.
50. For further information on *Comœdia Illustré* and its representation of the Ballets Russes, see Mary E. Davis, *Ballets Russes Style: Diaghilev's Dancers and Paris Fashion* (London: Reaktion Books, 2010).
51. Ibid., 49.
52. Ballets Russes, ed., *Théâtre National de l'Opéra, Juin 1910: La Saison Russe à l'Opéra, Ballets Russes, avec le concours d'artistes des Théâtres Impériaux*, souvenir program (Paris: Comœdia Illustré, 1910). Performing Arts Research Collections—Dance, NYPLPA.
53. Locke, "Scrapbooks / Gertrude Hoffman," 273:85, RLC, BRTD, NYPLPA.
54. Lynn Garafola, *Diaghilev's Ballets Russes* (New York: Da Capo Press, 2009), 32–33.
55. Locke, "Scrapbooks / Gertrude Hoffman," 273:89, RLC, BRTD, NYPLPA.
56. George Jean Nathan, "Trying It on the Dog Days," *Smart Set*, September 1911, Hathitrust, 145–52, 148.
57. The foundational book discussing this cultural shift is Lawrence Levine, *Highbrow/Lowbrow: The Emergence of Cultural Hierarchy in America* (Cambridge, Mass.: Harvard University Press, 1990). Janice Radway theorized the middlebrow in *A Feeling for Books: The Book-of-the-Month Club, Literary Taste, and Middle-Class Desire* (Chapel Hill: University of North Carolina Press, 1999). David Savran uses these terms to think about the transformation of theater into a high art in *Highbrow/Lowdown: Theater, Jazz, and the Making of a New Middle Class* (Ann Arbor: University of Michigan Press, 2009).
58. For a list of shows performed at the Casino Theatre, see "Casino Theatre," Internet Broadway Database, https://www.ibdb.com/theatre/casino-theatre-1085. "Clorindy" is not included on that list, perhaps because it was one act or because it was performed on the theater's roof garden. It is an important show in the history of African American performance, both for its authors and because it was

the first show with an all-black cast to play to a white Broadway audience. Bernard L. Peterson, *A Century of Musicals in Black and White: An Encyclopedia of Musical Stage Works by, about, or involving African Americans* (Westport, Conn.: Greenwood Press, 1993), 84–85.

59. Ralph E. Renaud, "Gertrude Hoffman in Sublime Art Captivates Senses with Her Ballets," *San Francisco Chronicle*, October 17, 1911, 2.

60. Foster Hirsch, *The Boys from Syracuse: The Shuberts' Theatrical Empire* (New York: Cooper Square Press, 2000), 83.

61. Ibid.

62. "Big Broadway Music Hall and Cafe on American Horse Exchange Site," *New York Times*, June 19, 1910, Society Fashion Drama Automobiles Real Estate, X14.

63. Sayler and Barkentin, "On Your Toes—America!" 23.

64. "Worst Theatrical Summer for Over Twenty Years," *Variety*, July 15, 1911, 5.

65. Locke, "Scrapbooks / Gertrude Hoffman," 273:90, RLC, BRTD, NYPLPA; "Business Falling Off," *Variety*, July 8, 1911, 6.

66. Sayler and Barkentin, "On Your Toes—America! 23.

67. Locke, "Scrapbooks / Gertrude Hoffman," 273:95, RLC, BRTD, NYPLPA.

68. "Act II, Article Transcripts and Notes on Polaire."

69. Sayler and Barkentin, "On Your Toes—America!" 25.

70. "Russian Dancers Quit Miss Hoffmann," *New York Times*, September 20, 1911.

71. "Ballet to the Coast," *Variety*, September 23, 1911, 4.

72. Sayler and Barkentin, "On Your Toes—America!" 25.

73. Ibid., 24.

74. Hohman, *Russian Culture*, 83.

75. Sayler and Barkentin, "On Your Toes—America!" 25.

76. Ibid., 26.

77. Anthony Walter, "The Thousand and Second Tale," *San Francisco Call*, October 22, 1911, Editorial/Dramatic/Society, 27.

78. Julian Johnson, "Kitty Hayes the Dreamer" *Los Angeles Sunday Times*, October 29, 1911, Art and Artists.

79. Renaud, "Gertrude Hoffman in Sublime Art."

80. Julian Johnson, "Mimodramas: Hoffmann Has Real Climate," *Los Angeles Daily Times*, October 30, 1911, box 11, folder 6, GMHP.

81. Ashton Stevens, "Miss Hoffmann as Imitator Stages Satires Cruel and Great," *Chicago American*, December 13, 1911, box 11, folder 6, GMHP.

82. Ibid.

83. Quoted in Sayler and Barkentin, "On Your Toes—America!" 27.

Chapter 9

1. Robinson Locke, "Scrapbooks / Gertrude Hoffman," series 1, reel 24, vols. 273–74, 274:58, RLC, BRTD, NYPLPA.

2. Ibid.

3. "Gertrude Hoffmann, New Star at Shuberts' Winter Garden," *Variety*, June 15, 1912, 12.

4. Foster Hirsch, *The Boys from Syracuse: The Shuberts' Theatrical Empire* (New York: Cooper Square Press, 2000), 27.

5. "Gertrude Hoffmann's Mission," *Variety*, April 6, 1912.

6. Ibid.

7. Here it is likely that the French play Hoffmann reportedly traveled to see is the same as the "one-act piece called 'The Beast' referenced in the letter, which she "also wanted to produce." Letter to Gertrude Hoffmann, December 2, 1912, Correspondence Re: From Broadway to Paris, General Correspondence 1910–1926, box 373, folder 1228, TSA.

8. "La Bete," *Variety*, April 27, 1912, 15.

9. Ibid.

10. Ibid.

11. Ship manifest, S.S. *La Provence*, under "Gertrude Hoffmann," May 4, 1912. Statue of Liberty—Ellis Island Foundation.

12. "La Bete," 15. Letter to Gertrude Hoffmann, December 2, 1912.

13. They try to "graft opera and ballet on to the revue format" (Hirsch, *Boys from Syracuse*, 89).

14. "The Ballet of 1830," Internet Broadway Database, https://www.ibdb.com/broadway-show/the-ballet-of-1830-478286.

15. Gerald Bordman and Thomas S. Hischak, "The Passing Show," in *The Oxford Companion to American Theatre* (Oxford: Oxford University Press, 2004).

16. "Programs: The Passing Show of 1912," The Passing Show of 1912 Clippings File, TSA.

17. "Lots of Agility in Winter Garden Skit," *New York Times*, July 23, 1912, 9.

18. "Hoffmann Co. Rehearsing," *Variety*, July 26, 1912, 13; "Musical Comedy Houses Permanent on Broadway," *Variety*, August 23, 1912, 13.

19. "Musical Comedy Houses Permanent on Broadway," 13; "Rita Gould and Jas. T. Duffy . . . ," *Variety*, August 30, 1912, 9.

20. "Winter Garden Does $25,000," *Variety*, August 2, 1912, 11.

21. "Musical Comedy Houses Permanent on Broadway," 13.

22. "Your Stockings Painted On!" *Chicago Examiner*, September 29, 1912, 65.

23. Polaire, "Make Your Feet a Feast for the Eye," *Times Dispatch*, March 23, 1913, 23.

24. See Anne Anlin Cheng, *Second Skin: Josephine Baker and the Modern Surface* (Oxford: Oxford University Press, 2010).

25. Homer Croy, "Watching Our Funny World Go By," *Judge*, May 3, 1913.

26. Thomas J. Gaffney, *Birds of a Feather: A Play in Four Acts* (Boston: Gorham Press, 1915), 57, http://hdl.handle.net/2027/mdp.39015059404239.

27. Ibid.

28. Hirsch, *Boys from Syracuse*, 136.

29. "Rita Gould and Jas. T. Duffy . . . ," 9.

30. Letter to Gertrude Hoffmann, December 2, 1912.

31. "Garden Gets Ahearn's Act," *Variety*, June 28, 1912, 5.

32. Letter to Gertrude Hoffmann, December 2, 1912.

33. "Clippings: Broadway to Paris," TSA.

34. "Broadway to Paris" (script), Ole Olsen Collection, Ned Wayburn material, box 1, folder 58, Cinematic Arts Library, University of Southern California.

35. Ibid., 24.

36. Ibid.

37. Max Hoffmann, "Paree's a Branch of Broadway," sheet music (New York: T. B. Harms; Francis, Day & Hunter; Jerome Remick & Co., 1912).

38. "Broadway to Paris" (script), 19.

39. "Trelawny of the 'Wells,'" Internet Broadway Database, https://www.ibdb.com/broadway-production/trelawny-of-the-wells-7262.

40. While Held was said to have rescued a man from a runaway carriage, Hoffmann's character rides on a runaway carriage pulled by a pantomime horse. "Broadway to Paris" (script), 16.

41. Max Hoffmann, "The Gertrude Hoffmann Glide," sheet music (1912), 53.196.6A-B, MCNY.

42. Ibid.

43. Gertrude and Max Hoffmann, box 11, folder 6, GMHP.

44. Ibid.

45. Gertrude and Max Hoffmann, box 2, folder 21: Personal notebooks, Red notebook, GMHP.

46. Letter to Gertrude Hoffmann, December 2, 1912.

47. Letter from Max Hoffmann to J. J. Shubert, Correspondence Re: From Broadway to Paris, General Correspondence 1910–1926, box 373, folder 1228, TSA.

48. Letter to Gertrude Hoffmann, December 2, 1912.

49. Locke, "Scrapbooks / Gertrude Hoffman," 274:11, RLC, BRTD, NYPLPA.

50. Letter to Gertrude Hoffmann, December 2, 1912.

51. Ibid.

52. Ibid.

53. Locke, "Scrapbooks / Gertrude Hoffman," 274:11, RLC, BRTD, NYPLPA.

54. Letters from Gilman Haskell to J. J. Shubert, November 21, 1912, and November 22, 1912, General Correspondence 1910–1926, File 1540, TSA.

55. Marilyn S. Kushner, Kimberly Orcutt, and Casey Nelson Blake, eds., *The Armory Show at 100: Modernism and Revolution* (New York: New-York Historical Society; in association with D. Giles, 2013).

56. "'Cubist' Dress Follows March of Latest Art," *Inter Ocean*, March 18, 1913, Tuesday Morning ed.

57. Ibid.

58. Amy Leslie, "Hoffmann in Gay Whirl: Dancer Surrounded by Swiftly Moving Ensemble at American Music Hall. Art Is of Decadent Kind. In Strong Contrast to Her Sensuous Method Is the Restful Acting of Louise Dresser," *Chicago Daily News*, March 24, 1913, Broadway to Paris Clippings, folder 1, TSA.

59. School of the Art Institute of Chicago (SAIC), "SAIC and the Armory Show | 150 Years of SAIC," http://www.saic.edu/150/saic-and-armory-show.

60. Peter Wollen, *Raiding the Icebox: Reflections on Twentieth-Century Culture* (Bloomington: Indiana University Press, 1993), 13.

61. Elizabeth Carlson, "Cubist Fashion: Mainstreaming Modernism after the Armory," *Winterthur Portfolio* 48, no. 1 (March 1, 2014): 1–28.

62. For other recent work that considers how modernism was transmitted to America through popular media, see Karen Leick, *Gertrude Stein and the Making of an American Celebrity* (New York: Routledge, 2009); Leonard Diepeveen, *Mock Modernism: An Anthology of Parodies, Travesties, Frauds, 1910–1935* (Toronto: University of Toronto Press, 2014).

Chapter 10

1. All of the information in this paragraph was take from "C-File, Max Hoffmann," n.d., C-480840, U.S. Citizenship and Immigration Services Genealogy Program, Department of Homeland Security, https://www.uscis.gov/genealogy.

2. "$90,000 Vaudeville Offer for Gertrude Hoffmann," *Variety*, June 6, 1913, 3.

3. "Road Show's $10,000 Salary List for 3-Star Combine," *Variety*, July 5, 1913, 7; "Act II, Article Transcripts and Notes on Polaire and Gertrude Hoffman, 1913, Undated," series 1, box 2, folder 5, MGP.

4. "Act II, Scene Ten (They Believed Their Publicity!), Undated," series 1, box 2, folder 2, MGP.

5. "Lyric Theatre," Jerome Robbins Dance Division, the New York Public Library, NYPL Digital Collections, http://digitalcollections.nypl.org/items/510d47da-5e01-a3d9-e040-e00a18064a99. In chapter 11, I expand on the idea that "barefoot dancing" came to be associated with wealth and leisure.

6. Gertrude and Max Hoffmann, box 2, folder 23: Performance Notes, Brown notebook, GMHP.

7. Ibid.

8. Ibid.

9. All descriptions in this paragraph are taken from "Lyric Theatre," JRDD, the New York Public Library, NYPL Digital Collections, http://digitalcollections.nypl.org/items/510d47da-5e01-a3d9-e040-e00a18064a99.

10. "Act II, Article Transcripts and Notes on Polaire and Gertrude Hoffman, 1913, Undated," series 1, box 2, folder 5, MGP.

11. "Act II, Scene Ten (They Believed Their Publicity!)."

12. "Act II, Article Transcripts and Notes on Polaire."

13. Ibid.

14. Letter from Max Hoffmann to J. J. Shubert, February 16, General Correspondence 1910–1926, box 373, folder 1228, TSA.

15. The historian Kathy Peiss notes the presence of over five hundred dance halls and one hundred dancing schools in the city during the decade. Kathy Peiss, *Cheap Amusements: Working Women and Leisure in Turn-of-the-Century New York* (Philadelphia: Temple University Press, 1986), 88. For other discussions of the dance craze in the early 1910s, see Lewis A. Erenberg, *Steppin' Out: New York Nightlife and the Transformation of American Culture, 1890–1930* (Chicago: University of Chicago Press, 1984); Susan C. Cook, "Passionless Dancing and Passionate Reform: Respectability, Modernism, and the Social Dancing of Irene and Vernon Castle," in *The Passion of Music and Dance: Body, Gender and Sexuality* (Oxford: Berg, 1998), 133–50.

16. "The Gertrude Hoffman Show," *Macon News*, Loose scrapbook pages of newspaper clippings, box 3, page 43, GHC.

17. Susan Cook discusses how these types of social dance were associated with working-class and minority cultures. See Cook, "Passionless Dancing and Passionate Reform."

18. Priya Srinivasan, *Sweating Saris: Indian Dance as Transnational Labor* (Philadelphia: Temple University Press, 2011), 88.

19. Krystyn R. Moon, *Yellowface: Creating the Chinese in American Popular Music and Performance, 1850s–1920s* (New Brunswick, N.J.: Rutgers University Press, 2005), 82–83.

20. On the conflation of Asianness and ragtime in performance of this period, see Robert Lancefield, "Hearing Orientality in (White) America, 1900–1930," *Dissertations*, January 1, 2004, 746, http://wesscholar.wesleyan.edu/etd_diss/2.

21. According to Kristyn Moon, Chinese vaudevillians "blended aspects of Chinese culture with American stereotypes to give white audiences what they wanted and expected, while simultaneously challenging those stereotypes." Moon, *Yellowface*, 144.

22. "Lyric Theatre," Jerome Robbins Dance Division, the New York Public Library. For a profile of Ben Ali and the acrobats he trained, see "Hassan Ben Ali, Manager: A Marabout from North Africa in the Vaudeville Business in New York," *Sun*, May 28, 1911, Old Fulton NY Postcards.

23. Susan Nance, *How the Arabian Nights Inspired the American Dream, 1790–1935* (Chapel Hill: University of North Carolina Press, 2009), 130.

24. Alan Dale, "A Diaphanous Dancer," *Cosmopolitan* 56 (December 1913): 117–19.

25. Srinivasan, *Sweating Saris*, 71.

26. An important early essay of ethnic humor and vaudeville is Lawrence E. Mintz, "Humor and Ethnic Stereotypes in Vaudeville and Burlesque," *MELUS* 21, no. 4 (1996): 19–28. This has been a topic of great interest in recent work on American vaudeville. See Rick DesRochers, *The New Humor in the Progressive Era: Americanization and the Vaudeville Comedian* (New York: Palgrave Macmillan, 2014); Moon, *Yellowface*; Jennifer Mooney, *Irish Stereotypes in Vaudeville, 1865–1905* (New York: Palgrave Macmillan, 2015); Nance, *How the Arabian Nights Inspired the American Dream*.

27. "Gertrude Hoffmann Coming," *Times-Democrat*, December 3, 1913, 4.

28. "Gertrude Hoffmann's Show Is Bewildering; Program Embraces Much That Is Wonderful," *Times-Democrat*, December 8, 1913, 4.

29. For a history of the Leo Frank case and its aftermath, see Steve Oney, *And the Dead Shall Rise: The Murder of Mary Phagan and the Lynching of Leo Frank* (New York: Vintage Books, 2004).

30. For an analysis of the hate group's political ascent in this era, see Linda Gordon, *The Second Coming of the KKK: The Ku Klux Klan of the 1920s and the American Political Tradition* (New York: Liveright, 2017).

31. "Hoffmann Show Closing?" *Variety*, January 30, 1914, 3.

32. "Colonial Theatre," Jerome Robbins Dance Division, the New York Public Library, NYPL Digital Collections, http://digitalcollections.nypl.org/items/510d47da-5c34-a3d9-e040-e00a18064a99.

33. Robinson Locke, "Scrapbooks / Gertrude Hoffman," series 1, reel 24, vols. 273–74, 274:44, RLC, BRTD, NYPLPA.

34. See Joel Dinerstein, *Swinging the Machine: Modernity, Technology, and African American Culture between the World Wars* (Amherst: University of Massachusetts Press, 2003).

35. Robert Grau, "How the Vaudeville Uplift Affects Stars Salaries," *Lippincott's Monthly Magazine: A Popular Journal of General Literature*, April 1914, 506.

36. Robert W. Snyder, *The Voice of the City: Vaudeville and Popular Culture in New York* (New York: Oxford University Press, 1989), 82.

37. After it opened in 1913, "Performing at the Palace soon became the goal of every vaudevillian." Arthur Wertheim, *Vaudeville Wars: How the Keith-Albee*

and Orpheum Circuits Controlled the Big-Time and Its Performers (New York: Palgrave Macmillan, 2006), 209.

38. Locke, "Scrapbooks / Gertrude Hoffman," 274:43, RLC, BRTD, NYPLPA.

Chapter 11

1. Alan Dale, "A Diaphanous Dancer," *Cosmopolitan* 56 (December 1913): 117–19, 118.

2. M. Alison Kibler, *Rank Ladies: Gender and Cultural Hierarchy in American Vaudeville* (Chapel Hill: University of North Carolina Press, 1999).

3. Leonard Diepeveen, *Mock Modernism: An Anthology of Parodies, Travesties, Frauds, 1910–1935* (Toronto: University of Toronto Press, 2014).

4. Karen Leick, *Gertrude Stein and the Making of an American Celebrity* (New York: Routledge, 2009), 66.

5. Michael Murphy, "'One Hundred Per Cent Bohemia': Pop Decadence and the Aestheticization of Commodity in the Rise of the Slicks," in *Marketing Modernisms: Self-Promotion, Canonization, Rereading*, ed. Kevin J. H. Dettmar and Stephen Watt, 61–89 (Ann Arbor: University of Michigan Press, 1996), 76.

6. Isadora Duncan, "The Dance of the Future," in *The Art of the Dance* (New York: Theatre Arts Books, 1970), 54–63.

7. Mary Simonson, *Body Knowledge: Performance, Intermediality, and American Entertainment at the Turn of the Twentieth Century* (Oxford: Oxford University Press, 2013), 50–68.

8. Ibid., 53. Some of the most important and interesting performance studies work in recent years has concerned itself with reconstructing and interrogating the influence of Delsarte on American performance, particularly by women. For an early essay on Delsarte's influence on American dance, see Nancy Chalfa Ruyter, "American Delsartism: Precursor of an American Dance Art," *Educational Theatre Journal* 25, no. 4 (1973): 421–35. Julia Walker considers Delsarte among the nineteenth-century influences against which American Expressionism reacts: Julia A. Walker, *Expressionism and Modernism in the American Theatre: Bodies, Voices, Words* (Cambridge: Cambridge University Press, 2005). Carrie Preston relates Delsarte to the history of modern women's solo performance, see Carrie J. Preston, *Modernism's Mythic Pose: Gender, Genre, Solo Performance* (Oxford: Oxford University Press, 2011). Marian Kimber focuses on Delsarte's influence in the realm of elocution in *The Elocutionists: Women, Music, and the Spoken Word* (Urbana: University of Illinois Press, 2017).

9. Gertrude Hoffmann, "The Well-Watered Woman," *Times Dispatch*, September 7, 1913, Features, 8.

10. Harry Reichenbach and David Freedman, *Phantom Fame* (London: Noel Douglas, 1932), 213.

11. Hoffmann, "Well-Watered Woman."

12. For a history of *Vanity Fair*'s genesis and early development as a "smart" magazine, see George H. Douglas, *The Smart Magazines: 50 Years of Literary Revelry and High Jinks at Vanity Fair, the New Yorker, Life, Esquire, and the Smart Set* (Hamden, Conn.: Archon Books, 1991).

13. Daniel Tracy, "Investing in 'Modernism': Smart Magazines, Parody, and Middlebrow Professional Judgment," *Journal of Modern Periodical Studies* 1, no. 1 (2010): 38–63, 44.

14. Douglas, *Smart Magazines*.

15. For the elite audience, see ibid., 99–101. For the aspirational audience, see Tracy, "Investing in 'Modernism,'" 40.

16. Gertrude Hoffmann, "Dancing, and the Magic of the Sea," *Vanity Fair*, July 1914, 24–26, 25. My understanding of *Vanity Fair* as a magazine invested in modeling and teaching sophistication to a mostly middle-class readership is influenced by the history of the magazine in Faye Hammill, *Sophistication: A Literary and Cultural History* (Liverpool: Liverpool University Press, 2010), 154–63.

17. G. Hoffmann, "Dancing, and the Magic of the Sea," 25.

18. Ibid.

19. Ibid.

20. "Dancing on the Sand Dunes," *Indianapolis News*, February 15, 1915, 12.

21. Robinson Locke, "Scrapbooks / Gertrude Hoffman," series 1, reel 24, vols. 273–74, 274:21, RLC, BRTD, NYPLPA.

22. "Several American Acts Booked for England," advertisement, *Variety*, April 16, 1915, 2.

23. Ibid.

24. Locke, "Scrapbooks / Gertrude Hoffman," 274:48, RLC, BRTD, NYPLPA.

25. Ibid., 274:49.

26. Ibid.

27. "History of the Provincetown Playhouse," http://www.provincetownplayhouse.com/history.html.

28. Gertrude and Max Hoffmann, box 2, folder 37, Scripts: Sumuran script, n.d., 37, GMHP.

29. Robert S. Bader, *Four of the Three Musketeers: The Marx Brothers on Stage* (Evanston, Ill.: Northwestern University Press, 2016), 139.

30. Locke, "Scrapbooks / Gertrude Hoffman," 274:52, RLC, BRTD, NYPLPA.

31. W. L. Sowers, "Pantomime in America," *Texas Review* 2, no. 3 (1916): 235–47, 237.

32. Ibid.

33. Media studies has a long history of considering the relationship between vaudeville and film. See Robert Clyde Allen, *Vaudeville and Film, 1895–1915: A Study in Media Interaction*, Dissertations on Film 1980 (New York: Arno Press, 1980); Henry Jenkins, *What Made Pistachio Nuts? Early Sound Comedy and the Vaudeville Aesthetic*, Film and Culture (New York: Columbia University Press, 1992). For a more recent approach to relations between stage and screen in this era, see Kaveh Askari et al., eds., *Performing New Media, 1890–1915* (New Barnet, Hertfordshire: John Libbey, 2015).

34. "Ordynski: The Man Behind 'Sumurun,'" *New York Dramatic Mirror*, September 8, 1915, 19.

35. Priya Srinivasan, *Sweating Saris: Indian Dance as Transnational Labor* (Philadelphia: Temple University Press, 2011), 80.

36. Kibler, *Rank Ladies*, 113.

37. Jeanne Scheper, *Moving Performances: Divas, Iconicity, and Remembering the Modern Stage* (New Brunswick, N.J.: Rutgers University Press, 2016), 63.

38. Locke, "Scrapbooks / Gertrude Hoffman," 274:52, RLC, BRTD, NYPLPA.

39. Ibid.

40. Gertrude and Max Hoffmann, box 2, folder 37, Scripts: Sumuran script, GMHP.
41. Gertrude and Max Hoffmann, box 2, folder 38: Sumuran scenario, GMHP.
42. Ibid.
43. Locke, "Scrapbooks / Gertrude Hoffman," 274:51, 52, RLC, BRTD, NYPLPA.
44. Ibid., 274:49.
45. Heywood Broun, "Public Bathing and the Drama," *New York Tribune*, September 8, 1915, 7.
46. Sime Silverman, "New Acts: Gertrude Hoffman and Co., 'Sumurun,'" *Variety*, August 20, 1915, 14.
47. "Palace," *Variety*, August 27, 1915, 13.
48. Ibid.
49. "B. F. Keith's Palace," advertisement, *New York Tribune*, September 5, 1915, sec. III, 5.
50. Frederick James Smith, "Vaudeville: 'Sumurun' Undergoes Changes, Fannie Brice's New Songs, Burt and Stanford Return," *New York Dramatic Mirror*, September 15, 1915, 18.
51. "Trouble in the Harem: Tank Affords Comic Relief in 'Sumurun,' at the Palace," *New York Times*, September 7, 1915, 13.
52. "Lots of Agility in Winter Garden Skit," *New York Times*, July 23, 1912, 9.
53. "'Sumurun' at Orpheum Gertrude Hoffman in Great Act," *Sacramento Union*, March 10, 1916, 5.
54. For a discussion of these vaudeville circuits, the United Booking Office, and their impact on vaudeville touring practices, see Arthur Frank Wertheim, *Vaudeville Wars: How the Keith–Albee and Orpheum Circuits Controlled the Big-Time and Its Performers* (New York: Palgrave Macmillan, 2006). What is most important to keep in mind for Hoffmann's tour is her familiarity with the West Coast Orpheum venues. Not all "big-time" vaudeville players would travel that far west.
55. Locke, "Scrapbooks / Gertrude Hoffman," 274:56, RLC, BRTD, NYPLPA. "Correspondence: Majestic," *Variety*, December 3, 1915, 24.
56. "From 'Movies' to Vaudeville for Facial Art," *New York Herald*, August 15, 1915, sec. 3, 9.
57. J. C. Jessen, "In and Out of West Coast Studios," *Motion Picture News* (January–March 1917), January 27, 1917, 554, http://archive.org/details/motionpicturenew15moti_1.
58. Locke, "Scrapbooks / Gertrude Hoffman," 274:56, RLC, BRTD, NYPLPA.
59. Grace Kingsley, "Rialto," *Los Angeles Daily Times*, March 23, 1916, part 3, 4.
60. Guy Price, "Coast Picture News," *Variety*, April 7, 1916, 20.
61. Kingsley, "Rialto."
62. For an overview of Weber's career, see Shelley Stamp, *Lois Weber in Early Hollywood* (Oakland: University of California Press, 2015).
63. Gillian B. Anderson, "Synchronized Music: The Influence of Pantomime on Moving Pictures," *Music and the Moving Image* 8, no. 3 (2015): 3–39.
64. Richard Koszarski, *An Evening's Entertainment: The Age of the Silent Feature Picture, 1915–1928* (Berkeley: University of California Press, 1994), 1–8.
65. "Pacific Coast Notes," *Motography*, April 15, 1916, 890.

66. An account of Bambrick's recruitment can be found in Linda Arvidson, *When the Movies Were Young* (New York: E. P. Dutton, 1925), 210–13.

67. David Mayer, "Architecture and Art Dance Meet in the Ancient World," in *The Ancient World in Silent Cinema*, ed. Pantelis Michelakis and Maria Wylke, 91–108 (New York: Cambridge University Press, 2013), 105.

68. Ibid., 105.

69. See ibid., 106–7; and Preston, *Modernism's Mythic Pose*, 87–88.

70. "Stars Twinkle at Actor Ball," *Los Angeles Daily Times*, March 23, 1916, part 2, 7.

71. Locke, "Scrapbooks / Gertrude Hoffman," 274:63, RLC, BRTD, NYPLPA.

72. Dorothy Ferris, "The Rage for Barefoot Dancing," *Vanity Fair*, April 1916, 68.

73. Ibid.

74. "New Hoffmann Act," *Variety*, August 11, 1916, 5.

75. "Max Hoffmann Leading," *Variety*, September 15, 1916, 5.

76. "Sues Gertie Hoffmann," *Variety*, December 1, 1916, 7.

77. "News Item: 'On Hand, One Oriental Dancer,'" *Variety*, October 13, 1916, 9.

78. *Passport Applications, January 2, 1906–March 31, 1925*, U.S. Passport Applications, 1795–1925, under "Gertrude Hoffmann," microfilm roll no. 336, December 5, 1916, National Archives and Records Administration: Washington, D.C. Accessed through ancestry.com.

79. Locke, "Scrapbooks / Gertrude Hoffman," 273:32–33, RLC, BRTD, NYPLPA.

80. See Marlis Schweitzer, *Transatlantic Broadway: The Infrastructural Politics of Global Performance* (Basingstoke, Eng.: Palgrave Macmillan, 2015).

81. "Obituary: H. B. Marinelli," *Variety*, January 10, 1924, 7.

Chapter 12

1. "The Century Girl," Internet Broadway Database, https://www.ibdb.com/broadway-production/the-century-girl-8469; "Cabarets," *Variety*, October 20, 1916, 18.

2. "Midnight in the Cocoanut Grove," *Vanity Fair*, April 1917, 65.

3. Service during the interval is discussed in "Cabarets: 'Dance and Grow Thin,'" *Variety*, January 26, 1917, 13. For Reisenweber's reputation, see "Reisenweber's Cafe: Glamour, Late Nights and Hot Jazz," *The Bowery Boys: New York City History* (blog), February 26, 2010, http://www.boweryboyshistory.com/2010/02/reisenwebers-cafe-glamour-late-nights.html.

4. "There's Something Nice about the South" was sung by Van and Schenck. Tin Pan Alley songs praising the South are described in John Bush Jones, *Reinventing Dixie: Tin Pan Alley's Songs and the Creation of the Mythic South* (Baton Rouge: Louisiana State University Press, 2015).

5. Lewis A. Erenberg, *Steppin' Out: New York Nightlife and the Transformation of American Culture, 1890–1930* (Chicago: University of Chicago Press, 1984), 123.

6. "Cabarets: 'Dance and Grow Thin,'" 13.

7. Ibid.

8. Ibid.

9. For Vernon and Irene Castle's tango, see Cook, "Passionless Dancing and Passionate Reform: Respectability, Modernism, and the Social Dancing of Irene

and Vernon Castle," in *The Passion of Music and Dance: Body, Gender and Sexuality*, 133–50 (Oxford: Berg, 1998), 141.

10. A. E. Weed, American Mutoscope and Biograph Company, *Princess Rajah dance* (1904), Library of Congress, Washington, D.C., https://www.loc.gov/item/96520235/.

11. "Snake Dancer at Victoria," *New York Times*, January 20, 1909, 2.

12. Gertrude and Max Hoffmann, box 2, folder 21: Personal notebooks, Red notebook, GMHP.

13. Ibid.

14. Robinson Locke, "Scrapbooks / Gertrude Hoffman," series 1, reel 24, vols. 273–74, 274:70, RLC, BRTD, NYPLPA.

15. Gertrude and Max Hoffmann, box 2, folder 21: Personal notebooks, Red notebook, GMHP. Zittel would later found *Zit's Theatrical Newspaper*, an important trade paper for striptease and burlesque acts in the 1920s and 1930s. See Rachel Shteir, *Striptease: The Untold History of the Girlie Show* (New York: Oxford University Press, 2005), 197.

16. "Gertrude Hoffman," *Vanity Fair*, April 1917, 64.

17. Peter Jensen Brown, "Early Sports and Pop Culture History Blog: The Colorful History and Etymology of 'Pink Elephant,'" *Early Sports and Pop Culture History Blog* (blog), August 20, 2014, https://esnpc.blogspot.com/2014/08/the-colorful-history-and-etymology-of.html.

18. "Gertie Strikes for Amber Lights," *Day Book*, February 3, 1917, 27.

19. Details in the previous three sentences are taken from "Cabarets: Enrico Muris," *Variety*, February 23, 1917, 8.

20. "Bushwick," *New York Clipper*, February 28, 1917, 8.

21. Sime Silverman, "Gertrude Hoffmann and Co.: 'Revue,'" *Variety*, March 2, 1917, 18.

22. Ibid.

23. Ibid.

24. Ibid.

25. Ibid.

26. For the discussion of fashion shows as politicized theatrical events in this era, see Marlis Schweitzer, "Patriotic Acts of Consumption: Lucile (Lady Duff Gordon) and the Vaudeville Fashion Show Craze," *Theatre Journal* 60, no. 4 (2008): 585–608.

27. Silverman, "Gertrude Hoffmann and Co.," 18.

28. "Cover," *Theatre*, January 1917. This image was also the cover of the 1917 calendar provided for new subscribers to *Theatre Magazine* that year. For the historical associations of Columbia with the United States and the Americas more broadly, see Kirsten Silva Gruesz, "America," in *Keywords for American Cultural Studies*, ed. Bruce Burgett and Glenn Hendler (New York: New York University Press, 2014), 21–25.

29. Neil Gould, *Victor Herbert: A Theatrical Life* (Oxford: Oxford University Press, 2011), 512.

30. See Leigh Woods, "American Vaudeville, American Empire," in *Performing America: Cultural Nationalism in American Theater*, ed. Jeffrey D. Mason and J. Ellen Gainor (Ann Arbor: University of Michigan Press, 1999), 73–90.

31. Barbara Stratyner, *Ned Wayburn and the Dance Routine: From Vaudeville to the Ziegfeld Follies* (Madison: University of Wisconsin Press, 1996).

32. David Monod, "'I Didn't Raise My Boy to Be a Soldier': Popular Song and American Neutrality, 1914–1917," *War in History* 24, no. 4 (November 1, 2017): 438–57, 454.

33. The first quote comes from a speech Wilson gave at a naturalization ceremony on May 10, 1915. See "Wilson's 'Too Proud to Fight' Speech," the Lusitania Resource, http://www.rmslusitania.info/primary-docs/too-proud-to-fight/.

34. Marlis Schweitzer, *When Broadway Was the Runway: Theater, Fashion, and American Culture* (Philadelphia: University of Pennsylvania Press, 2011), 211–12.

35. Abel Green and Joe Laurie, *Show Biz, from Vaude to Video* (New York: Garland, 1985), 116.

36. Ibid.

37. "Vaudeville's 'Honor' War Record," *Western Magazine* 13, no. 1 (January 1919): 33–34, 33.

38. Schweitzer, *When Broadway Was the Runway*, 211–12.

39. Ibid., 192–93.

40. "True Patriotism!," *Theatre*, June 1917, 322.

41. Fred, "Palace," *Variety*, April 20, 1917, 13.

42. "Gertrude Hoffmann Revue," *New York Times*, April 10, 1917, 17. For references to audiences mistakenly standing for the flag when this number went on tour, see Giles P. Cain, "Little Stories of Plays and Players," *The Independent*, December 22, 1917, 3.

43. Dorothy Parker, "The Star-Spangled Drama," *Vanity Fair*, August 1918, 29.

44. Ibid.

45. "With the Press Agents," *Variety*, April 27, 1917, 10.

46. For the background of the "Christy Girl" and the way she functions in opposition to the "Gibson Girl," Annessa Ann Babic, *America's Changing Icons: Constructing Patriotic Women from World War I to the Present* (Lanham, Md.: Rowman and Littlefield, 2018), 34–37. For an analysis of the poster, see Andrew J. Huebner, "Gee! I Wish I Were a Man: Gender and the Great War," in *The Routledge History of Gender, War, and the US Military*, ed. Kara D. Vuic (New York: Routledge, 2017), 84–102. For the poster itself, see Howard Chandler Christy, "Gee!! I Wish I Were a Man, I'd Join the Navy Be a Man and Do It—United States Navy Recruiting Station," color lithograph, 1917, Library of Congress, Washington, D.C., www.loc.gov/pictures/item/2002712088/.

47. Percy Hammond, "Gertrude Hoffmann as Artist and Patriot," *Chicago Daily Tribune*, May 22, 1917, 15.

48. Ibid.

49. "Askum," advertisement, *Chicago Daily Tribune*, June 24, 1917, 14.

50. Ibid.

51. Kerry Segrave, *Endorsements in Advertising: A Social History* (Jefferson, N.C.: McFarland, 2005), 5.

52. See "Collecting on Picture 'Names,'" *Variety*, February 14, 1919, 56.

53. Robert Birchard, *Cecil B. DeMille's Hollywood* (Lexington: University Press of Kentucky, 2004), 112.

54. "$75,000 for Hoffmann Films," *Variety*, August 31, 1917, 5.

55. "Hoffmann Prefers Vaudeville," *Variety*, September 14, 1917, 8.

56. "Players Collect Smokes," *New York Clipper*, November 28, 1917, 6; "Correspondence," *Variety*, November 2, 1917, 34.

57. Cain, "Little Stories of Plays and Players," 3.

58. Ibid.

59. "More or Less in the Spotlight," *New York Times*, December 26, 1926, Drama, X4.

60. Cain, "Little Stories of Plays and Players," 3.

61. Monod, "'I Didn't Raise My Boy to Be a Soldier,'" 439.

62. For a discussion of "enlistment dramas" see Susan Zeiger, "She Didn't Raise Her Boy to Be a Slacker: Motherhood, Conscription, and the Culture of the First World War," *Feminist Studies* 22, no. 1 (Spring 1996): 7–39, especially 20–28.

63. "Palace (Earl Steward, Mgr.; Orpheum)," *Variety*, November 9, 1917, 28.

64. Caroline Scurfield Caffin, *Vaudeville: The Book* (New York: M. Kennerley, 1914), 27.

65. Ibid., 102.

66. Locke, "Gertrude Hoffmann Scrapbooks," 274:71, RLC, BRTD, NYPLPA.

67. Ibid.

68. "Sees His Finish When Gertrude Hoffman Dances," *Daily Journal Gazette*, November 17, 1917, 4.

69. "News from the Dailies," *Variety*, November 23, 1917, 14.

70. "Gertrude Hoffman Is Acquitted of Indecency Charge," *St. Louis Post-Dispatch*, December 9, 1917, 16.

71. "Must Dress Up," *Variety*, December 21, 1917, 5.

72. See Katie N. Johnson, *Sex for Sale: Six Progressive-Era Brothel Dramas* (Iowa City: University of Iowa Press, 2015); Barbara Antoniazzi, *The Wayward Woman: Progressivism, Prostitution, and Performance in the United States, 1888–1917* (Madison, N.J.: Fairleigh Dickinson University Press, 2014).

73. Ronald Harold Wainscott, *The Emergence of the Modern American Theater, 1914–1929* (New Haven, Conn.: Yale University Press, 1997), 76.

74. For discussions of the theatrical censorship in this era, see ibid., 75–90; and Mae West, "The Case Against Mae West," in *Three Plays by Mae West*, ed. Lillian Schissel (New York: Routledge, 1997), 203–32.

75. W. J. Rorabaugh, *Prohibition: A Concise History* (New York: Oxford University Press, 2018), 53.

76. Ibid., 44.

77. Ibid., 54.

78. Gertrude and Max Hoffmann, box 2, folder 21: Personal notebooks, Red notebook, GMHP.

79. Ibid.

80. "Arrest Theatrical Troop [*sic*]," *Akron Beacon Journal*, December 25, 1917.

81. "Famous Dancer Needs Champagne," *Lincoln Star*, December 28, 1917, 7.

82. Carlton W. Miles, "'Is Celebrity Worth While' Asks Gertrude," *Minneapolis Journal*, October 5, 1919, Sunday ed., Amusement, box 1, Clippings, GMHP.

83. Ibid.

84. Elizabeth Siegel Watkins, "Stress and the American Vernacular: Popular Perceptions of Disease Causality," in *Stress, Shock, and Adaptation in the Twentieth Century*, ed. David Cantor and Edmund Ramsden (Rochester, N.Y.: University of Rochester Press, 2014), 49–70, 53–54.

85. Ibid., 56

86. Vernon Castle and Irene Castle, *Modern Dancing* (New York: Harper, 1914), 146.

87. Cook, "Passionless Dancing."

88. Locke, "Gertrude Hoffmann Scrapbooks," 274:76, RLC, BRTD, NYPLPA.

89. Patsy Smith, "Among the Women," *Variety*, April 12, 1918, 48.

90. "Max and Gertrude Hoffmann Are Now in Their New Home . . . ," *Variety*, August 16, 1918, 11.

91. Edward M. Coffman, *The War to End All Wars: The American Military Experience in World War I* (Lexington: University Press of Kentucky, 2014), 29.

92. World War I Selective Service System Draft Registration Cards, 1917–1918, under "Max Hoffmann," microfilm roll no. M1509, National Archives and Records Administration, Washington, D.C. Accessed through "U.S., World War I Draft Registration Cards, 1917–1918," ancestry.com.

93. Ibee, "Gertrude Hoffmann: Dances and Imitations," *Variety*, October 25, 1918, 18.

94. Ibid.

95. Patsy Smith, "Among the Women," *Variety*, June 6, 1919, 9.

96. Locke, "Gertrude Hoffmann Scrapbooks," 274:76, RLC, BRTD, NYPLPA.

97. Ibee, "Gertrude Hoffmann," 18.

98. For a history of the disease, see Alfred W. Crosby, *America's Forgotten Pandemic: The Influenza of 1918* (Cambridge: Cambridge University Press, 2003).

99. "Epidemic Casualties," *Variety*, October 25, 1918.

100. Gladys Hurlbut, *Next Week East Lynne! A Famous Stock Company Leading Lady Recounts Her Hilarious Experiences on the Gum-and-Gimlet Circuit* (New York: E. P. Dutton., 1950), 108.

101. "Epidemic Casualties," *Variety*, November 8, 1918, 5.

102. "Ill and Injured," *Variety*, November 15, 1918, 6.

103. "Gertrude Hoffman's Slip," *Variety*, January 10, 1919, 5.

104. Ibid.; "Alhambra's 'Hoodoo Week,'" *Variety*, January 10, 1919, 21.

Chapter 13

1. Arthur Frank Wertheim, *Vaudeville Wars: How the Keith-Albee and Orpheum Circuits Controlled the Big-Time and Its Performers* (New York: Palgrave Macmillan, 2006), 254.

2. Sheldon Cheney observes the "road-town problem" in 1917. DeAnna M. Toten Beard, *Sheldon Cheney's Theatre Arts Magazine: Promoting a Modern American Theatre, 1916–1921* (Lanham, Md.: Scarecrow Press, 2010), 37. George Jean Nathan discusses it in 1927, in "The Theatre," *American Mercury*, July 1927, 376–78. Theater historians have debated the cause and dates of this decline; see Roger Schultz, "Dating the Decline of the 'Road': The Verification of a New Hypothesis," *Theatre History Studies* 13 (1993): 163–79.

3. Abel Green and Joe Laurie, *Show Biz, from Vaude to Video* (New York: Garland, 1985), 268.

4. "For Sale—All Scenery and Equipment," advertisement, *Variety*, June 20, 1919, 38.

5. "For Sale—All Scenery and Effects," advertisement, *New York Clipper*, April 14, 1920, 33.

6. Robinson Locke, "Scrapbooks / Gertrude Hoffman," series 1, reel 24, vols. 273–74, 274:77, RLC, BRTD, NYPLPA.

7. "Seeks Gertrude Hoffmann," *New York Times*, July 26, 1919, 9.

8. "Gertrude Hoffmann Found," *New York Times*, July 27, 1919, 5.

9. Ibid.

10. Ibid.

11. Gertrude and Max Hoffmann, box 2, folder 21: Personal notebooks, Red notebook, GMHP.

12. Anne Harriet Fish, "Keeping on with the Dance," *Vanity Fair*, August 1919, 34–35, 34.

13. Ibid., 35.

14. Locke, "Scrapbooks / Gertrude Hoffman," 274:78, RLC, BRTD, NYPLPA.

15. Naima Prevots, *Dancing in the Sun: Hollywood Choreographers, 1915–1937* (Ann Arbor, Mich.: UMI Research Press, 1987), 155.

16. Suzanne Carbonneau, "Adolph Bolm in America," in *The Ballets Russes and Its World*, ed. Lynn Garafola and Nancy Van Norman Baer, 219–44 (New Haven, Conn.: Yale University Press, 1999), 223.

17. Ibid., 224.

18. For a description of Bolm's American career in its entirety, see ibid. For a source focusing on his late career work in California, see Prevots, *Dancing in the Sun*.

19. "Stadium Symphony to Start Next Week," *New York Times*, June 22, 1919, Drama, Music, 51.

20. John Dougherty, letter to Gertrude Hoffmann, July 12, 1963, box 1, folder 37, Adolph Bolm Collection, (S)*MGZMD 50, JRDD, NYPLPA.

21. This history is explored in Jessica Zeller, *Shapes of American Ballet: Teachers and Training before Balanchine* (New York: Oxford University Press, 2016).

22. For a discussion of "movie prologues" or "movie prologs," see ibid., 47–48. For a discussion from the period, see "'What's Wrong with the Movie Prolog?'" *Dance Magazine*, January 1927, 9.

23. "Stadium Symphony to Start Next Week."

24. "Moving Pictures: Rivoli," *Variety*, June 27, 1919, 45.

25. Ibid.

26. Mary Simonson, *Body Knowledge: Performance, Intermediality, and American Entertainment at the Turn of the Twentieth Century* (Oxford: Oxford University Press, 2013).

27. See Mary Simonson, "Visualizing Music in the Silent Era: The Collaborative Experiments of Visual Symphony Productions," *Journal of the Society for American Music* 12, no. 1 (2018): 2–36.

28. "Vaudeville Reviews by Special Wire: Majestic, Chicago," *Billboard*, September 6, 1919, 11.

29. Ibid.

30. "The Woman's Out-Door Companion," advertisement, *Greenfield Daily Reporter*, November 4, 1919, 8.

31. Discussions of women's mobility in this era have been particularly focused on women motorists. See Georgine Clarsen, *Eat My Dust: Early Women Motorists* (Baltimore: Johns Hopkins University Press, 2011); Cotten Seiler, *Republic of Drivers: A Cultural History of Automobility in America* (Chicago: University of Chicago Press, 2008), 36–68.

32. Carlton W. Miles, "'Is Celebrity Worth While' Asks Gertrude," *Minneapolis Journal*, October 5, 1919, Sunday ed., Amusement, box 1, Clippings, GMHP.

33. "One Native Opera among 4 Novelties," *New York Times*, September 22, 1919, 11. The one "native opera" due to be included was *Cleopatra's Night* by Henry Kimball Hadley. The two-act opera was based on a short story by Théophile Gautier. With its combination of orientalism, decadence, and an American pedigree, it is easy to imagine this opera appealing to Hoffmann. Norman Bel Geddes, best known as a set designer for the *Ziegfeld Follies*, did the sets for this opera as well.

34. Ibid.

35. M. Alison Kibler has discussed this strain as felt by actresses in vaudeville. "The pressures of aging and domesticity had a greater impact on women's careers in the theater than on men's, ending women's careers sooner than most men's and rendering them vulnerable to charges of disrepute for pursuing stage careers instead of staying within the confines of family life." M. Alison Kibler, *Rank Ladies: Gender and Cultural Hierarchy in American Vaudeville* (Chapel Hill: University of North Carolina Press, 1999), 88.

36. Miles, "'Is Celebrity Worth While?'"

37. Ibid.

38. Ibid.

39. *Fourteenth Census of the United States, 1920*, under "Margaret Hay," microfilm roll no. T625, RG 29, National Archives and Records Administration, Washington, D.C. Accessed through "1920 United States Federal Census," ancestry.com.

40. "More or Less in the Spotlight," *New York Times*, December 26, 1926, Drama, X4.

41. Ship manifest, S.S. *Mexico*, under "Max Hoffmann Jr.," November 5, 1919. Statue of Liberty—Ellis Island Foundation.

42. "Empress," advertisement, *Akron Evening Times*, September 16, 1919, 8.

43. Locke, "Scrapbooks / Gertrude Hoffman," 274:78, RLC, BRTD, NYPLPA.

44. Ibid.

45. "Warning!" advertisement, *Variety*, January 24, 1929, 61.

46. Herbert Howe, "Nazimova Speaks," *Picture-Play Magazine*, September 1920, 30.

47. Trav S.D. gives a quick overview of Petrova's life, "Olga Petrova: Vaudeville's Fake Russian," May 10, 2010, https://travsd.wordpress.com/2010/05/10/stars-of-vaudeville-155-olga-petrova/. Leigh Woods uses her career as a case study for American vaudeville: Leigh Woods, "American Vaudeville," in *Popular Performance*, ed. Adam Ainsworth, Oliver Double, and Louise Peacock (London: Bloomsbury, 2017), 55–74.

48. "Inside Stuff on Vaudeville," *Variety*, February 25, 1921, 7.

49. "Inside Stuff on Vaudeville," *Variety*, March 5, 1920, 8.

50. For information about Hoblitzelle and the Interstate Circuit, see Interstate Theatre Circuit, "Interstate Theatre Collection," MA77–1, Texas/Dallas History and Archives Division, Dallas Public Library. "The Hoblitzelle and Interstate Theater Collection," Harry Ransom Center, University of Texas at Austin, https://web.archive.org/web/20181107234159/http://www.hrc.utexas.edu/collections/film/holdings/interstate/.

51. "Gertrude Hoffman Rides into Trouble," *Wilkes-Barre Times Leader*, March 18, 1920, 44.

52. "'Speed' Is Motto of M. Hoffmann: Gertrude's Husband Is Fined," *Oregon Daily Journal*, May 9, 1920, 57.

53. "New Acts This Week: Palace," *Variety*, April 23, 1920, 33.

54. Ibid.

55. Ibid.

56. Ibid.

57. "Thirsty?—Try Dancing," *Topeka State Journal*, February 5, 1920, 2.

58. Ibid.

59. Zeller, *Shapes of American Ballet*, 26.

60. "Dancing for Children," *Daily News* (New York), May 1, 1920, 32.

61. Mark Franko, *The Work of Dance: Labor, Movement, and Identity in the 1930s* (Middletown, Conn.: Wesleyan University Press, 2002), 111. The interconnected nature of pre-1930s ballet and commercial dance is also central to Elizabeth Kendall, *Where She Danced: The Birth of American Art-Dance* (Berkeley: University of California Press, 1979).

62. Green and Laurie, *Show Biz, from Vaude to Video*, 269.

63. Ibid.

Chapter 14

1. *NYC Marriage Index—Manhattan 1920*, under "Max Hoffmann," December 21, 1920, https://archive.org/details/NYC_Marriage_Index_Manhattan_1920.

2. Jack O'Brian, "Voice of Broadway," *Springfield News Leader*, June 21, 1971, 8.

3. "More or Less in the Spotlight," *New York Times*, December 26, 1926, Drama, X4.

4. "Miss Hoffman and Son," *Variety*, April 15, 1921, 6.

5. *Asbury Park Evening News*, advertisement, June 10, 1921, 7.

6. Sime Silverman, "Junior and Terris," *Variety*, July 8, 1921, 14.

7. Lait, "Fifth Avenue," *Variety*, July 22, 1921, 19. For an introduction to eugenic discourse in the period's literature, see Beth Widmaier Capo, "Eugenics: Bad Blood and Better Babies," in *American Literature in Transition, 1910–1920*, ed. Mark W. Van Wienen (Cambridge: Cambridge University Press, 2017), 103–16.

8. *Harris County, Texas, Marriage Records*, under "Norma Blissbrook Terris," September 14, 1921, Harris County Clerk's Office, Houston, Texas. Accessed through "Houston, Texas Select County Marriage Records, 1837–2015," ancestry.com.

9. Ibid.

10. There are some discrepancies between the early listing of dances on the program and the act itself. Twelve dances are listed at the beginning of Sime Silverman, "Gertrude Hoffmann and Her American Ballet," *Variety*, October 7, 1921, 21. Later reviews note that some dances are performed without a separate line on the program. By the time they perform in Brooklyn, seventeen dances are

listed. Danni Bayles-Yeager, "Vaudeville / Orpheum / 12-5-1921," Performing Arts Archive, http://www.performingartsarchive.com.

11. "Orpheum," *Variety*, December 9, 1921, 23.

12. Details of the vaudeville act are taken from Silverman, "Gertrude Hoffmann and Her American Ballet," 21.

13. Bayles-Yeager, "Vaudeville / Orpheum."

14. "Orpheum," *Variety*, December 9, 1921, 23.

15. The Chicago review discusses the lighting scheme in most detail: "Miss Hoffman uses four spot lights, two from the wings, one from the flies, and the house spot." "'Loop' Majestic, Chicago," *Variety*, November 4, 1921, 8.

16. Cyril W. Beaumont, *Michel Fokine and His Ballets* (New York: Dance Horizons, 1981), 162.

17. "During the 1920s, the public's reactions to and understanding of ballet began to mature," writes Jessica Zeller in *Shapes of American Ballet: Teachers and Training before Balanchine* (New York: Oxford University Press, 2016), 23.

18. Ibid.

19. Beaumont, *Michel Fokine*, 162.

20. "Luescher's Keith's Staff," *Variety*, October 14, 1921, 7.

21. Ibid.

22. Coleman Harrison, "Pittsburgh," *Variety*, December 9, 1921, 31.

23. Gertrude and Max Hoffmann, box 1: Clippings, GMHP.

24. Arthur B. Waters, "Philadelphia," *Variety*, February 24, 1922, 33.

25. "Gertrude Hoffmann's Ambition Is to Found a Free Dancing School for Poor Children," *Vaudeville News*, October 21, 1921, 2.

26. Ibid.

27. Arthur Frank Wertheim, *Vaudeville Wars: How the Keith-Albee and Orpheum Circuits Controlled the Big-Time and Its Performers* (New York: Palgrave Macmillan, 2006), 242.

28. Foster Hirsch, *The Boys from Syracuse: The Shuberts' Theatrical Empire* (New York: Cooper Square Press, 2000), 129.

29. Jerry Stagg, *The Brothers Shubert* (Random House, 1968), 185.

30. Ibid., 86.

31. Robert S. Bader, *Four of the Three Musketeers: The Marx Brothers on Stage* (Evanston, Ill.: Northwestern University Press, 2016), 260.

32. For Dressler, see Arthur B. Waters, "Philadelphia," *Variety*, September 30, 1921, 31. For Bayes, see "Spotty Improvements in Business Some Comfort to Shubert Vaudeville," *Variety*, October 28, 1921, 5.

33. Suzanne Carbonneau, "Adolph Bolm in America," in *The Ballets Russes and Its World*, ed. Lynn Garafola and Nancy Van Norman Baer, 219–44 (New Haven, Conn.: Yale University Press, 1999), 228–29.

34. Like Charlie Chaplin, Krazy Kat was a pop culture hero across modernist culture, "reputed to have been read by Gertrude Stein, Ernest Hemingway, Pablo Picasso, Edmund Wilson, E. E. Cummings, Louis Zukovsky, and T. S. Eliot." Glenn Willmott, "Cat People," *Modernism/Modernity* 17, no. 4 (2010): 839–56, 845.

35. Carbonneau, "Adolph Bolm in America," 229.

36. Ibid.

37. Ibid.

38. David Savran, *Highbrow/Lowdown: Theater, Jazz, and the Making of a New Middle Class* (Ann Arbor: University of Michigan Press, 2009), 190.

39. See "Chauve-Souris," *Variety*, February 10, 1922, 16; and Valleri J. Hohman, *Russian Culture and Theatrical Performance in America, 1891–1933* (New York: Palgrave Macmillan, 2011).

40. Ralph Barton. "Chauve-Souris (Program)," National Portrait Gallery, Smithsonian Institution, http://npg.si.edu/object/npg_S_NPG.92.12.

41. "In and Out," *Variety*, February 3, 1922, 9.

42. "Change of Bills in Vaudeville," *Evening World*, February 4, 1922, 18.

43. "Gertrude Hoffmann and Her Ballet," *Brooklyn Daily Eagle*, February 5, 1922, C7.

44. Brenda D. Gottschild, *Digging the Africanist Presence in American Performance: Dance and Other Contexts* (Westport, Conn.: Praeger, 1998). See especially "Don't Take Away My Picasso: Cultural Borrowing and the Afro-Euro-American Triangle," 21–46.

45. "Gertrude Hoffmann and Her Ballet."

46. Brett Page, *Writing for Vaudeville: With Nine Complete Examples of Various Vaudeville Forms by Richard Harding Davis, Aaron Hoffman, Edgar Allan Woolf, Taylor Granville, Louis Weslyn, Arthur Denvir, and James Madison* (Springfield, Mass.: Home Correspondence School, 1915), 11.

47. Len Libbey, "Boston," *Variety*, January 20, 1922, 23.

48. Con, "Palace," *Variety*, April 7, 1922, 19.

49. Wertheim, *Vaudeville Wars*, 250.

50. Hirsch, *Boys from Syracuse*, 129.

51. "Gertrude Hoffman's Unit," *Variety*, June 30, 1922, 5.

52. Bader, *Four of the Three Musketeers*, 260–61.

53. Advertisement, *Variety*, October 13, 1922, 32–33.

54. "Central, J.C. Regular," *Variety*, September 15, 1922, 11.

55. "Shubert Crescent Theatre," Jerome Robbins Dance Division, the New York Public Library, NYPL Digital Collections, http://digitalcollections.nypl.org/items/510d47e3-87af-a3d9-e040-e00a18064a99.

56. "Remediation" is an important concept in media studies. It describes the process whereby one media form tries to mimic and thus incorporate the important elements of another media form. See J. David Bolter and Richard A. Grusin, *Remediation: Understanding New Media* (Cambridge, Mass.: MIT Press, 2000).

57. Max Hoffmann filed a complaint with the National Vaudeville Artists organization to stop the performance of Maurice Golden's "Movie Masque" act, another dance number with cinematic themes. After investigation, Hoffmann discovered that Golden's act predated theirs and shared the concept alone. He apologized in the *New York Clipper*. "Hoffmann Retracts Complaint," *New York Clipper*, January 10, 1923, 10.

58. A.H.D., "Hello Everybody," *New York Clipper*, September 20, 1922, 10.

59. Ibid.

60. Beaumont, *Michel Fokine*, 163.

61. "Queen O' Hearts," Internet Broadway Database, https://www.ibdb.com/broadway-show/queen-o-hearts-7318.

62. "Cabaret," *Variety*, January 12, 1923, 7.

63. "Hoffmann's $5,390," *Variety*, January 25, 1923, 5.
64. Wertheim, *Vaudeville Wars*, 224.
65. "Klein's Unit Going into Boston," *Variety*, February 22, 1923, 38.
66. "Nice Hotel People," *Variety*, March 1, 1923, 20.
67. Ibid.
68. Andrew L. Erdman, *Queen of Vaudeville: The Story of Eva Tanguay* (Ithaca, N.Y.: Cornell University Press, 2012), 184. Caroline Fraser discusses how this trend extended from vaudeville to Hollywood, where "Christian Science reigned supreme" in the 1930s and 40s. Caroline Fraser, *God's Perfect Child: Living and Dying in the Christian Science Church* (New York: Metropolitan Books), 204.
69. "Ends of Units and Season Looked For by March 17," *Variety*, March 1, 1923, 6.
70. "Klein's Unit Shut," *Variety*, March 22, 1923, 5.
71. "Shubert Vaudeville Circuit Ending Disastrous Season," *New York Clipper*, March 14, 1923, 5.
72. Wertheim, *Vaudeville Wars*, 244.
73. All these quotes are taken from "Gertrude Hoffman in Chi's Cabaret Shows," *Variety*, March 29, 1923, 5.
74. "Big Acts in Cabarets," *New York Clipper*, April 25, 1923, 8.
75. "Gertrude Hoffman at Marigold," *New York Clipper*, May 3, 1923, 6.

Chapter 15

1. Gertrude Hoffmann, "Gertrude Hoffmann: Experiences and Credits," box 1, folder 1, GHC.
2. Gertrude Hoffmann, Western Union telegram to Lee Shubert, May 9, 1923, General Correspondence 1910–1926, box 373, folder 1228, TSA.
3. Lee Shubert, telegram to Gertrude Hoffmann, May 10, 1923, General Correspondence 1910–1926, box 373, folder 1228, TSA.
4. "The Passing Show of 1923," Internet Broadway Database, https://www.ibdb.com/broadway-production/the-passing-show-of-1923–8344.
5. Cynthia Jane Krieg and Regina G. Feeney, *Freeport* (Charleston, S.C.: Arcadia, 2012), 29.
6. Fred Allen, *Much Ado about Me* (Boston: Little, Brown, 1956), 238.
7. Krieg and Feeney, *Freeport*, 29.
8. Ibid., 29, 32.
9. Allen, *Much Ado about Me*. 238.
10. For Max, see Krieg and Feeney, *Freeport*, 37. For Gertrude, see "'LIGHTS Will Shine Brighter than Ever' Flyer," Freeport Memorial Library, New York Digital Heritage.
11. "Real Estate News," *Brooklyn Standard Union*, June 4, 1921, 12; "Gertrude Hoffman Buys Plot," *Freeport News*, September 16, 1921, 1.
12. "Hoffman to Form Drum and Bugle Corps among Boys in Freeport," *Daily Review*, July 25, 1923, 2.
13. "Ground Broken for a New School," *Daily Review*, October 3, 1923, 8.
14. Advertisement, *Daily Review*, July 10, 1923, 10.
15. "Hoffman to Form Drum and Bugle Corps," 2.
16. "Ground Broken for a New School," 8.

17. Ibid.

18. According to several historians of popular theater, the 1920s were the decade when the revue's popularity exploded. See Robert Baral, *Revue: A Nostalgic Reprise of the Great Broadway Period* (New York: Fleet, 1962); Foster Hirsch, *The Boys from Syracuse: The Shuberts' Theatrical Empire* (New York: Cooper Square Press, 2000), 153.

19. See Susan A. Glenn, *Female Spectacle: The Theatrical Roots of Modern Feminism* (Cambridge, Mass.: Harvard University Press, 2000), 155–87.

20. For the importance of whiteness as a characteristic of chorus girls, see Joel Dinerstein, *Swinging the Machine: Modernity, Technology, and African American Culture between the World Wars* (Amherst: University of Massachusetts Press, 2003), 182–220.

21. "Follies Holds Forth until 2 O'Clock Sunday Morning," *Chicago Sunday Tribune*, October 28, 1923, sec. 8, 1.

22. Gertrude and Max Hoffmann, box 2, folder 21: Personal notebooks, Red notebook, GMHP.

23. Ibid.

24. Ibid.

25. "Hip's American Girls Told to Dress Up," *Variety*, April 2, 1924, 3.

26. Jolo, "New Plays Produced in London: Leap Year," *Variety*, May 7, 1924, 18, 44.

27. Gertrude Hoffmann, letter to Barbara Vernon, undated 1951, box 2, folder 14, GMHP.

28. International Herald Tribune, "1915: Fire Destroys Moulin Rouge," *IHT Retrospective Blog*, February 27, 2015, https://iht-retrospective.blogs.nytimes.com/2015/02/27/1915-fire-destroys-moulin-rouge/.

29. "Finest Music Hall in Europe with Semi-American Revue," *Variety*, December 24, 1924, 3.

30. Gertrude and Max Hoffmann, box 1: Clippings, GMHP.

31. Ibid.

32. Susan Glenn discusses the troubling qualities of the chorus girl's uniformity, and especially the growing emphasis on "personality" that sets the star apart from the mere chorus member. Glenn, *Female Spectacle*, 184–87.

33. Siegfried Kracauer, "The Mass Ornament," in *The Mass Ornament: Weimar Essays*, trans., ed., and introduction, Thomas Y. Levin, 75–86 (Cambridge, Mass.: Harvard University Press, 1995), 76.

34. "Gertrude Hoffmann Girls Have Established New Standard of Dancing Abroad," Gertrude Hoffmann (Clippings folder), n.d., TSA.

35. André Levinson, "The Girls," *Theatre Arts Monthly* 12, no. 8 (August 1928): 597–605, 597. At least one of the Moulin Rouge routines was featured in the 1927 film *La revue des revues*, which also includes footage of the Tiller Girls and Josephine Baker. Joe Francis, *La revue des revues* (1927), http://www.imdb.com/title/tt0462506/.

36. Levinson, "The Girls," 602.

37. The Tiller Girls were associated with American identity in discussions of the many precision dance troupes performing in Weimar Era Berlin. Kate Elswit, *Watching Weimar Dance* (Oxford: Oxford University Press, 2014), 77.

38. Karl von Wiegand, "Magic of 'Dollar Land,' with Jazz Tempo, Speeds Continental Work and Play," *Bridgeport Telegram*, April 18, 1925, 10.

39. As the comparative literature scholar Michelle Clayton notes of other modern dancers, the Hoffmann Girls "not only mobilized modernism through the movements of their bodies across stages and settings, but themselves served as screens for local projections of modernity in the locales they visited." Michelle Clayton, "Modernism's Moving Bodies," *Modernist Cultures* 9, no. 1 (May 1, 2014): 27–45, 32.

40. Wiegand, "Magic of 'Dollar Land,'" 10.

41. For the disavowal of sexuality in depictions of Weimar Germany's precision dancers, see Elswit, *Watching Weimar Dance*, 77–80.

42. Rachel Shteir, *Striptease: The Untold History of the Girlie Show* (New York: Oxford University Press, 2005), 76–77.

43. Gertrude Hoffmann, "Artists and Models 1925," Programs, JRDD, NYPLPA.

44. "Artists and Models (Winter Garden)," (June 25, 1925), *Artists and Models*, Paris ed., 3rd ed., Clippings, TSA.

45. Ibid.

46. American painters of the 1920s and 1930s made burlesque performers iconic figures of American performance culture. The *Artists and Models* shows were part of the same impulse. Kathleen Spies, "Baseball, Apple Pie, and Burlesque Queens: Nationalism in Walt Kuhn's Portraits of Showgirls," *Journal of American Culture* 31, no. 1 (February 10, 2008): 34–48.

47. Glenn, *Female Spectacle*, 193–94.

48. Hortense Saunders, "No Drinks, Smokes, or Dates for Modern Chorus Girls: That's The Formula of Gertrude Hoffmann, Who Lives in Freeport," *Daily Review*, November 16, 1925, 3.

49. Gladys Sanville, "Raising the Roof on Acrobatics; William J. Herrmann, Dean of Acrobatic Teachers, Makes a New Departure.," *Dance Magazine* 16, no. 2 (June 1931): 45, 55.

50. Tiny Kline, *Circus Queen and Tinker Bell: The Memoir of Tiny Kline*, ed. Janet M. Davis (Urbana: University of Illinois Press, 2008), 176.

51. "Screenland's Directory for Studios for Dance Instruction," advertisement, *Screenland*, May 1926, 102.

52. Ibid.

53. Jessica Zeller, *Shapes of American Ballet: Teachers and Training before Balanchine* (New York: Oxford University Press, 2016), 43.

54. "Screenland's Directory," 102.

55. Alvin J. Katon, "In the Theatres on Broadway," *Daily Star*, April 12, 1926, 14.

56. Advertisement, *New York Daily News*, February 25, 1926, 101.

57. Ibid.

58. J. J. Shubert, letter to J. M. Sneckenberger, November 12, 1925, General Correspondence 1910–1926, File 1791, January 1925–April 1926, TSA.

59. Ibid.

60. "At the Play in Brooklyn," *Brooklyn Daily Eagle*, December 27, 1925, 8.

61. "A Night in Paris," 1926, Program folder, TSA.

62. "Chorus: Precision Troupes (Hoffman Girls): Clippings," n.d., BRTD, NYPLPA.

63. Susan Rix, newspaper article shared with author, November 29, 2017.

64. "Mrs. Katherine Brogan Hay, 74, Dies in Freeport," *Nassau Daily Review*, July 29, 1926, 1.

65. Ibid.

66. Gertrude and Max Hoffmann, box 2, folder 21: Personal notebooks, Red notebook, GMHP.

67. G. Hoffmann, letter to Barbara Vernon.

68. "A Night in Spain," 1927, Program folder, TSA.

69. "Artists and Models (Winter Garden)."

70. "A Night in Spain," Internet Broadway Database, https://www.ibdb.com/broadway-production/a-night-in-spain-10316.

71. "Murray Anderson's Almanac," Playbill, http://www.playbill.com/production/murray-andersons-almanac-erlangers-theatre-vault-0000004278. Hoffmann harbored deep resentment against John Murray Anderson, the producer of the show. Not only did he mock her work, but he later stole her webbing concept for a circus routine. Gertrude and Max Hoffmann, box 2, folder 21: Personal Notebooks, Red notebook, GMHP. For the webbing routine in a Ringling Brothers Circus act, see "RB Given 'Theater' Tinge," *Billboard*, April 18, 1942, 30.

72. "Gertrude Hoffmann Stage School of Dancing," advertisement, *Nassau Daily Review*, March 30, 1929, 2.

Chapter 16

1. "Gertrude Hoffmann Stage School of Dancing," advertisement, *Nassau Daily Review*, March 30, 1929, 2.

2. Chubby Jackson, "Chubby's Doghouse," *The Leader*, May 25, 1961, 11.

3. Gary Marmorstein, *A Ship without a Sail: The Life of Lorenz Hart* (New York: Simon and Schuster, 2012), 293.

4. See Noel Brown, "'How Much Do You Love Me?' The Child's Obligations to the Adult in 1930s Hollywood," in *Entertaining Children: The Participation of Youth in the Entertainment Industry*, ed. Gillian Arrighi and Victor Emeljanow (New York: Palgrave Macmillan, 2014), 93–110.

5. "Obituary 4—No Title," *New York Times*, December 3, 1930, 23.

6. Richard Silvester, letter to Otto Kahn, November 8, 1930, Dancers' Club, box 62, folder 17, Otto H. Kahn Papers, Manuscripts Division, Department of Rare Books and Special Collections, Princeton University Library, Princeton, N.J.

7. "The Dancers' Club News 1930–1931," March 19, 1931, Performing Arts Research Collections—Dance, NYPLPA.

8. "Palace," *Variety*, January 20, 1926, 15.

9. Gertrude and Max Hoffmann, box 2, folder 21: Personal notebooks, Red notebook, GMHP.

10. Marcia B. Siegel, *Days on Earth: The Dance of Doris Humphrey* (Durham, N.C.: Duke University Press, 1993), especially 43, 53–69. Hoffmann attended the Dance Repertory Theater programs in February 1931.

11. Gertrude and Max Hoffmann, box 2, folder 21: Personal notebooks, Red notebook, GMHP.

12. Susan Manning, *Ecstasy and the Demon: The Dances of Mary Wigman* (Minneapolis: University of Minnesota Press, 2006), 257–65.

13. John Martin, "The Dance: Dynamic Art," *New York Times*, January 4, 1931, Arts and Leisure, X4.

14. Manning, *Ecstasy and the Demon*, 257.

15. Gertrude and Max Hoffmann, box 10, folder 44: Music Manuscripts—"Wigman Notes," GMHP.

16. Ibid.

17. Manning, *Ecstasy and the Demon*, 257.

18. "Monster Dance Performance," program, December 11, 1932, Dancers' Club New York (Clippings), NYPLPA.

19. Ibid.

20. Gertrude Hoffmann, telegram to John Martin, December 15, 1932, box 1, folder 1, JMP, JRDD, NYPLPA.

21. Advertisement, *Nassau Daily Review*, October 10, 1932, 13.

22. Anthony Slide, *The Encyclopedia of Vaudeville* (Jackson: University Press of Mississippi, 2012), 386–87.

23. Siegfried Kracauer, "Girls and Crisis," in *The Weimar Republic Sourcebook*, ed. Anton Kaes and Edward Dimendberg (Berkeley: University of California Press, 1994), 565–66.

24. "Paramount, New York, This Week," advertisement, *Variety*, March 25, 1933, 38.

25. Eugene Burr, "Paramount, New York," *Billboard*, April 29, 1933, 8.

26. Burr, "RKO Roxy," *Variety*, May 9, 1933, 16.

27. Char, "RKO Roxy," *Variety*, May 16, 1933, 16.

28. For a description of *Water Study* and its development, see Siegel, *Days on Earth*, 85–89.

29. Rasch combined ballet, jazz, and vaudeville in her choreographic work much the way Hoffmann did. See Frank W. D. Ries, "Albertina Rasch: The Broadway Career," *Dance Chronicle* 6, no. 2 (January 1, 1982): 95–137; Carrie Gaiser Casey, "The Ballet Corporealities of Anna Pavlova and Albertina Rasch," *Dance Chronicle* 35, no. 1 (January 1, 2012): 8–29.

30. Gerald Martin Bordman and Richard Norton, *American Musical Theatre: A Chronicle* (Oxford: Oxford University Press, 2010), 534–35.

31. Ibid.

32. Advertisement, *New York Daily News*, October 19, 1933, 50.

33. Rachel Shteir, *Striptease: The Untold History of the Girlie Show* (New York: Oxford University Press, 2005), 134.

34. "Paramount Grill, N.Y.," *Variety*, October 24, 1933, 46.

35. Ibid.

36. Kate Elswit, *Watching Weimar Dance* (Oxford: Oxford University Press, 2014), xviii.

37. Mark Franko, *The Work of Dance: Labor, Movement, and Identity in the 1930s* (Middletown, Conn.: Wesleyan University Press, 2002), 158–61.

38. "Hoffman, Gertrude—Clippings" (n.d.), Performing Arts Research Collections—Music, NYPLPA.

39. Art Arthur, "Reverting to Type," *Brooklyn Daily Eagle*, December 18, 1933, M3.

40. James Aswell, "New York—Pot Pourri," *Minneapolis Star*, December 21, 1933, 8.

41. Gertrude and Max Hoffmann, box 2, folder 4, Correspondence and Contracts 1934, GMHP.

42. Mary Rita Halpin, "No Fooling, Theatrical Ban Brings Success to Troupe," *Nassau Daily Review*, December 4, 1934, 5.

43. Gertrude and Max Hoffmann, box 2, folder 21: Personal notebooks, Red notebook, GMHP.

44. Gertrude and Max Hoffmann, box 1: Clippings, GMHP.

45. Ibid.

46. "2 Paris Transient Spots, Casino and Folies, Best of Dull Legits," *Variety*, July 24, 1934, 55.

47. "'Cat's Paw' Hits Detroit for $26,500," *Motion Picture Daily*, September 14, 1934; "'Servants' Is Detroit Smash with $24,600," *Motion Picture Daily*, September 20, 1934.

48. Halpin, "No Fooling."

49. Gertrude and Max Hoffmann, box 2, folder 5, Correspondence: Letters, 1935, GMHP.

50. "Bookers Eye South America; Field for Bands and Flashes," *Billboard*, April 20, 1935, 13.

51. Advertisement, *Press and Sun-Bulletin*, April 12, 1935, 34; "Stage Show at Capitol Sunday," *Daily Sentinel*, April 13, 1935, 5.

52. "Str.-Vode Show Grosses $2,700; Actors' Peanuts," *Variety*, September 11, 1935, 51.

53. Hallie Flanagan, *Arena: The History of the Federal Theatre* (New York: B. Blom, 1965), 27.

54. Ibid., 318, 386–87.

55. Gertrude and Max Hoffmann, box 2, folder 21: Personal notebooks, Red notebook, GMHP.

56. Kenneth Campbell, "Her Dancing Girls Take Time Out to Watch Salome Step as of Yore," *New York World-Telegram*, July 13, 1936, 2.

57. *The Proceedings of the First National Dance Congress and Festival* (New York: National Dance Congress and Festival, 1936), 7.

58. John Martin, "The Dance: A Convention," *New York Times*, May 17, 1936, 1; Edna Ocko, "Reviewing on the Left: The Dance Criticism of Edna Ocko," selected and introduced by Stacey Prickett, in "Of, By, and For the People: Dancing on the Left in the 1930s," ed. Lynn Garafola, special issue, *Studies in Dance History* 5, no. 1 (1994): 65–103, 93.

59. Foster Hirsch, *The Boys from Syracuse: The Shuberts' Theatrical Empire* (New York: Cooper Square Press, 2000), 140.

60. "The Student Prince," advertisement, *Brooklyn Daily Eagle*, July 13, 1936, 9; "'Blossom Time' Blooms Anew at Jones Beach," *Daily News*, July 30, 1936, 39.

61. "'Blossom Time' Blooms Anew at Jones Beach."

62. "Chi Variety Is Mostly in Nite Clubs; Floor Shows Read Like '26 Vaude Bills," *Variety*, October 7, 1936, 46.

63. For a detailed description of *Bassa Moona* and its reception by Federal Theatre Project audiences, see Susan Manning, *Modern Dance, Negro Dance: Race in Motion* (Minneapolis: University of Minnesota Press, 2004), 88–93.

64. Ibid., 81.

65. Ibid., 88.

66. "Theatre Notes," *New York Age*, January 2, 1937, 9.

67. Gertrude and Max Hoffmann, box 13, folder 11: Katherine Dunham, GMHP.

68. For a description of this nightclub's layout and floor show, see Burton William Peretti, *Nightclub City: Politics and Amusement in Manhattan* (Philadelphia: University of Pennsylvania Press, 2007), 201–3.

69. "Broadway (West 44th Street–West 45th Street)," Irma and Paul Milstein Division of United States History, Local History and Genealogy, the New York Public Library, NYPL Digital Collections, http://digital.gallery.nypl.org/items/510d47e2-cc31-a3d9-e040-e00a18064a99.

70. Gertrude and Max Hoffmann, box 2, folder 7: Letters, Telegrams, Contracts, 1939, GMHP; "Int'l's Show on P.A. Tour After Night Club Folds," *Variety*, January 18, 1939, 40.

71. This term is of course taken from Henry Jenkins, *What Made Pistachio Nuts? Early Sound Comedy and the Vaudeville Aesthetic*, Film and Culture (New York: Columbia University Press, 1992). For radio and television, see Rick DesRochers, *The Comic Offense from Vaudeville to Contemporary Comedy: Larry David, Tina Fey, Stephen Colbert, and Dave Chappelle* (New York: Bloomsbury, 2014).

72. "Spectacular Fire Destroys Famed Lights Clubhouse," *Nassau Daily Review*, February 9, 1939, 1.

73. "Sailings," *Variety*, August 9, 1939, 2; "New 'Crazy' Show Clicks in Tryout," *Variety*, August 30, 1939, 12.

74. Ship manifest, S.S. *Manhattan*, under "Gertrude Hoffman," September 30, 1939. Statue of Liberty—Ellis Island Foundation; "Naughty or Nice? The War Over England's Wartime Stage," *Minneapolis Star*, March 3, 1940.

Chapter 17

1. Gertrude and Max Hoffmann, box 2, folder 26: Performance and Music Notes, GMHP.

2. Ibid.

3. Gertrude and Max Hoffmann, box 2, folder 24: Costume and Performance Notes, GMHP.

4. Lee Mortimer, "Bright Light Invasion," *Sunday Mirror*, November 24, 1940, Magazine. Found in Gertrude and Max Hoffmann, box 2, folder 24: Costume and Performance Notes, GMHP.

5. Gertrude and Max Hoffmann, box 2, folder 26: Performance and Music Notes, GMHP.

6. Ibid.

7. Ibid.

8. Ibid.

9. Gertrude and Max Hoffmann, box 2, folder 24: Costume and Performance Notes, GMHP.

10. Eleanor King, *Transformations: The Humphrey-Weidman Era: A Memoir* (Trenton, N.J.: Dance Horizons, 1978), 277.

11. Ibid.

12. Donna Perlmutter, *Shadowplay: The Life of Antony Tudor* (New York: Viking, 1991), 136.

13. De Mille and Hoffmann both served on the reception committee for an Arnold Genthe exhibit of dance photographs. See "In the Galleries: News and Comments," *Brooklyn Daily Eagle*, December 24, 1933, 28.

14. Dorothy Bird and Joyce Greenberg, *Bird's Eye View: Dancing with Martha Graham and on Broadway* (Pittsburgh, Pa.: University of Pittsburgh Press, 2002), 166.

15. Ibid.

16. As Anthea Kraut discusses, de Mille was a vocal advocate for the intellectual property rights of Broadway choreographers. Anthea Kraut, *Choreographing Copyright: Race, Gender, and Intellectual Property Rights in American Dance* (Oxford: Oxford University Press, 2015), 167.

17. Gertrude and Max Hoffmann, box 2, folder 21: Personal notebooks, Red notebook, GMHP.

18. Agnes de Mille, *Dance to the Piper* (Boston: Little, Brown, 1952), 51.

19. Bird and Greenberg, *Bird's Eye View*, 166.

20. Ibid.

21. Gertrude and Max Hoffmann, box 2, folder 23: Performance Notes, GMHP.

22. Ibid.

23. Uno, "Burlesque Bits," *Billboard*, April 26, 1952, 50.

24. Uno, "Burlesque Bits," *Billboard*, April 11, 1953, 46.

25. For a history from the end of the decade that makes that claim see, George Amberg, *Ballet in America: The Emergence of an American Art* (New York: Duell, Sloan and Pearce, 1949), especially 72–81, 165–73.

26. "Dancing through Two Centuries, 1740–1940 (February 11–May 3, 1942)," Theater Collection, MCNY.

27. Ibid.

28. Gertrude and Max Hoffmann, box 2, folder 21: Personal notebooks, Brown notebook, GMHP, with the first line "You darlings." She seems to have started writing down the ideas for this project in 1941; the lyrics to a song from "Lady in the Dark" (which premiered in January 1941) are written on the page after her Fokine Ballet notes. Later ideas appear in a notebook the first page of which is dated July 19, 1942. It is possible that Hoffmann's return to the project was inspired by Fokine's death, but this cannot be conclusively stated.

29. Gertrude and Max Hoffmann, box 2, folder 21: Personal notebooks, Brown notebook, GMHP, with the first line "You darlings."

30. Ibid.

31. Charlotte Canning, "Feminist Performance as Feminist Historiography," *Theatre Survey* 45, no. 2 (November 2004): 227–33.

32. Gertrude and Max Hoffmann, box 2, folder 21: Personal notebooks, Brown notebook with the first line "July 19—42 Christian Science Lesson," GMHP.

33. Gertrude and Max Hoffmann, box 2, folder 21: Personal notebooks, Brown notebook with the first line "You darlings," GMHP.

34. Gertrude and Max Hoffmann, box 2, folder 21: Personal notebooks, Brown notebook with the first line "July 19—42 Christian Science Lesson," GMHP.

35. "Morris Gest Dead: A Noted Showman," *New York Times*, May 17, 1942, 45.

36. "Fokine Dies Here: Father of Ballet," *New York Times*, August 22, 1942, 13.

37. Raymond Hubbell, letter to Max Hoffmann, July 21, 1942, box 2, folder 8, Correspondence: Letters, 1940–1942, GMHP.

38. Sol Bloom, letter to Max Hoffmann, October 8, 1943, box 2, folder 9: Letters, 1943, GMHP.

39. The same was true of film culture. Martha Shearer discusses the cinematic "nostalgia musicals" of the 1940s in *New York City and the Hollywood Musical: Dancing in the Streets* (London: Palgrave Macmillan, 2016), 75–111.

40. Richard Hasbany, "Irene: Considering the Nostalgic Sensibility," *Journal of Popular Culture* 9, no. 4 (March 1, 1976): 816–26, 817.

41. Max Hoffmann seems to have been involved in the orchestra for *Oklahoma!* for most of its initial run at the St. James Theatre. He is reported as "playing a fiddle in the 'Oklahoma' pit orchestra" in Danton Walker, "New York Letter," *Philadelphia Inquirer*, July 2, 1943, 18. By 1947 he was conducting the show. Walter Winchell, "Walter Winchell on Broadway," *Courier-Post*, September 9, 1947, 18.

42. Gertrude and Max Hoffmann, box 1: Clippings, GMHP.

43. Gertrude and Max Hoffmann, box 2, folder 24: Costume and Performance Notes, Black notebook with "Record" cover, GMHP.

44. Gertrude and Max Hoffmann, box 2, folder 25: Performance Notes, GMHP.

45. Gertrude and Max Hoffmann, box 2, folder 24: Costume and Performance Notes, Brown spiral-bound notebook, GMHP.

46. Gertrude and Max Hoffmann, box 2, folder 24: Costume and Performance Notes, Brown spiral-bound notebook, GMHP, includes a list of characters she would play and costumes she would need for each; costs are in Gertrude and Max Hoffmann, box 2, folder 23: Performance Notes, GMHP.

47. Jeanne Scheper, *Moving Performances: Divas, Iconicity, and Remembering the Modern Stage* (New Brunswick, N.J.: Rutgers University Press, 2016), 161.

48. "Gertrude Hoffman Readies Comeback," *Variety*, August 9, 1944, 1.

49. Ibid.

50. Gertrude and Max Hoffmann, box 2, folder 24: Costume and Performance Notes, Black notebook with "Record" cover, GMHP.

51. Pannill Camp, "The Poetics of Performance Nonevents," *Journal of Dramatic Theory and Criticism* 32, no. 2 (July 17, 2018): 141–50.

52. Gertrude and Max Hoffmann, box 2, folder 24: Costume and Performance Notes, Brown spiral-bound notebook, GMHP.

53. Ibid.

54. Cecil Smith, "It May Be Low, but This Farce Is Very Funny," *Chicago Daily Tribune*, April 13, 1942, 15.

55. John Chapman, "'Good Night Ladies' Is Chicago's Idea of a Wow; Good Night, Now," *New York Daily News*, January 19, 1945, 39.

56. "Max Hoffmann Jr., 43, Dies after Collapse," *New York Times*, April 1, 1945, 38.

57. Ibid.

58. Alexander Sheldon Ware, letter to Gertrude and Max Hoffmann, March 30, 1945, box 2, folder 10, Letters, 1945, GMHP.

59. Reina (Belasco) Gest, letter to Gertrude and Max Hoffmann, April 2, 1945, box 2, folder 10, Letters, 1945, GMHP.

60. Ann Cary, note to Max Hoffmann, April 2, 1945, box 2, folder 10, Letters, 1945, GMHP.

61. Julia L. Foulkes, *A Place for Us: "West Side Story" and New York* (Chicago: University of Chicago Press, 2016), 33.

62. Ibid., 45.

63. "Obituaries: Mrs. Rose Marie Waite," *Van Nuys News*, November 29, 1951, 12.

64. Agnes McCloskey, "Chaperones Must Come Along If Ballet Girls Have Dates," *Nassau Daily Review*, August 5, 1936, 12.

65. Maryverne Tupper Jones, letter to Gertrude Hoffmann, December 28, 1948, box 2, folder 12: Letters, 1948–1949, GMHP.

66. Ibid.

67. Starr West Jones, *Hello God, Can We Talk? Discoveries That Challenge Modern Thinking* (Hollywood, Fla.: Frederick Fell, 1988), 163–64.

68. Maryverne "Polly" Jones, letter to Gertrude Hoffmann, May 8, 1951, box 2, folder 14: Letters, 1951, GMHP.

69. Starr West Jones, letter to "Kitty" [Gertrude Hoffmann], May 15, 1951, box 2, folder 14: Letters, 1951, GMHP.

70. Gertrude and Max Hoffmann, Max Hoffmann: Apartment Inventory and Packing Lists, 1953, box 2, folder 33, GMHP.

71. Jones, letter to Gertrude Hoffmann, May 8, 1951.

72. "Obituaries: Mrs. Rose Marie Waite."

73. Rose Marie Waite, card to Gertrude Hoffmann, December 1949, box 2, folder 12: Letters, 1948–1949, GMHP.

74. Charlotte Schley, letter to Mr. and Mrs. Max Hoffmann, September 21, 1953, box 2, folder 15: Letters, 1952–1954, GMHP.

75. The sale of the Hoffmann property "minus houses at Bayview avenue and Johnson place" is noted in July. "Jottings," *Nassau Daily Review-Star*, July 16, 1952, 10.

76. Schley, letter to Mr. and Mrs. Max Hoffmann.

77. "The I Don't Care Girl," Internet Movie Database, https://www.imdb.com/title/tt0045898/.

78. Ibid.

79. Gertrude and Max Hoffmann, box 2, folder 21, Brown notebook with first line "To Al Roon—Hotel Ansonia," GMHP.

80. George Frederick Custen, *Bio/Pics: How Hollywood Constructed Public History* (New Brunswick, N.J.: Rutgers University Press, 1992), 47.

81. Gertrude and Max Hoffmann, box 2, folder 23: Performance Notes, Brown notebook with "Cards/Christmas List" cover.

82. Mrs. John Hammet, letter to Max Hoffmann, n.d., box 2, folder 16: Letters, 1956, GMHP.

83. John N. W. Johnson, "Gertrude Hoffman Theater Posters—the Totality—ZSR Library: Comments," https://zsr.wfu.edu/2010/gertrude-hoffman-theater-posters-the-totality/.

84. "Week's TV Programs," *New York Daily News*, March 17, 1957, 179.

85. Gertrude and Max Hoffmann, box 2, folder 21: Personal notebooks, Red notebook, GMHP.

86. Ibid.

87. Ibid.

88. Ibid.

89. Ibid.

90. Frank Cullen, *Vaudeville, Old and New: An Encyclopedia of Variety Performers in America*, 2 vols. (New York: Routledge, 2006), 1:317.

91. Gary Chapman, *The Delectable Dollies: The Dolly Sisters, Icons of the Jazz Age* (Stroud: Sutton, 2006), 13–14.

92. Gertrude and Max Hoffmann, box 2, folder 21: Personal notebooks, Red notebook, GMHP.

93. Ibid.

94. Grant Hayter-Menzies, *Charlotte Greenwood: The Life and Career of the Comic Star of Vaudeville, Radio and Film* (Jefferson, N.C.: McFarland, 2007).

95. Gertrude Hoffmann, draft of a letter to Lucille Ball, n.d., box 2, folder 18, Clippings, photos, and notes from correspondence, unsorted, GMHP.

96. Dorothy Hechtlinger, "Inter-Department Communication to Mr. Bert Granet. Subject: LUCY SOLO Possibilities," January 18, 1960, Margaret Herrick Library, Academy of Motion Picture Arts and Sciences, Beverly Hills California.

97. Hoffmann, draft of a letter to Lucille Ball.

98. Ibid.

99. Max Hoffmann, letter to J. J. Shubert, n.d., John Shubert Correspondence (1962), box 2, folder 1: "G"–"H," TSA.

100. Gertrude Hoffmann, letter to John Shubert, September 14, 1962, John Shubert Correspondence (1962), box 2, folder 1: "G"–"H," TSA.

101. Ibid.

102. "Convalescent Home in Valley Started," *Los Angeles Times*, January 12, 1958, sec. VI, 16.

103. Certificate of Death, Max Hoffmann, May 21, 1963, County of Los Angeles Registrar-Recorder/County Clerk.

104. "Obituary: Hoffman, Max—1963 (d. May 21) Age 88," *Variety*, May 29, 1963, Special Collections, NYPLPA.

105. Ibid.

106. John Dougherty, letter to Gertrude Hoffmann, July 12, 1963, box 1, folder 37, Adolph Bolm Collection, (S)*MGZMD 50, JRDD, NYPLPA.

107. Stephen Gottschalk, *The Emergence of Christian Science in American Religious Life* (Berkeley: University of California Press, 1978), 168–69.

108. "First Church of Christ, Scientist," *New-Messenger*, October 22, 1966, 6.

109. "Obituary: Gertrude Hoffman," *Variety*, November 2, 1966, Hoffman, Gertrude. Clippings, JRDD, NYPLPA.

110. "She came into dance prominence when she presented what the programs called La Saison des Ballets Russes, at the Winter Garden, New York, beginning Sept. 4, 1911," the obituary reads. The program premiered on June 14, 1911. "G. Hoffmann Dies on Coast," *Dance News*, December 1966, 12.

111. "Obituary: Gertrude Hoffman."

112. Ibid.

113. Agnes de Mille, *Dance to the Piper* (Boston: Little, Brown, 1952), 45.

114. "Obituary: Gertrude Hoffman."

115. Ibid.

116. "G. Hoffmann Dies on Coast." "Sic" was in the original.

117. Certificate of Death, Max Hoffmann; Certificate of Death, Gertrude Hoffmann, October 21, 1966, County of Los Angeles Registrar-Recorder/County Clerk.

Conclusion

1. Henry Jenkins, *What Made Pistachio Nuts? Early Sound Comedy and the Vaudeville Aesthetic*, Film and Culture (New York: Columbia University Press, 1992).

2. Susan A. Glenn, *Female Spectacle: The Theatrical Roots of Modern Feminism* (Cambridge, Mass.: Harvard University Press, 2000), 8.

3. Katherine Newey, "Feminist Historiography and Ethics," in *Theatre History and Historiography*, 85–102 (London: Palgrave Macmillan, 2016).

4. The ideas in this paragraph are influenced by Rebecca Schneider, *Performing Remains: Art and War in Times of Theatrical Reenactment* (New York: Routledge, 2011), 29–30.

5. The coda to *Choreographing Copyright* discusses Beyoncé's appropriation of the Belgian choreographer Anne Teresa De Keersmaeker's *Rosas danst Rosas*, as well as De Keersmaeker's subsequent invitation to the public to post their own versions of the dance online, is a fascinating case study of the "circulation of choreography in the age of Youtube." Anthea Kraut, *Choreographing Copyright: Race, Gender, and Intellectual Property Rights in American Dance* (Oxford: Oxford University Press, 2015), 265.

6. These re-creations are sometimes called "Sweded" versions, a term that comes from the Michel Gondry movie *Be Kind, Rewind* in which video store clerks re-create the films on VHS tapes that have been erased and then claim the versions of the film have been imported from Sweden. See John Finlay Kerr, "'Rereading' Be Kind Rewind (USA 2008): How Film History Can Be Remapped through the Social Memories of Popular Culture," *Screening the Past*, no. 24 (April 26, 2009); Pelin Aytemiz, "Thoughts on the New Dadaist Tactic of Our Era: 'Sweded Films' and Michel Gondry's *Be Kind Rewind*," *Turkish Online Journal of Design Art and Communication* 6, no. 1 (January 2016).

7. Celeste Barber (@celestebarber). https://www.instagram.com/celestebarber/.

SELECTED BIBLIOGRAPHY

Archival Collections

Belknap Playbills and Programs Collection. Special and Area Studies Collection, George A. Smathers Library, University of Florida, Gainesville

Morris Gest Papers. Harry Ransom Center, University of Texas at Austin

Gertrude Hoffmann Collection. Brooklyn Public Library, Brooklyn Collection

Gertrude and Max Hoffmann Papers (MS 608). Z. Smith Reynolds Library Special Collections and Archives, Wake Forest University, Winston-Salem, N.C.

Museum of the City of New York

The New York Public Library for the Performing Arts, Dorothy and Lewis B. Cullman Center

- Billy Rose Theatre Division
- John Martin Papers, Jerome Robbins Dance Division
- Robinson Locke Collection, NAFR+, Billy Rose Theatre Division

The Shubert Archive, New York

Publications

"Agent's Own 'Girl Act.'" *Variety*, September 1, 1906.

A. H. D. "Hello Everybody." *New York Clipper*, September 20, 1922.

"Alhambra's 'Hoodoo Week.'" *Variety*, January 10, 1919.

Allen, Fred. *Much Ado about Me*. Boston: Little, Brown, 1956.

———. "A Tribute to Vaudeville's Golden Era." *Life*, November 12, 1956.

Allen, Robert Clyde. *Vaudeville and Film, 1895–1915: A Study in Media Interaction*. Dissertations on Film 1980. New York: Arno Press, 1980.

Amberg, George. *Ballet in America: The Emergence of an American Art*. New York: Duell, Sloan and Pearce, 1949.

Anderson, Gillian B. "Synchronized Music: The Influence of Pantomime on Moving Pictures." *Music and the Moving Image* 8, no. 3 (2015): 3–39.

Antoniazzi, Barbara. *The Wayward Woman: Progressivism, Prostitution, and Performance in the United States, 1888–1917*. Madison, N.J.: Fairleigh Dickinson University Press, 2014.

Araneo, Margaret. "Nervous Salomes: New York Salomania and the Neurological Condition of Modernité." Ph.D. diss., City University of New York, 2017. ProQuest Dissertations and Theses Full Text (1899182112).

Arthur, Art. "Reverting to Type." *Brooklyn Daily Eagle*, December 18, 1933.

"Artists and Models (Winter Garden)." June 25, 1925. *Artists and Models*. Paris ed., 3rd ed. Clippings. The Shubert Archive, New York.

"Artist's Forum." *Variety*, January 25, 1908.

Arvidson, Linda. *When the Movies Were Young*. New York: E. P. Dutton, 1925.

Askari, Kaveh, Scott Curtis, Frank Gray, Louis Pelletier, Tami Williams, and Joshua Yumibe, eds. *Performing New Media, 1890–1915*. New Barnet, Hertfordshire, Eng.: John Libbey, 2015.

Aswell, James. "New York—Pot Pourri." *Minneapolis Star*, December 21, 1933.

"At the Local Theaters: The Alcazar." *San Francisco Dramatic Review*, December 9, 1899.

Aytemiz, Pelin. "Thoughts on the New Dadaist Tactic of Our Era: 'Sweded Films' and Michel Gondry's Be Kind Rewind." *Turkish Online Journal of Design Art and Communication* 6, no. 1 (January 2016).

Babic, Annessa Ann. *America's Changing Icons: Constructing Patriotic Women from World War I to the Present*. Lanham, Md.: Rowman and Littlefield, 2018.

"Baby Steals Buggy and Tries Auto: Maxmillion Hoffmann, Three Years Old, Has Penchant for Free Rides." *San Francisco Chronicle*, March 17, 1905. Box 1, folder 2, Gertrude Hoffmann Collection, Brooklyn Public Library, Brooklyn Collection.

"Back from a Road Tour of Twenty-Seven Weeks." *Variety*, March 2, 1912.

Bader, Robert S. *Four of the Three Musketeers: The Marx Brothers on Stage*. Evanston, Ill.: Northwestern University Press, 2016.

"The Ballet of 1830." Internet Broadway Database. https://www.ibdb.com/broadway-show/the-ballet-of-1830-478286.

"Ballet to the Coast." *Variety*, September 23, 1911.

Ballets Russes, ed. *Théâtre National de l'Opéra, Juin 1910: La Saison Russe à l'Opéra, Ballets Russes, avec le concours d'artistes des Théâtres Impériaux*. Souvenir program. Paris: Comœdia Illustré, 1910.

Baral, Robert. *Revue: A Nostalgic Reprise of the Great Broadway Period*. New York: Fleet, 1962.

Barber, Celeste (@celestebarber). https://www.instagram.com/celestebarber/.

Barton, Ralph. "Chauve-Souris (Program)." National Portrait Gallery, Smithsonian Institution. http://npg.si.edu/object/npg_S_NPG.92.12.

Bayles-Yeager, Danni. "Vaudeville / Orpheum / 12-5-1921." Performing Arts Archive. http://www.performingartsarchive.com.

Beard, DeAnna M. Toten. *Sheldon Cheney's Theatre Arts Magazine: Promoting a Modern American Theatre, 1916–1921*. Lanham, Md.: Scarecrow Press, 2010.

Beaumont, Cyril W. *Michel Fokine and His Ballets*. New York: Dance Horizons, 1981.

Berlin, Edward A. *Ragtime: A Musical and Cultural History*. Berkeley: University of California Press, 1984.

Birchard, Robert. *Cecil B. DeMille's Hollywood*. Lexington: University Press of Kentucky, 2004.

Bird, Dorothy, and Joyce Greenberg. *Bird's Eye View: Dancing with Martha Graham and on Broadway*. Pittsburgh, Pa.: University of Pittsburgh Press, 2002.

Bolter, J. David, and Richard A. Grusin. *Remediation: Understanding New Media*. Cambridge, Mass.: MIT Press, 2000.

"Bookers Eye South America; Field for Bands and Flashes." *Billboard*, April 20, 1935.

Bordman, Gerald, and Thomas S. Hischak. "The Passing Show." In *The Oxford Companion to American Theatre*, 490–91. Oxford: Oxford University Press, 2004.

Bordman, Gerald Martin, and Richard Norton. *American Musical Theatre: A Chronicle*. Oxford: Oxford University Press, 2010.

Boyle, Peyton. *The Federal Reporter*. St. Paul: West, 1908.

Brechin, Gray. *Imperial San Francisco: Urban Power, Earthly Ruin*. With a new preface. Berkeley: University of California Press, 2006.

"Broadway to Paris." Script. Ole Olsen Collection, Ned Wayburn material, box 1, folder 58. Cinematic Arts Library, University of Southern California.

"Broadway (West 44th Street–West 45th Street)." Photograph. Irma and Paul Milstein Division of United States History, Local History and Genealogy, the New York Public Library, New York Public Library Digital Collections. http://digital.gallery.nypl.org/items/510d47e2-cc31-a3d9-e040-e00a18064a99.

Brooks, Lori Lynne. "'To Be Black Is to Be Funny': 'Coon-Shouting' and the Melancholic Production of the White Comedienne." *Women and Performance: A Journal of Feminist Theory* 25, no. 1 (January 2, 2015): 1–22.

Broun, Heywood. "Public Bathing and the Drama." *New York Tribune*, September 8, 1915.

Brown, Noel. "'How Much Do You Love Me?' The Child's Obligations to the Adult in 1930s Hollywood." In *Entertaining Children: The Participation of Youth in the Entertainment Industry*, edited by Gillian Arrighi and Victor Emeljanow, 93–110. New York: Palgrave Macmillan, 2014.

Brown, Peter Jensen. "Early Sports and Pop Culture History Blog: The Colorful History and Etymology of 'Pink Elephant.'" *Early Sports and Pop Culture History Blog* (blog), August 20, 2014. https://esnpc.blogspot.com/2014/08/the-colorful-history-and-etymology-of.html.

Brown v. Select Theatres Corporation. 56 F. Supp. 438 (D. Mass. 1944). https://www.leagle.com/decision/194449456fsupp4381384.

Burr. "RKO Roxy." *Variety*, May 9, 1933.

Burr, Eugene. "Paramount, New York." *Billboard*, April 29, 1933.

"Business Falling Off." *Variety*, July 8, 1911.

"Cabaret." *Variety*, January 12, 1923.

"Cabarets." *Variety*, October 20, 1916.

"Cabarets: 'Dance and Grow Thin.'" *Variety*, January 26, 1917.

"Cabarets: Enrico Muris." *Variety*, February 23, 1917.

Caffin, Caroline Scurfield. *Vaudeville: The Book*. New York: M. Kennerley, 1914.

Cain, Giles P. "Little Stories of Plays and Players." *The Independent*, December 22, 1917.

Camp, Pannill. "The Poetics of Performance Nonevents." *Journal of Dramatic Theory and Criticism* 32, no. 2 (July 17, 2018): 141–50.

Campbell, Kenneth. "Her Dancing Girls Take Time Out to Watch Salome Step as of Yore." *New York World-Telegram*, July 13, 1936.

Canning, Charlotte. "Feminist Performance as Feminist Historiography." *Theatre Survey* 45, no. 2 (November 2004): 227–33.

Cantu, Maya. "'Gilding the Guild': Art Theatre, the Broadway Revue and Cultural Parody in The Garrick Gaieties (1925–1930)." *Studies in Musical Theatre* 7, no. 1 (March 1, 2013): 45–60.

Capo, Beth Widmaier. "Eugenics: Bad Blood and Better Babies." In *American Literature in Transition, 1910–1920*, edited by Mark W. Van Wienen, 103–16. Cambridge: Cambridge University Press, 2017.

Carbonneau, Suzanne. "Adolph Bolm in America." In *The Ballets Russes and Its World*, edited by Lynn Garafola and Nancy Van Norman Baer, 219–44. New Haven, Conn.: Yale University Press, 1999.

Carlson, Elizabeth. "Cubist Fashion: Mainstreaming Modernism after the Armory." *Winterthur Portfolio* 48, no. 1 (March 1, 2014): 1–28.

Carlson, Marvin. *The Haunted Stage: The Theatre as Memory Machine*. Ann Arbor: University of Michigan Press, 2003.

Casey, Carrie Gaiser. "The Ballet Corporealities of Anna Pavlova and Albertina Rasch." *Dance Chronicle* 35, no. 1 (January 1, 2012): 8–29.

Casey, Kathleen B. *The Prettiest Girl on Stage Is a Man: Race and Gender Benders in American Vaudeville*. Knoxville: University of Tennessee Press, 2015.

"Casino Theatre." Internet Broadway Database. https://www.ibdb.com/theatre/casino-theatre-1085.

Castle, Vernon, and Irene Castle. *Modern Dancing*. New York: Harper, 1914.

"Catharine Beecher." National Women's History Museum. https://www.womenshistory.org/education-resources/biographies/catharine-esther-beecher.

"Central, J.C. Regular." *Variety*, September 15, 1922.

"The Century Girl." Internet Broadway Database. https://www.ibdb.com/broadway-production/the-century-girl-8469.

Certificate of Death, Gertrude Hoffmann. October 21, 1966. County of Los Angeles Registrar-Recorder/County Clerk.

Certificate of Death, Max Hoffmann. May 21, 1963. County of Los Angeles Registrar-Recorder/County Clerk.

C-File, Max Hoffmann. n.d. C-480840. U.S. Citizenship and Immigration Services Genealogy Program, Department of Homeland Security. https://www.uscis.gov/genealogy.

"'Chantecler' for New York." *Variety*, March 12, 1910.

Chapman, Gary. *The Delectable Dollies: The Dolly Sisters, Icons of the Jazz Age*. Stroud, [Eng.]: Sutton, 2006.

Chapman, John. "'Good Night Ladies' Is Chicago's Idea of a Wow; Good Night, Now." *New York Daily News*, January 19, 1945.

Chapman, Mary. *Making Noise, Making News: Suffrage Print Culture and U.S. Modernism*. Oxford: Oxford University Press, 2014.

Char. "RKO Roxy." *Variety*, May 16, 1933.

"Chauve-Souris." *Variety*, February 10, 1922.

Cheng, Anne Anlin. *Second Skin: Josephine Baker and the Modern Surface*. Oxford: Oxford University Press, 2010.

"Chi Variety Is Mostly in Nite Clubs; Floor Shows Read Like '26 Vaude Bills." *Variety*, October 7, 1936.

Chicot. "'Corks' on Girl Acts." *Variety*, December 23, 1905.

Chinitz, David E. *T. S. Eliot and the Cultural Divide*. Chicago: University of Chicago Press, 2005.

Christy, Howard Chandler. "Gee!! I Wish I Were a Man, I'd Join the Navy; Be a Man and Do It—United States Navy Recruiting Station." Color lithograph,

1917. Library of Congress Prints and Photographs Division, Washington, D.C. http://www.loc.gov/pictures/item/2002712088/.
Clarsen, Georgine. *Eat My Dust: Early Women Motorists*. Baltimore: Johns Hopkins University Press, 2011.
Clayton, Michelle. "Modernism's Moving Bodies." *Modernist Cultures* 9, no. 1 (May 1, 2014): 27–45.
Coffin, Harriet. "All Sorts and Kinds of Salomes." *Theatre*, April 1909.
Coffman, Edward M. *The War to End All Wars: The American Military Experience in World War I*. Lexington: University Press of Kentucky, 2014.
Cohen, Barbara Naomi. "The Borrowed Art of Gertrude Hoffmann." *Dance Data* 2 (1977): 2–11.
Cohen-Stratyner, Barbara. "Hoffman, Gertrude (1886–1966)." *Routledge Encyclopedia of Modernism*, 2016. https://www.rem.routledge.com/articles/hoffman-gertrude-1886-1966.
"Collecting on Picture 'Names.'" *Variety*, February 14, 1919.
Collins, Charles W. "The Mimic World." *Chicago Inter Ocean*, December 23, 1908.
"Colonial Theatre." 1913–23. Program. Jerome Robbins Dance Division, New York Public Library Digital Collections. http://digitalcollections.nypl.org/items/510d47da-5c34-a3d9-e040-e00a18064a99.
Con. "Palace." *Variety*, April 7, 1922.
Cook, Susan C. "Passionless Dancing and Passionate Reform: Respectability, Modernism, and the Social Dancing of Irene and Vernon Castle." In *The Passion of Music and Dance: Body, Gender and Sexuality*, edited by William Washabaugh, 133–50. Oxford: Berg, 1998.
"Correspondence." *Variety*, November 2, 1917.
"Correspondence: Majestic." *Variety*, December 3, 1915.
"Cover." *Theatre*, January 1917.
Cover of Souvenir Programme Benefit given by the Columbia, Orpheum, California, Alcazar, Tivoli, Grand Opera House and the Chutes Theater for the Reception of the Returning United States Volunteers at the Orpehum Theater on Thursday Aug. 17th 1899. Museum of Performance and Design, Performing Arts Library. Online Archive of California. http://oac.cdlib.org/ark:/13030/c8k935gc/?brand=oac4.
Coyle, Lee. *George Ade*. New York: Twayne, 1964.
Crosby, Alfred W. *America's Forgotten Pandemic: The Influenza of 1918*. Cambridge: Cambridge University Press, 2003.
Croy, Homer. "Watching Our Funny World Go By." *Judge*, May 3, 1913.
Cullen, Frank. *Vaudeville, Old and New: An Encyclopedia of Variety Performers in America*. With Florence Hackman and Donald McNeilly. 2 vols. New York: Routledge, 2006.
Custen, George Frederick. *Bio/Pics: How Hollywood Constructed Public History*. New Brunswick, N.J.: Rutgers University Press, 1992.
Dale, Alan. "A Diaphanous Dancer." *Cosmopolitan* 56 (December 1913): 117–19.
"Dancer a Sensation." *Variety*, March 5, 1910.
"The Dancers' Club News 1930–1931." March 19, 1931. Performing Arts Research Collections—Dance, New York Public Library for the Performing Arts.

Davis, Lee Allyn. *Scandals and Follies: The Rise and Fall of the Great Broadway Revue*. New York: Limelight Editions, 2000.

Davis, Mary E. *Ballets Russes Style: Diaghilev's Dancers and Paris Fashion*. London: Reaktion, 2010.

De Mille, Agnes. *Dance to the Piper*. Boston: Little, Brown, 1952.

Desmond, Jane. "Dancing Out the Difference: Cultural Imperialism and Ruth St. Denis's 'Radha' of 1906." *Signs* 17, no. 1 (1991): 28–49.

DesRochers, Rick. *The Comic Offense from Vaudeville to Contemporary Comedy: Larry David, Tina Fey, Stephen Colbert, and Dave Chappelle*. New York: Bloomsbury, 2014.

———. *The New Humor in the Progressive Era: Americanization and the Vaudeville Comedian*. New York: Palgrave Macmillan, 2014.

Dewberry, Eric Jay. "Jake Wells Enterprises and the Development of Urban Entertainments in the South, 1890–1925." Ph.D. diss., Georgia State University, 2010.

Diamond, Elin. *Unmaking Mimesis: Essays on Feminism and Theater*. New York: Routledge, 1997.

Diepeveen, Leonard. *Mock Modernism: An Anthology of Parodies, Travesties, Frauds, 1910–1935*. Toronto: University of Toronto Press, 2014.

Dierkes-Thrun, Petra. *Salome's Modernity: Oscar Wilde and the Aesthetics of Transgression*. Ann Arbor: University of Michigan Press, 2011.

Dinerstein, Joel. *Swinging the Machine: Modernity, Technology, and African American Culture between the World Wars*. Amherst: University of Massachusetts Press, 2003.

Douglas, George H. *The Smart Magazines: 50 Years of Literary Revelry and High Jinks at Vanity Fair, the New Yorker, Life, Esquire, and the Smart Set*. Hamden, Conn.: Archon Books, 1991.

"The Drama in the Law of Copyright." *Harvard Law Review* 44, no. 4 (1931): 628–33.

"The Dubious Past of 'The Merry Widow.'" *Current Literature* 44, no. 6 (June 1908): 651–52.

Duncan, Isadora. "The Dance of the Future." In Isadora Duncan, *The Art of the Dance*, 54–63. Edited with an introduction by Sheldon Cheney. New York: Theatre Arts Books, 1970.

"Eddie Leonard Objects." *Variety*, March 19, 1910.

Elswit, Kate. *Watching Weimar Dance*. Oxford: Oxford University Press, 2014.

"Ends of Units and Season Looked For by March 17." *Variety*, March 1, 1923.

"Epidemic Casualties." *Variety*, October 25, 1918.

"Epidemic Casualties." *Variety*, November 8, 1918.

Erdman, Andrew L. *Blue Vaudeville: Sex, Morals and the Mass Marketing of Amusement, 1895–1915*. Jefferson, N.C.: McFarland, 2004.

———. *Queen of Vaudeville: The Story of Eva Tanguay*. Ithaca, N.Y.: Cornell University Press, 2012.

Erenberg, Lewis A. *Steppin' Out: New York Nightlife and the Transformation of American Culture, 1890–1930*. Chicago: University of Chicago Press, 1984.

Estavan, Lawrence, and Edmond McAdoo Gagey, eds. *Theatre Buildings: Part 1*. San Francisco Theatre Research 15. San Francisco: Work Projects Administration, Northern California, 1940.

Farfan, Penny. *Performing Queer Modernism*. Oxford: Oxford University Press, 2017.

———. "The Picture Postcard Is a Sign of the Times." *Theatre History Studies* 32 (January 2012): 93–119.

Federal Writers Project of the Works Progress Administration. *San Francisco in the 1930s: The WPA Guide to the City by the Bay*. Berkeley: University of California Press, 2011.

Ferris, Dorothy. "The Rage for Barefoot Dancing." *Vanity Fair*, April 1916.

Fields, Armond. *Women Vaudeville Stars: Eighty Biographical Profiles*. Jefferson, N.C.: McFarland, 2012.

"Finest Music Hall in Europe with Semi-American Revue." *Variety*, December 24, 1924.

"First Church of Christ, Scientist." *New-Messenger*, October 22, 1966.

Fish, Anne Harriet. "Keeping on with the Dance." *Vanity Fair*, August 1919.

Flanagan, Hallie. *Arena: The History of the Federal Theatre*. New York: B. Blom, 1965.

"Florence Roberts Takes Opposite View to Mary Anderson." *San Francisco Dramatic Review*, February 6, 1909.

Foulkes, Julia L. *A Place for Us: "West Side Story" and New York*. Chicago: University of Chicago Press, 2016.

Fourteenth Census of the United States, 1920. Microfilm roll no. T625, RG 29. National Archives and Records Administration: Washington, D.C. Accessed through "1920 United States Federal Census." ancestry.com.

Franceschina, John. *Harry B. Smith: Dean of American Librettists*. New York: Routledge, 2003.

Francis, Joe. *La revue des revues*. 1927. http://www.imdb.com/title/tt0462506/.

Franko, Mark. *The Work of Dance: Labor, Movement, and Identity in the 1930s*. Middletown, Conn.: Wesleyan University Press, 2002.

Fraser, Caroline. *God's Perfect Child: Living and Dying in the Christian Science Church*. New York: Metropolitan Books, 1999.

Fred. "Palace." *Variety*, April 20, 1917.

Fyles, Franklin. "Broadway Roof Gardens Open in Summer Rivalry." *Chicago Sunday Tribune*, June 9, 1907, sec. Drama.

———. "The Critical First-Nighters." *Salt Lake Herald*, June 9, 1907, Magazine.

———. "New York Is Dancing Mad." *Washington Post*. July 26, 1908.

———. "New York's First Melodrama." *Salt Lake Herald*. August 4, 1907, Magazine.

"G. Hoffmann Dies on Coast." *Dance News*, December 1966.

Gaffney, Thomas J. *Birds of a Feather: A Play in Four Acts*. Boston: Gorham Press, 1915.

Garafola, Lynn. *Diaghilev's Ballets Russes*. New York: Da Capo Press, 2009.

———. "Ida Rubinstein." Jewish Women's Archive. https://jwa.org/encyclopedia/article/rubinstein-ida.

"Garden Gets Ahearn's Act." *Variety*, June 28, 1912.

Garelick, Rhonda K. *Electric Salome: Loie Fuller's Performance of Modernism*. Princeton, N.J.: Princeton University Press, 2007.

"Gertie Hoffmann's Surprise." *Variety*, June 10, 1911.

"Gertie Strikes for Amber Lights." *Day Book*. February 3, 1917.
"Gertrude Hoffman." *Vanity Fair*, April 1917.
"Gertrude Hoffman in Chi's Cabaret Shows." *Variety*, March 29, 1923.
"Gertrude Hoffmann, New Star at Shuberts' Winter Garden." *Variety*, June 15, 1912.
"Gertrude Hoffman Readies Comeback." *Variety*, August 9, 1944.
"The Gertrude Hoffman Show." *Macon News*, n.d. Loose scrapbook pages of newspaper clippings, box 3, p. 43, Gertrude Hoffmann Collection, Brooklyn Public Library, Brooklyn Collection.
"Gertrude Hoffmann's Mission." *Variety*, April 6, 1912.
"Gertrude Hoffman's Slip." *Variety*, January 10, 1919.
"Gertrude Hoffman's Unit." *Variety*, June 30, 1922.
Gibson, Charles Dana. "The Gibson Girl's America: Drawings by Charles Dana Gibson; Creating an Ideal." March 30, 2013. Online exhibition. The Library of Congress. http://www.loc.gov/exhibits/gibson-girls-america/creating-an-ideal.html.
Glenn, Susan A. *Female Spectacle: The Theatrical Roots of Modern Feminism*. Cambridge, Mass.: Harvard University Press, 2000.
Golden, Eve. *Anna Held and the Birth of Ziegfeld's Broadway*. Lexington: University Press of Kentucky, 2000.
Goldman, Jonathan. *Modernism Is the Literature of Celebrity*. Austin: University of Texas Press, 2011.
Goldstein, Paul. *Goldstein on Copyright*. New York: Aspen, 2005.
Gordon, Linda. *The Second Coming of the KKK: The Ku Klux Klan of the 1920s and the American Political Tradition*. New York: Liveright, 2017.
Gottschalk, Stephen. *The Emergence of Christian Science in American Religious Life*. Berkeley: University of California Press, 1978.
Gottschild, Brenda D. *Digging the Africanist Presence in American Performance: Dance and Other Contexts*. Westport, Conn.: Praeger, 1998.
Gould, Neil. *Victor Herbert: A Theatrical Life*. Oxford: Oxford University Press, 2011.
Grau, Robert. "How the Vaudeville Uplift Affects Stars Salaries." *Lippincott's Monthly Magazine*, April 1914.
Green, Abel, and Joe Laurie. *Show Biz, from Vaude to Video*. New York: Garland, 1985.
Gruesz, Kirsten Silva. "America." In *Keywords for American Cultural Studies*, edited by Bruce Burgett and Glenn Hendler, 21–25. New York: New York University Press, 2014.
Halpin, Mary Rita. "No Fooling, Theatrical Ban Brings Success to Troupe." *Nassau Daily Review*, December 4, 1934.
Hamera, Judith. *Unfinished Business: Michael Jackson, Detroit, and the Figural Economy of American Deindustrialization*. Oxford: Oxford University Press, 2017.
Hammill, Faye. *Sophistication: A Literary and Cultural History*. Liverpool, Eng.: Liverpool University Press, 2010.
Hammond, Percy. "Gertrude Hoffmann as Artist and Patriot." *Chicago Daily Tribune*, May 22, 1917.
Harris, Chas. K. (Charles Kassell). *After the Ball: Forty Years of Melody; An Autobiography*. New York: Frank-Maurice, 1926. http://archive.org/details/afterballfortyye00harr.

Harris County, Texas, Marriage Records. September 14, 1921. Harris County Clerk's Office: Houston, Texas. Accessed through "Houston, Texas Select County Marriage Records, 1837–2015." ancestry.com.

Harrison, Coleman. "Pittsburgh." *Variety*, December 9, 1921.

Hart, Jerome A. *In Our Second Century: From an Editor's Note-Book*. San Francisco: Pioneer Press, 1931. http://hdl.handle.net/2027/uc1.$b51352.

Hasbany, Richard. "Irene: Considering the Nostalgic Sensibility." *Journal of Popular Culture* 9, no. 4 (March 1, 1976): 816–26.

Hayter-Menzies, Grant. *Charlotte Greenwood: The Life and Career of the Comic Star of Vaudeville, Radio and Film*. Jefferson, N.C.: McFarland, 2007.

Hechtlinger, Dorothy. "Inter-Department Communication to Mr. Bert Granet. Subject: LUCY SOLO Possibilities." January 18, 1960. Margaret Herrick Library, Academy of Motion Picture Arts and Sciences, Beverly Hills, California.

Herbert, Victor. "Victor Herbert Defends 'Mlle. Modiste.'" *Evening Telegram*, October 28, 1907.

"Hip's American Girls Told to Dress Up." *Variety*, April 2, 1924.

Hirsch, Foster. *The Boys from Syracuse: The Shuberts' Theatrical Empire*. New York: Cooper Square Press, 2000.

"History of the Provincetown Playhouse." http://www.provincetownplayhouse.com/history.html.

"The Hoblitzelle & Interstate Theater Collection." Harry Ransom Center, University of Texas at Austin. https://web.archive.org/web/20181107234159/http://www.hrc.utexas.edu/collections/film/holdings/interstate/.

"Hoffman, Gertrude—Clippings." n.d. Performing Arts Research Collections—Music, New York Public Library for the Performing Arts.

Hoffmann, Gertrude. "Dancing, and the Magic of the Sea." *Vanity Fair*, July 1914.

———. "The Well-Watered Woman." *Times Dispatch*, September 7, 1913, Feature.

Hoffmann, Max. "Paree's a Branch of Broadway." Sheet music. New York: T. B. Harms; Francis, Day & Hunter; Jerome Remick & Co., 1912.

"Hoffmann Co. Rehearsing." *Variety*, July 26, 1912.

"Hoffmann Prefers Vaudeville." *Variety*, September 14, 1917.

"Hoffmann Show Closing?" *Variety*, January 30, 1914.

"Hoffmann's $5,390." *Variety*, January 25, 1923.

Hohman, Valleri J. *Russian Culture and Theatrical Performance in America, 1891–1933*. New York: Palgrave Macmillan, 2011.

Howe, Herbert. "Nazimova Speaks." *Picture-Play Magazine*, September 1920.

Huebner, Andrew J. "Gee! I Wish I Were a Man: Gender and the Great War." In *The Routledge History of Gender, War, and the U..S Military*, edited by Kara D. Vuic, 84–102. New York: Routledge, 2017.

Hurlbut, Gladys. *Next Week East Lynne! A Famous Stock Company Leading Lady Recounts Her Hilarious Experiences on the Gum-and-Gimlet Circuit*. New York: E. P. Dutton, 1950.

Ibee. "Gertrude Hoffmann: Dances and Imitations." *Variety*, October 25, 1918.

"The I Don't Care Girl (1953)." Internet Movie Database. https://www.imdb.com/title/tt0045898/?ref_=fn_al_tt_1.

"Ill and Injured." *Variety*, November 15, 1918.

"In and Out." *Variety*, February 3, 1922.

"In Manhattan." *Brooklyn Life*, September 6, 1902.

"Inside Stuff on Vaudeville." *Variety*, February 25, 1921.

"Inside Stuff on Vaudeville." *Variety*, March 5, 1920.

International Herald Tribune. "1915: Fire Destroys Moulin Rouge." *IHT Retrospective Blog*, February 27, 2015. https://iht-retrospective.blogs.nytimes.com/2015/02/27/1915-fire-destroys-moulin-rouge/.

Interstate Theatre Circuit. "Interstate Theatre Collection." MA77–1. Texas/Dallas History and Archives Division, Dallas Public Library.

"Int'l's Show on P.A. Tour After Night Club Folds." *Variety*, January 18, 1939.

Jackson, Chubby. "Chubby's Doghouse." *The Leader*, May 25, 1961.

Järvinen, Hanna. "Failed Impressions: Diaghilev's Ballets Russes in America, 1916." *Dance Research Journal* 42, no. 2 (2010): 76–108.

Jenkins, Henry. *What Made Pistachio Nuts? Early Sound Comedy and the Vaudeville Aesthetic*. Film and Culture. New York: Columbia University Press, 1992.

Jessen, J. C. "In and Out of West Coast Studios." *Motion Picture News* (January–March 1917), January 27, 1917. http://archive.org/details/motionpicturenew15moti_1.

J. L. "Is the Merry Widow as Young as She Says?" *Theatre*, May 1908.

Johnson, James Weldon. *The Autobiography of an Ex-Colored Man*. New York: Hill and Wang, 1991.

Johnson, John N. W. "Gertrude Hoffman Theater Posters—the Totality." ZSR Library. https://zsr.wfu.edu/2010/gertrude-hoffman-theater-posters-the-totality/.

Johnson, Julian. "Kitty Hayes the Dreamer." *Los Angeles Sunday Times*, October 29, 1911, Art and Artists.

———. "Mimodramas: Hoffmann Has Real Climate." *Los Angeles Daily Times*, October 30, 1911, box 11, folder 6, Gertrude and Max Hoffmann Papers (MS 608), Z. Smith Reynolds Library Special Collections and Archives, Wake Forest University, Winston-Salem, N.C.

Johnson, Katie N. *Sex for Sale: Six Progressive-Era Brothel Dramas*. Iowa City: University of Iowa Press, 2015.

Jolo. "New Plays Produced in London: Leap Year." *Variety*, May 7, 1924.

Jones, John Bush. *Reinventing Dixie: Tin Pan Alley's Songs and the Creation of the Mythic South*. Baton Rouge: Louisiana State University Press, 2015.

Jones, Starr West. *Hello God, Can We Talk? Discoveries That Challenge Modern Thinking*. Hollywood, Fla.: Frederick Fell, 1988.

"Just of Passing Interest." *San Francisco Dramatic Review*, August 18, 1900.

"Just of Passing Interest." *San Francisco Dramatic Review*, June 30, 1900.

Katon, Alvin J. "In the Theatres on Broadway." *Daily Star*, April 12, 1926.

Kendall, Elizabeth. *Where She Danced: The Birth of American Art-Dance*. Berkeley: University of California Press, 1979.

Kerr, John Finlay. "'Rereading' *Be Kind Rewind* (USA 2008): How Film History Can Be Remapped through the Social Memories of Popular Culture." *Screening the Past*, no. 24 (April 26, 2009).

Kibler, M. Alison. *Rank Ladies: Gender and Cultural Hierarchy in American Vaudeville*. Chapel Hill: University of North Carolina Press, 1999.

Kimber, Marian Wilson. *The Elocutionists: Women, Music, and the Spoken Word*. Urbana: University of Illinois Press, 2017.

King, Eleanor. *Transformations: The Humphrey-Weidman Era: A Memoir*. Trenton, N.J.: Dance Horizons, 1978.
Kingsley, Grace. "An All-Star Interview." *Los Angeles Sunday Times*, October 17, 1920, sec. 3.
———. "Rialto." *Los Angeles Daily Times*, March 14, 1916.
———. "Rialto." *Los Angeles Daily Times*, March 23, 1916.
Kirstein, Lincoln. *Dance: A Short History of Classic Theatrical Dancing*. Trenton, N.J.: Princeton Book, 1969.
"Klein's Unit Going into Boston." *Variety*, February 22, 1923.
"Klein's Unit Shut." *Variety*, March 22, 1923.
Kline, Tiny. *Circus Queen and Tinker Bell: The Memoir of Tiny Kline*. Edited by Janet M. Davis. Urbana: University of Illinois Press, 2008.
Koritz, Amy. "Dancing the Orient for England: Maud Allan's 'The Vision of Salome.'" *Theatre Journal* 46, no. 1 (1994): 63–78.
Koszarski, Richard. *An Evening's Entertainment: The Age of the Silent Feature Picture, 1915–1928*. Berkeley: University of California Press, 1994.
"K.-P. Employees Give Ball." *Variety*, March 28, 1908.
Kracauer, Siegfried. "Girls and Crisis." In *The Weimar Republic Sourcebook*, edited by Anton Kaes and Edward Dimendberg, 565–66. Berkeley: University of California Press, 1994.
———. "The Mass Ornament." In *The Mass Ornament: Weimar Essays*. Translated, edited, and with an introduction by Thomas Y. Levin, 75–86. Cambridge, Mass.: Harvard University Press, 1995.
Kraut, Anthea. *Choreographing Copyright: Race, Gender, and Intellectual Property Rights in American Dance*. Oxford: Oxford University Press, 2015.
Krieg, Cynthia Jane, and Regina G. Feeney. *Freeport*. Charleston, S.C.: Arcadia, 2012.
Kushner, Marilyn S., Kimberly Orcutt, and Casey Nelson Blake, eds. *The Armory Show at 100: Modernism and Revolution*. New York: New-York Historical Society, 2013.
"La Bete." *Variety*, April 27, 1912.
Lait. "Fifth Avenue." *Variety*, July 22, 1921.
Lancefield, Robert. "Hearing Orientality in (White) America, 1900–1930." *Dissertations*, January 1, 2004. http://wesscholar.wesleyan.edu/etd_diss/2.
Lavitt, Pamela Brown. "First of the Red Hot Mamas: 'Coon Shouting' and the Jewish Ziegfeld Girl." *American Jewish History* 87, no. 4 (1999): 253–90.
Leick, Karen. *Gertrude Stein and the Making of an American Celebrity*. New York: Routledge, 2009.
Levine, Lawrence. *Highbrow/Lowbrow: The Emergence of Cultural Hierarchy in America*. Cambridge, Mass.: Harvard University Press, 1990.
Levinson, André. "The Girls." *Theatre Arts Monthly* 12, no. 8 (August 1928): 597–605.
Levy, Eugene. *James Weldon Johnson: Black Leader, Black Voice*. Chicago: University of Chicago Press, 1976.
Libbey, Len. "Boston." *Variety*, January 20, 1922.
"'LIGHTS Will Shine Brighter than Ever' Flyer." Freeport Memorial Library. New York Digital Heritage. https://cdm16694.contentdm.oclc.org/digital/collection/p15281coll12/id/16158.

Lindvall, Terry. "Cinema Virtue, Cinema Vice: Race, Religion, and Film Exhibition in Norfolk, Virginia, 1908–1922." In *Hollywood in the Neighborhood: Historical Case Studies of Local Moviegoing*, edited by Kathryn Fuller-Seeley, 91–103. Berkeley: University of California Press, 2008.

"Loie Fuller." Special issue, *Dance Index* 1, no. 3 (March 1942). http://archive.org/details/danceindexunse_1.

"'Loop' Majestic, Chicago." *Variety*, November 4, 1921.

Lowrey, Carolyn. *The First One Hundred Noted Men and Women of the Screen*. New York: Moffat, Yard, 1920.

"Luescher's Keith's Staff." *Variety*, October 14, 1921.

"Lyric Theatre." Jerome Robbins Dance Division, the New York Public Library for the Performing Arts, New York Public Library Digital Collections. http://digitalcollections.nypl.org/items/510d47da-5e01-a3d9-e040-e00a18064a99.

Macgowan, Kenneth. *The Theatre of Tomorrow*. New York: Boni and Liveright, 1921. http://archive.org/details/theatreoftomorro00macgiala.

Macgowan, Kenneth, and Robert Edmond Jones. *Continental Stagecraft*. New York: Harcourt, Brace, 1922. http://archive.org/details/continentalstage00macg.

Manning, Susan. *Ecstasy and the Demon: The Dances of Mary Wigman*. Minneapolis: University of Minnesota Press, 2006.

———. *Modern Dance, Negro Dance: Race in Motion*. Minneapolis: University of Minnesota Press, 2004.

Marcus, Sharon. "Salomé!! Sarah Bernhardt, Oscar Wilde, and the Drama of Celebrity." *PMLA* 126, no. 4 (2011): 999–1021.

Marmorstein, Gary. *A Ship without a Sail: The Life of Lorenz Hart*. New York: Simon and Schuster, 2012.

Marotti, Frank. "Gibson Girl." In *Fashion and Merchandising Fads*, edited by Frank Hoffmann and Beulah B. Ramirez, 100–104. New York: Routledge, 2014.

Martin, John. "The Dance: A Convention." *New York Times*, May 17, 1936.

———. "The Dance: Dynamic Art." *New York Times*, January 4, 1931, Arts and Leisure.

"Max and Gertrude Hoffmann Are Now in Their New Home . . ." *Variety*, August 16, 1918.

"Max Hoffmann Leading." *Variety*, September 15, 1916.

Mayer, Charles S. "Ida Rubinstein: A Twentieth-Century Cleopatra." *Dance Research Journal* 20, no. 2 (1988): 33–51.

Mayer, David. "Architecture and Art Dance Meet in the Ancient World." In *The Ancient World in Silent Cinema*, edited by Pantelis Michelakis and Maria Wylke, 91–108. New York: Cambridge University Press, 2013.

———. "'Quote the Words to Prompt the Attitudes': The Victorian Performer, the Photographer, and the Photograph." *Theatre Survey* 43, no. 2 (2002): 223–51.

McCloskey, Agnes. "Chaperones Must Come Along If Ballet Girls Have Dates." *Nassau Daily Review*, August 5, 1936.

McIniss, Ian. Email message to the author. July 19, 2016.

"'Merry Widow' in Burlesque." *Variety*, January 4, 1908.

Metzger, Alfred. "History of the Tivoli Opera House, 1879–1899." *Pacific Coast Musical Review*, September 25, 1915.

"Midnight in the Cocoanut Grove." *Vanity Fair*, April 1917.

Miles, Carlton W. "'Is Celebrity Worth While?' Asks Gertrude." *Minneapolis Journal*, October 5, 1919, Sunday ed., Amusement, box 1, Clippings, Gertrude and Max Hoffmann Papers (MS 608), Z. Smith Reynolds Library Special Collections and Archives, Wake Forest University, Winston-Salem, N.C.

Miller, Bonnie M. *From Liberation to Conquest: The Visual and Popular Cultures of the Spanish-American War of 1898*. Amherst: University of Massachusetts Press, 2011.

Miller, Derek. *Copyright and the Value of Performance, 1770–1911*. Theatre and Performance Theory. Cambridge: Cambridge University Press, 2018.

Mintz, Lawrence E. "Humor and Ethnic Stereotypes in Vaudeville and Burlesque." *MELUS* 21, no. 4 (Winter 1996): 19–28.

"Miss Hoffman and Son." *Variety*, April 15, 1921.

"Mlle. Bianci." *Variety*, September 3, 1910.

Monod, David. "'I Didn't Raise My Boy to Be a Soldier': Popular Song and American Neutrality, 1914–1917." *War in History* 24, no. 4 (November 1, 2017): 438–57.

"Monster Dance Performance." Program. December 11, 1932. Dancers' Club New York (Clippings), New York Public Library for the Performing Arts.

Moon, Krystyn R. *Yellowface: Creating the Chinese in American Popular Music and Performance, 1850s–1920s*. New Brunswick, N.J.: Rutgers University Press, 2005.

Mooney, Jennifer. *Irish Stereotypes in Vaudeville, 1865–1905*. New York: Palgrave Macmillan, 2015.

Mordden, Ethan. *Ziegfeld: The Man Who Invented Show Business*. New York: St. Martin's Press, 2008.

Mortimer, Lee. "Bright Light Invasion." *Sunday Mirror*, November 24, 1940, Magazine.

"Moving Pictures: Rivoli." *Variety*, June 27, 1919.

"Mr. and Mrs. Max Hoffman." *Variety*, December 21, 1907.

Murphy, Michael. "'One Hundred Per Cent Bohemia': Pop Decadence and the Aestheticization of Commodity in the Rise of the Slicks." In *Marketing Modernisms: Self-Promotion, Canonization, Rereading*, edited by Kevin J. H. Dettmar and Stephen Watt, 61–89. Ann Arbor: University of Michigan Press, 1996.

"Murray Anderson's Almanac." Playbill. http://www.playbill.com/production/murray-andersons-almanac-erlangers-theatre-vault-0000004278.

"Musical Comedy Houses Permanent on Broadway." *Variety*, August 23, 1912.

"Must Dress Up." *Variety*, December 21, 1917.

Nance, Susan. *How the Arabian Nights Inspired the American Dream, 1790–1935*. Chapel Hill: University of North Carolina Press, 2009.

Nathan, George Jean. "The Theatre." *American Mercury*, July 1927.

———. "Trying It on the Dog Days." *Smart Set*, September 1911. https://hdl.handle.net/2027/njp.32101076380292.

Neville, Amelia Ransome. "Fin de Siècle." In *More San Francisco Memoirs, 1852–1899: The Ripening Years*, edited by Malcolm E. Barker, 289–93. San Francisco: Londonborn, 1996.

"New Acts of the Week: In the Swim." *Variety*, March 24, 1906.

"New Acts This Week: Palace." *Variety*, April 23, 1920.

"New 'Crazy' Show Clicks in Tryout." *Variety*, August 30, 1939.

"New Hoffmann Act." *Variety*, August 11, 1916.

"New York's Incredible Lost Rooftop Theatres." Messy Nessy Chic, March 17, 2017. http://www.messynessychic.com/2017/03/17/new-yorks-incredible-lost-rooftop-theatres/.

Newey, Katherine. "Feminist Historiography and Ethics." In *Theatre History and Historiography: Ethics, Evidence and Truth*, edited by Claire Cochrane and Jo Robinson, 85–102. London: Palgrave Macmillan, 2016.

"News from the Dailies." *Variety*, November 23, 1917.

"News Item: 'On Hand, One Oriental Dancer.'" *Variety*, October 13, 1916.

"Nice Hotel People." *Variety*, March 1, 1923.

"A Night in Spain." Internet Broadway Database. https://www.ibdb.com/broadway-production/a-night-in-spain-10316.

"$90,000 Vaudeville Offer for Gertrude Hoffmann." *Variety*, June 6, 1913.

"Notes." *Variety*, May 9, 1908.

NYC Marriage Index–Manhattan 1920. December 21, 1920. https://archive.org/details/NYC_Marriage_Index_Manhattan_1920.

"Obituary: H. B. Marinelli." *Variety*, January 10, 1924.

"Obituary: Hoffman, Max—1963 (d. May 21) Age 88." *Variety*, May 29, 1963. New York Public Library for the Performing Arts, Special Collections.

O'Brian, Jack. "Voice of Broadway." *Springfield News Leader*, June 21, 1971.

Ocko, Edna. "Reviewing on the Left: The Dance Criticism of Edna Ocko." Selected and introduced by Stacey Prickett. In "Of, By, and For the People: Dancing on the Left in the 1930s," edited by Lynn Garafola. Special issue, *Studies in Dance History* 5, no. 1 (1994): 65–103.

Oney, Steve. *And the Dead Shall Rise: The Murder of Mary Phagan and the Lynching of Leo Frank*. New York: Vintage Books, 2004.

"Orpheum." *Variety*, December 9, 1921.

"Pacific Coast Notes." *Motography*, April 15, 1916.

Page, Brett. *Writing for Vaudeville: With Nine Complete Examples of Various Vaudeville Forms by Richard Harding Davis, Aaron Hoffman, Edgar Allan Woolf, Taylor Granville, Louis Weslyn, Arthur Denvir, and James Madison*. Springfield, Mass.: Home Correspondence School, 1915.

Page, Max. *The Creative Destruction of Manhattan, 1900–1940*. Chicago: University of Chicago Press, 2001.

"Palace." *Variety*, August 27, 1915.

"Palace." *Variety*, January 20, 1926.

"Palace (Earl Steward, Mgr.; Orpheum)." *Variety*, November 9, 1917.

"Paramount Grill, N.Y." *Variety*, October 24, 1933.

Parker, Dorothy. "The Star-Spangled Drama." *Vanity Fair*, August 1918.

"The Passing Show of 1923." Internet Broadway Database. https://www.ibdb.com/broadway-production/the-passing-show-of-1923-8344.

Passport Applications, January 2, 1906–March 31, 1925. Microfilm roll no. 336. December 5, 1916. National Archives and Records Administration: Washington, D.C. Accessed through "U.S. Passport Applications, 1795–1925." ancestry.com.

Patterson, Ethel Lloyd. "'It Is So Silly, All This Fuss,' Says Anna Held, as She Tells about Her Full-Grown Daughter.'" *Evening World*, September 24, 1908.

Peiss, Kathy. *Cheap Amusements: Working Women and Leisure in Turn-of-the-Century New York*. Philadelphia: Temple University Press, 1986.

Peretti, Burton William. *Lift Every Voice: The History of African American Music*. Lanham, Md.: Rowman and Littlefield, 2009.

———. *Nightclub City: Politics and Amusement in Manhattan*. Philadelphia: University of Pennsylvania Press, 2007.

Perlmutter, Donna. *Shadowplay: The Life of Antony Tudor*. New York: Viking, 1991.

"Personal Mention." *San Francisco Dramatic Review*, December 9, 1899.

"Person to Person (Tommy Armour; Moss Hart & Kitty Carlisle)." CBS, May 8, 1959, Paley Center for Media. https://www.paleycenter.org/collection/item/?q=murrow&p=5&item=T:07497.

Peterson, Bernard L. *A Century of Musicals in Black and White: An Encyclopedia of Musical Stage Works by, about, or Involving African Americans*. Westport, Conn.: Greenwood Press, 1993.

"Plays and Players." *Theatre Magazine*, July 1904.

Polaire. "Make Your Feet a Feast for the Eye." *Times Dispatch*, March 23, 1913.

Preston, Carrie J. *Learning to Kneel: Noh, Modernism, and Journeys in Teaching*. New York: Columbia University Press, 2016.

———. *Modernism's Mythic Pose: Gender, Genre, Solo Performance*. Oxford: Oxford University Press, 2011.

Prevots, Naima. *Dancing in the Sun: Hollywood Choreographers, 1915–1937*. Ann Arbor, Mich.: UMI Research Press, 1987.

Price, Guy. "Coast Picture News." *Variety*, April 7, 1916.

The Proceedings of the First National Dance Congress and Festival. New York: National Dance Congress and Festival, 1936.

"The Pullman Girls." *Variety*, February 24, 1906.

"Queen O' Hearts." Internet Broadway Database. https://www.ibdb.com/broadway-show/queen-o-hearts-7318.

Radway, Janice A. *A Feeling for Books: The Book-of-the-Month Club, Literary Taste, and Middle-Class Desire*. Chapel Hill: University of North Carolina Press, 1999.

"RB Given 'Theater' Tinge." *Billboard*, April 18, 1942.

Reichenbach, Harry, and David Freedman. *Phantom Fame*. London: Noel Douglas, 1932.

"Reisenweber's Cafe: Glamour, Late Nights and Hot Jazz." *The Bowery Boys: New York City History* (blog), February 26, 2010. http://www.boweryboyshistory.com/2010/02/reisenwebers-cafe-glamour-late-nights.html.

Renaud, Ralph E. "Gertrude Hoffman in Sublime Art Captivates Senses with Her Ballet." *San Francisco Chronicle*, October 17, 1911.

Ries, Frank W. D. "Albertina Rasch: The Broadway Career." *Dance Chronicle* 6, no. 2 (January 1, 1982): 95–137.

"Rita Gould and Jas. T. Duffy . . ." *Variety*, August 30, 1912.

Rix, Susan. Newspaper article shared with author, November 29, 2017.

"Road Show's $10,000 Salary List for 3-Star Combine." *Variety*, July 5, 1913.

Robbins, Trina. *Nell Brinkley and the New Woman in the Early 20th Century*. Jefferson, N.C.: McFarland, 2001.

Rorabaugh, W. J. *Prohibition: A Concise History*. New York: Oxford University Press, 2018.

Rosen, Jody. "Vanishing Act: In Search of Eva Tanguay, the First Rock Star." *Slate*, December 1, 2009. http://www.slate.com/articles/arts/music_box/2009/12/vanishing_act.html.

Rush. "Virginia Earl." *Variety*, February 29, 1908.

Russo, Mary. "Aging and the Scandal of Anachronism." In *Figuring Age: Women, Bodies, Generations*, edited by Kathleen M. Woodward, 20–33. Theories of Contemporary Culture. Bloomington: Indiana University Press, 1999.

Ruyter, Nancy Chalfa. "American Delsartism: Precursor of an American Dance Art." *Educational Theatre Journal* 25, no. 4 (1973): 421–35.

"Sadie My Creole Lady." Sheet music. Duke University Libraries, Digital Collections. http://library.duke.edu/digitalcollections/hasm_b0438/.

"Sailings." *Variety*, August 9, 1939.

Sanville, Gladys. "Raising the Roof on Acrobatics: William J. Herrmann, Dean of Acrobatic Teachers, Makes a New Departure." *Dance Magazine* 16, no. 2 (June 1931): 45, 55.

Saunders, Hortense. "No Drinks, Smokes, or Dates for Modern Chorus Girls: That's the Formula of Gertrude Hoffmann, Who Lives in Freeport." *Daily Review*, November 16, 1925.

Savage v. Hoffmann. 159 F. 584 (C. C. S. D. N. Y 1908). https://www.ravellaw.com/opinions/48bdbd192738073a5f25a22d06a3b143.

Savran, David. *Highbrow/Lowdown: Theater, Jazz, and the Making of a New Middle Class*. Ann Arbor: University of Michigan Press, 2009.

Sayler, Oliver M., and Marjorie Barkentin. "On Your Toes—America! The Story of the First Ballet Russe." *Dance Data*, no. 2 (1977): 20–27.

Scheper, Jeanne. *Moving Performances: Divas, Iconicity, and Remembering the Modern Stage*. New Brunswick, N.J.: Rutgers University Press, 2016.

Schiecke, Konrad. *Downtown Chicago's Historic Movie Theatres*. Jefferson, N.C.: McFarland, 2011.

Schmidt, Jennifer. "Unruly Reproductions: The Embodied Art of Mimicry in Vaudeville." *Journal of American Drama and Theatre* 31, no. 3 (Spring 2019). https://jadtjournal.org/2019/05/13/unruly-reproductions-the-embodied-art-of-mimicry-in-vaudeville/.

Schneider, Rebecca. *Performing Remains: Art and War in Times of Theatrical Reenactment*. New York: Routledge, 2011.

School of the Art Institute of Chicago (SAIC). "SAIC and the Armory Show: 150 Years of SAIC." http://www.saic.edu/150/saic-and-armory-show.

Schultz, Roger. "Dating the Decline of the 'Road': The Verification of a New Hypothesis." *Theatre History Studies* 13 (1993): 163–79.

Schweitzer, Marlis. "'Darn That Merry Widow Hat': The On- and Offstage Life of a Theatrical Commodity, circa 1907–1908." *Theatre Survey* 50, no. 2 (November 2009): 189–221.

———. "Patriotic Acts of Consumption: Lucile (Lady Duff Gordon) and the Vaudeville Fashion Show Craze." *Theatre Journal* 60, no. 4 (2008): 585–608.

———. "The Salome Epidemic." In *The Oxford Handbook of Dance and Theater*, edited by Nadine George-Graves, 890–921. Oxford: Oxford University Press, 2015.

———. *Transatlantic Broadway: The Infrastructural Politics of Global Performance*. Basingstoke, Eng.: Palgrave Macmillan, 2015.

———. *When Broadway Was the Runway: Theater, Fashion, and American Culture*. Philadelphia: University of Pennsylvania Press, 2011.

Schweitzer, Marlis, and Daniel Guadagnolo. "Feeling Scottish: Affect, Mimicry, and Vaudeville's 'Inimitable' Harry Lauder." *Journal of Dramatic Theory and Criticism* 26, no. 2 (July 13, 2012): 145–60.

S.D., Trav. *No Applause—Just Throw Money: The Book That Made Vaudeville Famous*. New York: Faber and Faber, 2005.

———. "Olga Petrova: Vaudeville's Fake Russian." May 10, 2010. https://travsd.wordpress.com/2010/05/10/stars-of-vaudeville-155-olga-petrova/.

Segrave, Kerry. *Endorsements in Advertising: A Social History*. Jefferson, N.C.: McFarland, 2005.

Seiler, Cotten. *Republic of Drivers: A Cultural History of Automobility in America*. Chicago: University of Chicago Press, 2008.

"$75,000 for Hoffmann Films." *Variety*, August 31, 1917.

Shearer, Martha. *New York City and the Hollywood Musical: Dancing in the Streets*. London: Palgrave Macmillan, 2016.

Sheean, Vincent. *The Amazing Oscar Hammerstein: The Life and Exploits of an Impresario*. London: Weidenfeld and Nicolson, 1956.

Shields, David S. "Frank C. Bangs | Broadway Photographs." https://www.broadway.cas.sc.edu/content/frank-c-bangs.

———. "Studio, Elite | Broadway Photographs." Broadway Photographs. https://www.broadway.cas.sc.edu/content/studio-elite.

Ship manifest. S.S. *Kronprinzessin Cecilie*. June 30, 1909. Statue of Liberty—Ellis Island Foundation.

Ship manifest. S.S. *La Provence*. May 4, 1912. Statue of Liberty—Ellis Island Foundation.

Ship manifest. S.S. *Manhattan*. September 30, 1939. Statue of Liberty—Ellis Island Foundation.

Ship manifest. S.S. *Mexico*. November 5, 1919. Statue of Liberty—Ellis Island Foundation.

"Shows of the Week: Metropolis Roof." *Variety*, August 4, 1906.

"Shows of the Week: Metropolis Roof." *Variety*, August 11, 1906.

Shteir, Rachel. *Striptease: The Untold History of the Girlie Show*. New York: Oxford University Press, 2005.

"Shubert Crescent Theatre." Jerome Robbins Dance Division, the New York Public Library for the Performing Arts, New York Public Library Digital Collections. http://digitalcollections.nypl.org/items/510d47e3–87af-a3d9-e040-e00a18064a99.

Siegel, Marcia B. *Days on Earth: The Dance of Doris Humphrey*. Durham, N.C.: Duke University Press, 1993.

Silverman, Sime. "Danses Classique Russe." *Variety*, September 10, 1910.

———. "Gertrude Hoffmann and Co.: 'Revue.'" *Variety*, March 2, 1917.

———. "Gertrude Hoffmann and Her American Ballet." *Variety*, October 7, 1921.

———. "The Girl Question." *Variety*, January 11, 1908.

———. "Junior and Terris." *Variety*, July 8, 1921.

———. "Mabel Hite Soon." *Variety*, January 11, 1908.

———. "New Acts: Gertrude Hoffman and Co., 'Sumurun.'" *Variety*, August 20, 1915.

Simonson, Mary. *Body Knowledge: Performance, Intermediality, and American Entertainment at the Turn of the Twentieth Century*. Oxford: Oxford University Press, 2013.

———. "Visualizing Music in the Silent Era: The Collaborative Experiments of Visual Symphony Productions." *Journal of the Society for American Music* 12, no. 1 (2018): 2–36.

Slide, Anthony. *The Encyclopedia of Vaudeville*. Jackson: University Press of Mississippi, 2012.

Smith, Cecil. "It May Be Low, but This Farce Is Very Funny." *Chicago Daily Tribune*, April 13, 1942.

Smith, Frederick James. "Vaudeville: 'Sumurun' Undergoes Changes, Fannie Brice's New Songs, Burt and Stanford Return." *New York Dramatic Mirror*, September 15, 1915, 18.

Smith, James R. *San Francisco's Lost Landmarks*. Fresno, Calif.: Quill Driver Books, 2005.

Smith, Patsy. "Among the Women." *Variety*, April 12, 1918.

———. "Among the Women." *Variety*, June 6, 1919.

Snyder, Robert W. *The Voice of the City: Vaudeville and Popular Culture in New York*. New York: Oxford University Press, 1989.

Sowers, W. L. "Pantomime in America." *Texas Review* 2, no. 3 (1916): 235–47.

Sparks, Edith. *Capital Intentions: Female Proprietors in San Francisco, 1850–1920*. Chapel Hill: University of North Carolina Press, 2006.

Spies, Kathleen. "Baseball, Apple Pie, and Burlesque Queens: Nationalism in Walt Kuhn's Portraits of Showgirls." *Journal of American Culture* 31, no. 1 (February 10, 2008): 34–48.

Spoo, Robert. *Without Copyrights: Piracy, Publishing, and the Public Domain*. Oxford: Oxford University Press, 2016.

"Spotty Improvements in Business Some Comfort to Shubert Vaudeville." *Variety*, October 28, 1921.

Srinivasan, Priya. *Sweating Saris: Indian Dance as Transnational Labor*. Philadelphia: Temple University Press, 2011.

"Stage Gossip: Last Week of Dunne and Ryley's Comedians." *Argonaut*, August 6, 1900.

Stagg, Jerry. *The Brothers Shubert*. New York: Random House, 1968.

Stamp, Shelley. *Lois Weber in Early Hollywood*. Oakland: University of California Press, 2015.

State Population Census Schedules, 1905. New York State Archives, Albany. Accessed through "New York State Census, 1905." ancestry.com.

Stein, Gertrude. *Last Operas and Plays*. Baltimore: Johns Hopkins University Press, 1995.

Stevens, Ashton. "Miss Hoffmann as Imitator Stages Satires Cruel and Great." *Chicago American*, December 13, 1911. Box 11, folder 6, Gertrude and Max Hoffmann Papers (MS 608), Z. Smith Reynolds Library Special Collections and Archives, Wake Forest University, Winston-Salem, N.C.

———. "Our Own Little Theatrical Monopoly." *San Francisco Call*, December 19, 1897.

Stevens-Garmon, Morgan. "Gertrude Hoffman and the Dance That Offended Public Decency." Museum of the City of New York, August 1, 2017. https://www.mcny.org/story/gertrude-hoffman.

Stratyner, Barbara. *Ned Wayburn and the Dance Routine: From Vaudeville to the Ziegfeld Follies*. Madison: University of Wisconsin Press, 1996.

"Str.-Vode Show Grosses $2,700; Actors' Peanuts." *Variety*, September 11, 1935.

"Sues Gertie Hoffmann." *Variety*, December 1, 1916.

"Summer Shows at the Roof Gardens: Hammerstein's Roof. Gertrude Hoffman and Variety." *Theatre*, August 1908.

Taussig, Michael T. *Mimesis and Alterity: A Particular History of the Senses*. New York: Routledge, 1993.

Titterton, W. R. "The Maud Allan Myth." *New Age: A Weekly Review of Politics, Literature, and Art* 3, no. 9 (June 27, 1908): 171–72.

Tracy, Daniel. "Investing in 'Modernism': Smart Magazines, Parody, and Middlebrow Professional Judgment." *Journal of Modern Periodical Studies* 1, no. 1 (2010): 38–63.

"Trelawny of the 'Wells.'" 1911. Internet Broadway Database. https://www.ibdb.com/broadway-production/trelawny-of-the-wells-7262.

"True Patriotism!" *Theatre*, June 1917.

Twelfth Census of the United States, 1900. Microfilm roll no. T623, RG 29, National Archives and Records Administration, Washington, D.C. Accessed through "1900 United States Federal Census," ancestry.com.

"2 Paris Transient Spots, Casino and Folies, Best of Dull Legits." *Variety*, July 24, 1934.

"United's Unsettled State." *Variety*, February 29, 1908.

University of Toronto. "Sartorial." *Varsity*, November 24, 1908.

Uno. "Burlesque Bits." *Billboard*, April 11, 1953.

———. "Burlesque Bits." *Billboard*, April 26, 1952.

U.S. Bureau of the Census. "Availability of 1890 Census." https://www.census.gov/history/www/genealogy/decennial_census_records/availability_of_1890_census.html.

———. *Twelfth Census of the United States, 1900*. Ancestry.com

Van Vechten, Carl. "Anna Pavlowa a Wonderful Dancer." *New York Times*, March 1, 1910.

———. "Russian Dancers in Amazing Feats." *New York Times*, March 2, 1910.

Variety Protected Materials Department Collection. Collection MSS 017. Emerson College Archives and Special Collections. http://atom.emerson.edu/index.php/variety-protected-materials-department-collection-2.

"Vaudeville Reviews by Special Wire: Majestic, Chicago." *Billboard*, September 6, 1919.

"Vaudeville's 'Honor' War Record." *Western Magazine* 13, no. 1 (January 1919): 33–34.

Wainscott, Ronald Harold. *The Emergence of the Modern American Theater, 1914–1929*. New Haven, Conn.: Yale University Press, 1997.

Walker, Danton. "New York Letter." *Philadelphia Inquirer*, July 2, 1943.

Walker, Julia A. *Expressionism and Modernism in the American Theatre: Bodies, Voices, Words*. Cambridge: Cambridge University Press, 2005.

Walter, Anthony. "The Thousand and Second Tale." *San Francisco Call*, October 22, 1911, Editorial/Dramatic/Society.

Waters, Arthur B. "Philadelphia." *Variety*, February 24, 1922.

———. "Philadelphia." *Variety*, September 30, 1921.

Watkins, Elizabeth Siegel. "Stress and the American Vernacular: Popular Perceptions of Disease Causality." In *Stress, Shock, and Adaptation in the Twentieth Century*, edited by David Cantor and Edmund Ramsden, 49–70. Rochester, N.Y.: University of Rochester Press, 2014.

Weed, A. E., American Mutoscope and Biograph Company. *Princess Rajah dance*. United States: American Mutoscope and Biograph Company, 1904. Video. The Library of Congress, Washington, D.C. https://www.loc.gov/item/96520235/.

Wertheim, Arthur Frank. *Vaudeville Wars: How the Keith-Albee and Orpheum Circuits Controlled the Big-Time and Its Performers*. New York: Palgrave Macmillan, 2006.

West, Mae. *Three Plays by Mae West*. Edited by Lillian Schissel. New York: Routledge, 1997.

"What's Wrong with the Movie Prolog?" *Dance Magazine*, January 1927.

White, Matthew Jr. "'The Merry Widow' Travestied." *Munsey's Magazine* 38, no. 6 (March 1908): 820–21.

"White Rats' Ball." *Variety*, March 21, 1908.

Wiegand, Karl von. "Magic of 'Dollar Land,' with Jazz Tempo, Speeds Continental Work and Play." *Bridgeport Telegram*, April 18, 1925.

Willmott, Glenn. "Cat People." *Modernism/Modernity* 17, no. 4 (2010): 839–56.

"Wilson's 'Too Proud to Fight' Speech." The Lusitania Resource. http://www.rmslusitania.info/primary-docs/too-proud-to-fight/.

Winchell, Walter. "Walter Winchell on Broadway." *Courier-Post*, September 9, 1947.

Winter, William. *The Life of David Belasco*. New York: Moffat, Yard, 1918.

"Winter Garden Does $25,000." *Variety*, August 2, 1912.

"With the Press Agents." *Variety*, April 27, 1917.

Witmark, Isidore, and Isaac Goldberg. *The Story of the House of Witmark: From Ragtime to Swingtime*. New York: L. Furman, 1939.

Wollen, Peter. *Raiding the Icebox: Reflections on Twentieth-Century Culture*. Bloomington: Indiana University Press, 1993.

Woods, Leigh. "American Vaudeville." In *Popular Performance*, edited by Adam Ainsworth, Oliver Double, and Louise Peacock, 55–74. London: Bloomsbury, 2017.

———. "American Vaudeville, American Empire." In *Performing America: Cultural Nationalism in American Theater*, edited by Jeffrey D. Mason and J. Ellen Gainor, 73–90. Ann Arbor: University of Michigan Press, 1999.

Woolf, Vicki. *Dancing in the Vortex: The Story of Ida Rubinstein*. New York: Routledge, 2013.

World War I Selective Service System Draft Registration Cards, 1917–1918. Microfilm roll no. M1509. National Archives and Records Administration: Washington, D.C. Accessed through "U.S., World War I Draft Registration Cards, 1917–1918," under "Max Hoffmann." ancestry.com.

"Worst Theatrical Summer for Over Twenty Years." *Variety*, July 15, 1911.

Yohalem, John. “The Salome Scandals of 1907.” *Opera News*. https://www.operanews.com/operanews/issue/article.aspx?id=174&issueID=9&archive=true.

Young, Jeremy C. *The Age of Charisma: Leaders, Followers, and Emotions in American Society, 1870–1940*. Cambridge: Cambridge University Press, 2016.

Zeiger, Susan. “She Didn't Raise Her Boy to Be a Slacker: Motherhood, Conscription, and the Culture of the First World War.” *Feminist Studies* 22, no. 1 (Spring 1996): 7.

Zeller, Jessica. *Shapes of American Ballet: Teachers and Training before Balanchine*. New York: Oxford University Press, 2016.

INDEX

Page numbers in italic refer to illustrations.